Anaerobic Infections in Childhood

Anaerobic Infections in Childhood

Itzhak Brook, M.Sc., M.D.

Associate Professor of Pediatrics and of Surgery
Uniformed Services University of the Health Sciences

School of Medicine
Senior Investigator
Medical Microbiology Branch
Naval Medical Research Institute
National Naval Medical Center
Bethesda, Maryland

YEAR BOOK MEDICAL PUBLISHERS, INC.
Chicago • London • Boca Raton

Designed by Jack Schwartz.

Copyedited by Susan Glick under the direction of Lucie Ferranti.

Produced by Carole Rollins.

Composed in Baskerville by P & M Typesetting, Inc.

0 9 8 7 6 5 4 3 2 1

Brook, Itzhak
  Anaerobic infections in childhood.

  Bibliography.
  Includes index.
  1. Bacterial diseases in children. 2. Bacteria, Anaerobic. I. Title.
[DNLM: 1. Bacterial infections—In infancy and childhood.
WC 200 B871a]
RJ406.B32B76 1983   618.92'92   83-196
ISBN 0-8161-2246-6

The author and publisher have worked to ensure that all information in this book concerning drug dosages, schedules, and routes of administration is accurate at the time of publication. As medical research and practice advance, however, therapeutic standards may change. For this reason, and because human and mechanical errors will sometimes occur, we recommend that our readers consult the *PDR* or a manufacturer's product information sheet prior to prescribing or administering any drug discussed in this volume.

To my children Dafna, Dan, Tamar, and Yonatan

CONTENTS

PREFACE

This book was written for physicians who diagnose and treat children with infections. Its purpose is to present—in one volume—the clinical, microbiological, and therapeutic data necessary for the diagnosis and treatment of anaerobic infections in children.

To this end, the book is divided into five parts: Introduction to Anaerobes, Neonatal Infections, Anaerobic Infections of Specific Organ Sites, Other Types of Anaerobic Infections, and Principles of Management. The first part offers background information on anaerobes as normal flora and pathogens, and on laboratory and clinical diagnosis of anaerobic infections. Neonatal anaerobic infections—because they differ from those presenting in older children—are discussed separately in Part II. Parts III and IV, which encompass most anaerobic infections of later childhood, are divided into the following convenient subdivisions within each disease category: microbiological etiology, pathogenesis, diagnosis, management, complications, and, where appropriate, prevention. Part V discusses general principles of treatment. References are provided for those readers interested in more in-depth study.

General books on pediatric infectious disease offer inadequate coverage of anaerobes. Advances in laboratory identification, an increased awareness of the role of anaerobes in childhood, the frustrations of failed attempts to diagnose and treat anaerobic and mixed aerobic-anaerobic infections, and the aforementioned dearth of information on anaerobes available in book form—all prompted the undertaking of this volume. Most of the data herein was derived from clinical and microbiological experience with children. In several instances, however, sufficient data were unavailable in the pediatric literature, and adult data were substituted, which is proof that further work in childhood anaerobic infections is necessary.

I hope that this book will assist physicians and other health care professionals in the treatment of children with infections, and will prompt further studies in the role of anaerobic bacterial infectious diseases.

Itzhak Brook, M.Sc., M.D.

ACKNOWLEDGMENTS

I am most grateful to those who have made this book possible.

I would like to express my deepest gratitude to my parents, Haya and Baruch, who worked so hard to ensure that I would have a proper education. They have always encouraged the development of my scientific curiosity and capabilities. I would also like to thank my children and especially my wife, Joyce, for their patience, assistance, and understanding.

I am indebted to many of my teachers in the Hareali Haivri High School in Haifa, Israel, for their devotion and enthusiastic teaching, which were instrumental in promoting my scientific, professional, and ethical development. I am especially grateful to my biology teacher, Mr. Z. Zilberstein, for his enthusiastic recognition of nature's role in human life, and to my physics teacher, Mr. L. Green, for teaching me an analytical and scientific approach to my studies. I am grateful to many of my teachers in the Hebrew University Hadassah School of Medicine in Jerusalem and especially to the late Professor H. Berenkoff, who introduced me to the wonders of microbiology; to Dr. T. Sacks, who taught me clinical microbiology; and to Dr. S. Levine from Kaplan Hospital, Rehovot, Israel, who taught me general pediatrics.

I owe special gratitude to my teacher and mentor at UCLA, Dr. S. M. Finegold, for sharing his knowledge of anaerobic microbiology and clinical infectious diseases. Dr. Finegold has served over the years as a constant source of support and encouragement. Other teachers who provided invaluable help are Drs. W. J. Martin and V. L. Sutter from UCLA, and Drs. C. V. Sumaya, G. D. Overturf, and P. Wherle, who taught me about pediatric infectious diseases.

I am also grateful to my friends and collaborators who assisted in many of the clinical and laboratory studies: K. S. Bricknel for his excellent gas liquid chromatography work, and L. Calhoun and P. Yocum for their dedication and laboratory support.

Finally, I would like to thank the many medical students, house officers, infectious diseases fellows, and faculty members of the University of California, Los Angeles; University of California, Irvine; and George Washington University, for their collaboration in clinical studies. I am especially grateful to Drs. J. C. Coolbaugh and R. I. Walker from the Naval Medical Research Institute, for their outstanding support of my research efforts. I am indebted also to Mrs. Carol Cairns for her excellent secretarial assistance in typing this manuscript.

PART I

Introduction to Anaerobes

CHAPTER 1

Anaerobes as Normal Flora in Children

The human body mucosal and epithelial surfaces are covered with aerobic and anaerobic microorganisms.[1] Differences in the environment, such as oxygen tension and pH and variations in the ability of bacteria to adhere to these surfaces, account for changing patterns of colonization. Microflora also vary in different sites within the body system, as in the oral cavity; for example, the microorganisms present in the buccal folds vary in their concentration and types of strains from those isolated from the tongue or gingival sulci. However, the organisms that prevail in one body system tend to belong to certain major bacterial species, and their presence in that system is predictable. The relative and total counts of organisms can be affected by various factors, such as age, diet, illness, and antimicrobial therapy.

Knowledge of the composition of the flora at certain sites is useful for predicting which organisms may be involved in an infection adjacent to that site and can assist in the selection of a logical antimicrobial therapy, even before the exact microbial etiology of the infection is known. Recognition of the normal flora can also help the clinical microbiology laboratory to choose proper culture media that will be selective in inhibiting certain organisms regarded as contaminants. Furthermore, proper media can be used to enhance the growth of expected pathogens that reside as part of the indigenous flora at the proximity of the infectious site. The usefulness of such information is apparent during investigation of bacteremia of unknown origin, for which the presence of certain organisms can suggest a possible port of entry (i.e. *Clostridium* and *Bacteroides fragilis* usually originate from the gastrointestinal tract).[2]

The Skin

The anaerobic microflora of the total body skin usually is made up of the genus *Propionibacterium*.[3] The majority of the isolates of the genus *Propionibacterium* are *Propionibacterium acnes,* while *Propionibacterium granulosum* and *Propionibacterium avidum* can be recovered less frequently. Species of *Eubacterium* and *Peptococcus* also are sometimes encountered.

These organisms grow within the openings of the sebaceous glands, and consequently their distribution is proportional to the number of glands, the amount of sebum produced, and the composition of skin surface lipids.[4] Because of their prevalence in the skin these organisms can contaminate blood cultures and aspirates of abscesses and inner ear fluid.

The Oral Cavity

Establishment of Normal Oral Flora in the Newborn

The establishment of the normal oral flora is initiated at birth. Certain organisms such as lactobacilli and anaerobic streptococci, which establish themselves at an early date, reach high numbers within a few days. *Actinomyces, Fusobacterium,* and *Nocardia* are acquired by age six months. Following that time, *Bacteroides, Leptotrichia, Propionibacterium,* and *Candida* also are established as part of the oral flora.[5] *Fusobacterium* populations reach high numbers after dentition, and reach maximal numbers at age one year.

The microflora of the oral cavity is complex and contains many kinds of obligate anaerobes. The differences in numbers of the anaerobic microflora probably are due to variations in the oxygen concentration in parts of the oral cavity; the ratio of anaerobic bacteria to aerobic bacteria in saliva is approximately 10:1. The total count of anaerobic bacteria is 1.1×10^8/ml.

The number of strains of anaerobes varies. The incidence of *Clostridium* organisms was found to be 10% of the flora of periodontal pockets, 38% in normal gingival crevices, and 44% in carious teeth.[6] Fusobacteria also are a predominant part of the oral flora,[7] as are treponemas.[8] *Bacteroides melaninogenicus* represent less than 1% of the coronal tooth surface, but constitute 4% to 8% of gingival crevice flora. Veillonellae represent 1% to 3% of the coronal tooth surface, 5% to 15% of the gingival crevice flora, and 10% to 15% of the tongue flora. Microaerophilic streptococci predominate in all areas of the oral cavity, and they reach high numbers in the tongue and cheek.[9] Other anaerobes prevalent in the mouth are *Actinomyces,*[10] anaerobic cocci, *Leptotrichia buccalis, Bifidobacterium, Eubacterium,* and *Propionibacterium.*[11]

The Gastrointestinal Tract

The gastrointestinal tract becomes contaminated with organisms during the delivery process, when the newborn aspirates material from the cervical canal.[12] Streptococci, enterococci, and staphylococci usually are present in the first days of life.[13]

There are differences in bacterial flora between breast-fed and bottle-fed infants. In breast-fed infants, *Bifidobacterium* becomes the predominant anaerobe.[14] In full-term infants delivered by the vaginal route, *Bacteroides fragilis* is established by the first week in 22% of breast-fed infants as compared to 61% of formula-fed infants.[15] *Veillonella* organisms were more commonly found in infants delivered by cesarean section. As the child grows and is weaned, the numbers of *Bifidobacterium* organisms decrease, while the numbers of *Bacteroides* organisms increase until they outnumber *Bifidobacterium* organisms by a ratio of 3:1.

The fate of swallowed bacteria and their ability to colonize the gut depends on a number of factors: ability to adhere to mucosa, and environmental factors of diet, nutrient availability, chemical and pH conditions, secretory immunoglobulins, intestinal motility, and interference by other bacteria.[16–19] The stomach is seeded constantly with bacteria from the drainage of nasopharyngeal and salivary secretions, and usually contains less than 1000 organisms per milliliter. Only a few of these organisms are anaerobic.[20, 21] The bacterial counts in the small intestine are relatively low, with total counts of 10^4 to 10^5 organisms per milliliter. The organisms that predominate up to the ileocecal valve are Gram-positive facultative, while below that structure *Bacteroides* organisms (mostly *B. fragilis*), *Bifidobacterium* organisms, *Lactobacillus* organisms, and coliform bacteria are the major isolates.[22]

The normal colonic microflora tends to be relatively constant in an individual,[13, 23] and constitutes an important defense mechanism against infection. Organisms belonging to the normal flora, such as *B. fragilis*, are capable of protecting against infection by *Shigella flexneri*[24] and *Pseudomonas aeruginosa*.[25]

Vaginal and Cervical Flora

The normal vaginal flora is fairly homogeneous. The aerobic components consist of lactobacilli, group B and D streptococci, *Staphylococcus epidermidis*, *Staphylococcus aureus*, and Gram-negative enteric rods such as *Escherichia coli*.[26]

Studies of the anaerobic flora of the cervical canal show it to be composed of mixed aerobic and anaerobic flora.[27–31] Different strains of anaerobes were recovered in 49% to 92% of the subjects. Peptococci were reported in 7% to 57% of the cultures and peptostreptococci in

50%. One study reported the predominance of *Peptococcus asaccharolyticus* and *Peptostreptococcus anaerobius*.[29]

Bacteroides organisms were recovered from most of the cultures; their isolation rates were between 57% and 65%. The predominant strains were *B. fragilis, B. melaninogenicus,* and *Bacteroides oralis. Veillonella* organisms were recovered from 27%, bifidobacteria species from 10% to 72%, and eubacteria species from 15%. *Clostridium* species were recovered from 17%; these were isolates of *Clostridium bifermentans, Clostridium perfringens, Clostridium ramosum,* and *Clostridium difficile.*

Variations in cervical-vaginal flora are related to the effects of age, pregnancy, and menstrual cycle. The microflora in females before puberty, during childbearing years, pregnancy, and after menopause are not uniform. Colonization with lactobacilli is low in children and in postclimactic women, and high in pregnant women and those in their reproductive years. Although differences in colonization between age groups occur in organisms other than *Lactobacillus,* the vaginal flora of children contains many of the aerobic strains recovered from adult women. One study reported the recovery of *B. fragilis* in 24%, *B. melaninogenicus* in 56%, and *C. perfringens* in 32% of the children in the sample.[32] Although the isolation rate of these organisms is not different from those found in adult women by other investigators, this study did not include such a group for comparison.

The influence of pregnancy on the vaginal flora is of particular interest, since the newborn is exposed to that flora during passage through the birth canal or through exposure to infected amniotic fluid.[12] Most reports[12, 33-35] indicate that the bacterial component of the vaginal flora during pregnancy generally is identical to that found prior to pregnancy; the major change is an increase in the colonization by lactobacilli. This increase in the number of avirulent lactobacilli at the expense of the more virulent groups of microorganisms may serve to protect the fetus, so that the infant is exposed to benign organisms while passing through the heavily colonized birth canal.

Data collected from animals[36, 37] have indicated that estrogen can increase the bacterial population of the female genital tract, while progesterone decreases it. The influence of these hormonal changes on the quantitative isolation of anaerobes in the menstrual cycle has not been studied.

The Urogenital Tract

Finegold and colleagues[38] isolated anaerobes from the urethra of 8 of 17 normal male subjects; however, the bacterial counts were between 10^2 and 10^4/ml. The anaerobes isolated were *B. fragilis, B. melaninogenicus, Fusobacterium necrophorum,* and anaerobic Gram-positive cocci. Headington and Beyerlein[39] studied 15,250 midstream samples and recovered anaerobes from 158 of them. These included lactobacilli, Gram-negative rods, cocci, and clostridia. Since these studies indicate that anaerobes may colonize the urethra in many individuals, urine sampled for anaerobic bacteria should be obtained via another route (e.g., suprapubic aspiration).

The Eye

Anaerobes were recovered from up to 80% of the conjunctival cultures obtained from normal individuals.[40-42] The predominant isolates in descending order of frequency were *Propionibacterium acnes, P. avidum, P. granulosum, Peptococcus anaerobius, Bacteroides* species, *Actinomyces* species, and *Eubacterium* species. These organisms were recovered also from parts adjacent to the conjunctiva such as the eyelids and lacrimal sac. *P. acnes* was recovered also from normal uninflamed conjunctiva of children.[43] This organism was isolated from 18.5% of the children studied, as compared to 46.2% of adults.[41]

REFERENCES

1. Socransky, S. S., and Manganiello, S. D. The oral microflora of man from birth to senility. *J. Periodontol.* 42:485, 1971.

2. Brook, I. et al. Anaerobic bacteremia in children. *Am. J. Dis. Child.* 134:1052, 1980.

3. Evans, C. A. et al. Bacterial flora of the normal human skin. *J. Invest. Dermatol.* 15:305, 1950.

4. McGinley, K. J. et al. Regional variation in density of cutaneous *Propionibacterium*: correlation of *Propionbacterium acnes* populations with sebaceous secretions. *J. Clin. Microbiol.* 12:672, 1980.

5. Gibbons, R. J. et al. Studies of the predominant cultivable microbiota of dental plaque. *Arch. Oral Biol.* 9:365, 1964.

6. Loesche, W. J.; Hockett, R. N.; and Syed, S. A. The predominant cultivable flora of tooth surface plaque removed from institutionalized subjects. *Arch. Oral Biol.* 17:1311, 1972.

7. Baird-Parker, A. C. The classification of fusobacteria from the human mouth. *J. Gen. Microbiol.* 22:458, 1960.

8. Smibert, R. M. Spirochaetales, a review. *CRC Crit. Rev. Microbiol.* 2:491, 1973.

9. Gibbons, R. J. Aspects of the pathogenicity and ecology of the indigenous oral flora of man. In *Anaerobic bacteria: role in disease*, eds. A. Balows et al. Springfield, Ill.: Charles C Thomas, 1974, p. 267.

10. Rasmussen, E. G.; Gibbons, R. J.; and Socransky, S. S. A taxonomic study of fifty Gram-positive anaerobic diphtheroides isolated from the oral cavity of man. *Arch. Oral Biol.* 11:573, 1966.

11. Gibbons, R. J. et al. The microbiota of the gingival crevice of man. II. The predominant cultivable organisms. *Arch. Oral Biol.* 8:281, 1963.

12. Brook, I. et al. Aerobic and anaerobic bacterial flora of the maternal cervix and newborn gastric fluid and conjunctiva: a prospective study. *Pediatrics* 63:451, 1979.

13. Mitsuoka, R., and Hayakawa, K. The fecal flora of man. I. Communication: the composition of the fecal flora of different age groups. *Zentralbl. Bakteriol.* 223(3):333, 1973.

14. Mata, L. J.; Carillo, C; and Villatoro, E. Fecal microflora in healthy persons of a preindustrial region. *Appl. Microbiol.* 17:596, 1969.

15. Long, S. S., and Swenson, R. M. Development of anaerobic fecal flora in healthy newborn infants. *J. Pediatr.* 91:298, 1977.

16. Gorbach, S. L. Intestinal microflora. *Gastroenterology* 60:1110, 1971.

17. Barbero, G. J. et al. Investigations on the bacterial flora, pH and sugar content in the intestinal tract of infants. *J. Pediatr.* 40:152, 1952.

18. Donaldson, R. M. Normal bacterial populations of the intestine and their relation to intestinal function. *N. Engl. J. Med.* 270:938, 1964.

19. Williams, R. C., and Gibbons, R. J. Inhibition of bacterial adherence by secretory immunoglobulin A: a mechanism of antigen disposal. *Science* 177:697, 1972.

20. Franklin, M. A., and Skorna, S. C. Studies on natural gastric flora. I. Bacterial flora of fasting human subjects. *Can. Med. Assoc. J.* 95:1349, 1966.

21. Nelson, D. P., and Mata, L. J. Bacterial flora associated with the human gastrointestinal mucosa. *Gastroenterology* 58:56, 1970.

22. Gorbach, S. L. et al. Studies of intestinal microflora. II. Microorganisms of the small intestine and their relation to oral and fecal flora. *Gastroenterology* 53:856, 1967.

23. Zubryzycki, L., and Spaulding, E. H. Studies on the stability of the normal human fecal flora. *J. Bacteriol.* 83:968, 1962.

24. Bohnohoff, M.; Miller, C. P.; and Martin, W. R. Resistance of the mouse's intestinal tract to experimental *Salmonella* infection. I. Factors which interfere with the initiation of infection by oral inoculation. *J. Exp. Med.* 120:805, 1964.

25. Levison, M. E. Effect of colon flora and short-chain fatty acids on growth in vitro of *Pseudomonas aeruginosa* and Enterobacteriaceae. *Infect. Immun.* 8:30, 1973.

26. Larsen, B., and Galask, R. P. Vaginal microbial flora and theoretic relevance. *Obstet. Gynecol.* 55(suppl):1005, 1980.

27. Mead, P. B., and Louria, D. B. Antibiotics in pelvic infections. *Clin. Obstet. Gynecol.* 12:219, 1969.

28. Gorbach, S. L. et al. Anaerobic microflora of the cervix in healthy women. *Am. J. Obstet. Gynecol.* 117:1053, 1973.

29. Ohm, M. J., and Galask, R. P. Bacterial flora of the cervix from 100 prehysterectomy patients. *Am. J. Obstet. Gynecol.* 12:683, 1975.

30. Sanders, C. V. et al. Anaerobic flora of the endocervix in women with normal versus abnormal Papanicolaou (Pap) smears. *Clin. Res.* 23:30A, 1975.

31. Bartizal, F. J. et al. Microbial flora found in the products of conception in spontaneous abortions. *Obstet. Gynecol.* 43:109, 1974.

32. Goplerud, C. P.; Ohm, M. J.; and Galask, R. P. Aerobic and anaerobic flora of the cervix during pregnancy and the puerperium. *Am. J. Obstet. Gynecol.* 126:858, 1976.

33. Tashjian, J. H.; Coulan, C. B.; and Washington, J. A. II. Vaginal flora in asymptomatic women. *Mayo Clin. Proc.* 51:557, 1976.

34. Hammerschlag, M. R.; Albert, S.; and Onderdonketal, A. B. Anaerobic microflora of the vagina in children. *Am. J. Obstet. Gynecol.* 131:853, 1978.

35. Moberg, P. et al. Cervical bacterial flora in infertile and pregnant women. *Med. Microbiol. Immunol.* 165:139, 1978.

36. Larsen, B.; Markovetz, A. J.; and Galask, R. P. The role of estrogen in controlling the genital microflora of female rats. *Appl. Environ. Microbiol.* 34:534, 1977.

37. Larsen, B.; Markovetz, A. J.; and Galask, R. P. The bacterial flora of the female rat genital tract. *Proc. Soc. Exp. Biol. Med.* 151:571, 1976.

38. Finegold, S. M. et al. Significance of anaerobic and capnophilic bacteria isolated from the urinary tract. In *Progress in pyelonephritis,* ed. E. H. Kass. Philadelphia: Davis, 1965, p. 159.

39. Headington, J. T., and Beyerlein, B. Anaerobic bacteria in routine urine culture. *J. Clin. Pathol.* 19:573, 1966.

40. Matsura, H. Anaerobes in the bacterial flora of the conjunctival sac. *Jpn. J. Ophthalmol.* 15:116, 1971.

41. Perkins, R. E. et al. Bacteriology of normal and infected conjunctiva. *J. Clin. Microbiol.* 1:147, 1975.

42. Brook, I. et al. Anaerobic and aerobic bacteriology of acute conjunctivitis. *Ann. Ophthalmol.* 11:389, 1979.

43. Brook, I. Anaerobic and aerobic bacterial flora of acute conjunctivitis in children. *Arch. Ophthalmol.* 98:833, 1980.

CHAPTER 2

Collection and Transportation of Specimens for Culture

Since anaerobic bacteria frequently are involved in various infections, all properly collected specimens should be cultured for these organisms. The physician should make special efforts to isolate these organisms from infections from which they frequently are recovered; such infections include abscesses, wounds in and around the oral and anal cavities, chronic otitis media, sinusitis, and aspiration pneumonia.

The most acceptable documentation of an anaerobic infection is through culture of these microorganisms from the infected site. This procedure requires the cooperation of the physician and the microbiology laboratory. Three essential requirements are needed for appropriate documentation of anaerobic infection: collection of appropriate specimens, expeditious transportation of the specimen, and careful laboratory processing.

Collection of Specimens

Specimens must be obtained free of contamination so that saprophytic organisms or normal flora are excluded, and culture results can be interpreted correctly. Since indigenous anaerobes often are present on the surfaces of skin and mucous membranes in large numbers, even minimal contamination of a specimen with the normal flora can give misleading results. On this basis, specimens can be designated according to their acceptability for anaerobic culture to either the acceptable or unacceptable category. Materials that are appropriate for anaerobic cultures should be obtained using a technique that bypasses the normal flora. Unacceptable or inappropriate specimens can be expected to yield normal flora also and therefore have no diagnostic value. Unacceptable specimens include coughed sputum, bronchoscopy aspirates, gingival and throat swabs, feces, gastric aspirates, voided urine, and vaginal swabs. Exceptions to these guidelines can be made when the clinical condition warrants such a culture, such as the use of selective media to detect only a possible pathogen, such as *Clostridium difficile,* in stool obtained from a patient with colitis.

Acceptable specimens include blood specimens, aspirates of body fluids (pleural, pericardial, cerebrospinal, peritoneal, and joint fluids), urine collected by percutaneous suprapubic bladder aspiration, abscess contents, deep aspirates of wounds, and specimens collected by special techniques such as transtracheal aspirates or direct lung puncture. Direct needle aspiration probably is the best method of obtaining a culture, while use of swabs is much less desirable. Specimens obtained from sites that normally are sterile may be collected after thorough skin decontamination, as for collection of blood, spinal joint, or peritoneal fluids.

Cultures of coughed sputum and specimens obtained from bronchial brushing or bronchoscopy generally are contaminated with normal oral and nasal aerobic and anaerobic flora and are therefore unsuitable for culture. Because the trachea below the thyroglossal area is sterile in the absence of pulmonary infection, transtracheal aspiration (TTA), which is done below this site, is a reliable procedure for obtaining suitable culture material for the diagnosis of pulmonary infection.[1,2] An alternative procedure is direct lung puncture. These procedures, when performed by experienced operators, yield important data, and the complication rates are very low. TTA usually is not recommended in patients with severe hypoxia, hemorrhagic diathesis, or severe cough.[3] Rare complications such as hypoxia, bleeding, subsequent emphysema, or arrhythmia rarely have been reported in adult patients.[4] TTA has been used successfully also for the diagnosis of aspiration pneumonia and lung abscess in children.[2] Cultures obtained by TTA contained fewer pathogens than did cultures of expectorated sputum. Side effects of this procedure in children included mild hemoptysis and, in rare instances, subcutaneous emphysema.

Transportation of Specimens

The ability to recover anaerobes is influenced by the care applied to transportation and laboratory processing of specimens. Unless proper precautionary measures are taken during collection, transport, and laboratory processing, pronounced changes can occur in the aerobic and anaerobic microbial population of a clinical specimen.[5] Sensitivity to oxygen causes some obligate anaerobes to die rapidly on exposure to air. In clinical samples, obligate anaerobes can be overgrown by facultative anaerobes unless the sample is processed rapidly after collection. The organisms must be protected, therefore, from the deleterious effects of oxygen during the time between the collection of the specimen until they are inoculated into the proper anaerobic medium in the

.microbiology laboratory. Failure to take proper precautions can result in misleading data, which may be detrimental to the patient.[5–9]

Anaerobes vary in the conditions they require for survival. In accordance with their oxygen sensitivity, some organisms are classified as "moderate" and some as "fastidious."[10] The moderate group is capable of growing in an oxygen concentration of 2% to 8%. *Bacteroides fragilis, Bacteroides oralis, Bacteroides melaninogenicus, Fusobacterium nucleatum,* and *Clostridium perfringens* belong to this group. Some fastidious anaerobes will grow at 0.5% oxygen levels, and some are extremely oxygen-sensitive, such as some strains of *B. fragilis* and peptococci.[11] Low oxidation-reduction potential is another basic requirement for growth of certain anaerobic bacteria, as for *Bacteroides vulgatus* and *Clostridium sporogenes.*[12] Such conditions usually exist in areas where anaerobes are present as part of the normal flora and at infected sites. The implication of these observations is that specimens must be carefully and rapidly handled in both transport and processing to ensure good recovery of anaerobes.

Figure 2.1. Commercial transport media used for the transportation of anaerobic specimens. *Left,* swab; *middle,* vial; *right,* syringe and needle. (Brook, I. Collection and transportation of specimens in anaerobic infections. *J. Fam. Pract.* 15:775–779, 1982. Copyright 1982, Appleton-Century-Crofts. Reprinted by permission.)

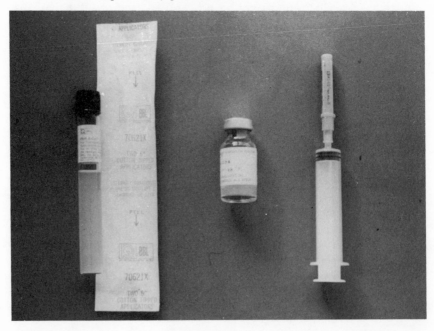

The specimens should be placed as soon as possible after their collection into an anaerobic transporter. Aspirates of liquid specimen or tissue are always preferred to swabs, although systems for the collection of all three culture forms are commercially available (fig. 2.1). Several versions of the anaerobic transport media also are commercially available (Baltimore Biological Laboratories, Cockeysville, Maryland; Marion Scientific Corporation, Kansas City, Missouri; Scott Laboratories, Fiskville, Rhode Island; and Becton-Dickinson, Rutherford, New Jersey).

These transport media are very helpful in preserving the anaerobes until the time of inoculation. Liquid specimens may be inoculated into a commercially available anaerobic transport vial, which is devoid of oxygen and sometimes contains an indicator. A plastic or glass syringe and needle also may be used for transport. After the specimen is collected and all air bubbles are expelled from the syringe and needle, the needle tip should be inserted into a sterile rubber stopper (fig. 2.2). Because air gradually diffuses through the wall of a plastic syringe, no more than 30 minutes should elapse before the specimen is processed. This inexpensive transport device for liquid specimens is especially useful in the hospital situation where it can be rapidly transported to the microbiology laboratory.[9]

Swabs may be placed in the sterilized tubes containing carbon dioxide or prereduced, anaerobically sterile Carey and Blair semisolid media. A preferred method is to use a swab that has been prepared in a prereduced anaerobic tube.

Figure 2.2. Corked syringe and needle used for the transportation of an anaerobic specimen. (Brook, I. Collection and transportation of specimens in anaerobic infections. *J. Fam. Pract.* 15:775–779, 1982. Copyright 1982, Appleton-Century-Crofts. Reprinted by permission.)

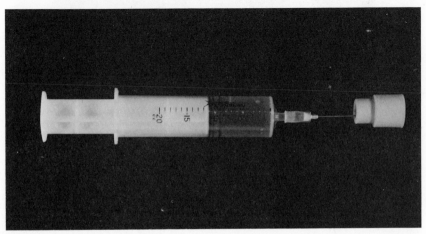

Tissue specimens or swabs can be transported anaerobically in an anaerobic jar or in a petri dish placed in a sealed plastic bag that can be rendered anaerobic by use of a catalyzer (Marion, Kansas City, Missouri) (fig. 2.3). Most of the common and clinically important anaerobic bacteria are moderate anaerobes, as shown by the examination of various types of clinical specimens for anaerobes.[11, 13]

Syed and Loesche studied the survival of human dental plaque flora in various transport media and concluded that because numbers and kinds of microorganisms in clinical materials vary widely, no transport device should be expected to give optimal protection for all anaerobes that may be encountered in specimens.[14] Even though some of

Figure 2.3. Commercial anaerobic bag system used for transportation of tissue or other specimens. (Brook, I. Collection and transportation of specimens in anaerobic infections. *J. Fam. Pract.* 15:775–779, 1982. Copyright 1982, Appleton-Century-Crofts. Reprinted by permission.)

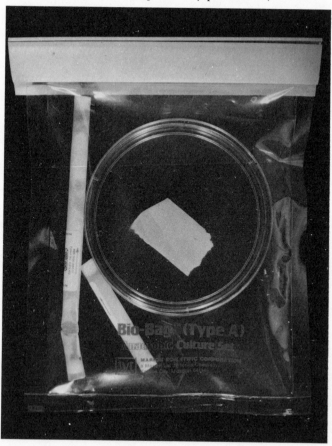

the transport systems can support the viability of anaerobic organisms for up to 24 hours,[15, 16] all specimens should be transported and processed as rapidly as possible after collection to avoid loss of fastidious oxygen-sensitive anaerobes and overgrowth of facultative bacteria.

When delay in transportation is expected, refrigeration of the sample may prevent overgrowth of some organisms and preserve their distribution. Unfortunately, several investigators have found this procedure to be of little benefit.[15]

Processing of Specimens in the Laboratory

Laboratory diagnosis of anaerobic infections begins with the examination of a Gram-stained smear of the specimen. The appearance of the Gram-stained organisms will give important preliminary information regarding types of organisms present and will suggest appropriate initial therapy. It also serves as a quality control on the final culture analysis. The laboratory should be able to recover all of the morphological types in the approximate ratio in which they are seen.

The techniques for cultivation of anaerobes should provide optimal anaerobic conditions throughout processing. Detailed procedures of these methods can be found in microbiology manuals.[8, 9] Briefly, these methods could be the prereduced tube method or the anaerobic glove box technique, which provides an anaerobic environment throughout processing, or the GasPak system (Becton Dickinson Co., Cockeysville, Md.) or the Bio-Bag system (Marion Scientific Corp., Kansas City, Mo.), which is a more simplified method.

As a minimum requirement for the recovery of anaerobes, specimens should be inoculated onto enriched blood agar medium (containing vitamin K_1 and hemin); for *Bacteroides* species, a selective medium such as laked sheep blood agar with kanamycin and vancomycin should be used.

Cultures should be placed immediately under anaerobic conditions and incubated for 48 hours or longer. Plates are then examined for approximate number and types of colonies present. Each colony type is isolated, tested for aero-tolerance, and identified.

Conclusion

It is imperative that the physician treating a patient with suspected anaerobic infection use appropriate methods of obtaining samples of the infected site. Proper procedure allows the physician to bypass areas of the normal flora and assures appropriate and rapid transportation of the sample. Reliable microbiological data can be obtained only when proper procedures are followed.

REFERENCES

1. Pecora, D. V. A method of securing uncontaminated tracheal secretions for bacterial examination. *J. Thorac. Surg.* 37:653, 1959.

2. Brook, I. Percutaneous transtracheal aspiration in the diagnosis and treatment of aspiration pneumonia in children. *J. Pediatr.* 90:1000, 1980.

3. Bartlett, J. G.; Rosenblatt, J. E.; and Finegold, S. M. Percutaneous transtracheal aspiration in the diagnosis of anaerobic pulmonary infection. *Ann. Intern. Med.* 22:535, 1973.

4. Spencer, C. D., and Beaty, H. N. Complications of transtracheal aspiration. *N. Engl. J. Med.* 286:304, 1972.

5. Dowell, V. R., Jr. Anaerobic infections. In *Diagnostic procedures for bacterial, mycotic and parasitic infections*, 5th edition, eds. H. L. Bodily, E. L. Updyke, and J. O. Mason. New York: American Public Health Association, 1970, p. 494.

6. Dowell, V. R., Jr., and Hawkins, T. M. *Laboratory methods in anaerobic bacteriology, CDC laboratory manual.* U.S. Department of Health, Education, and Welfare publ. no. (CDC) 74-8272. Atlanta: Center for Disease Control.

7. Finegold, S. M. *Anaerobic bacteria in human disease.* New York: Academic Press, 1977.

8. Holderman, L. V., and Moore, W. E. C., eds. *Anaerobe laboratory manual,* 4th edition. Blacksburg, Va.: Virginia Polytechnic Institute and State University, 1977.

9. Sutter, V. L.; Citron, D. M.; and Finegold, S. M. *Wadsworth anaerobic bacteriology manual,* 3rd ed. St. Louis: C. V. Mosby, 1980.

10. Loesche, W. J. Oxygen sensitivity by various anaerobic bacteria. *Appl. Microbiol.* 18:911, 1973.

11. Gorbach, S. L., and Bartlett, J. G. Anaerobic infections. *N. Engl. J. Med.* 190:1117, 1237, 1289, 1974.

12. Hankle, M. E., and Katz, Y. J. An electrolytic method for controlling oxidation-reducing potential and its application in the study of anaerobiosis. *Arch. Biochem. Biophys.* 2:183, 1943.

13. Tally, F. P. et al. Oxygen tolerance of fresh clinical anaerobic bacteria. *J. Clin. Microbiol.* 1:161, 1975.

14. Syed, S. A., and Loesche, W. J. Survival of human dental plaque flora in various transport media. *Appl. Microbiol.* 24:638, 1972.

15. Mena, E. et al. Evaluation of Port-A-Cal transport system for protection of anaerobic bacteria. *J. Clin. Microbiol.* 8:28, 1978.

16. McConville, J. H.; Timmons, R. F.; and Hansen, S. L. Comparison of three transport systems for recovery of aerobes and anaerobes from wounds. *Am. J. Clin. Pathol.* 72:968, 1979.

CHAPTER 3

Clinical Approach to Diagnosis of Anaerobic Infections

The diagnosis of anaerobic infections in children may be difficult, but is expedited by recognition of certain clinical signs[1]:

1. Necrotic gangrenous tissue;
2. Foul-smelling discharge;
3. Infection adjacent to a mucosal surface;
4. Free gas in tissue;
5. Bacteremia or endocarditis with no growth on aerobic blood cultures;
6. Infection related to the use of antibiotics effective against aerobes only;
7. Infection related to tumors or other destructive processes;
8. Infected thrombophlebitis;
9. Infection following bites;
10. Black discoloration of exudates containing *Bacteroides melaninogenicus,* which may fluoresce under ultraviolet light;
11. "Sulfur granules" in discharges caused by actinomycosis;
12. Clinical presentation of gas gangrene;
13. Clinical condition predisposing to anaerobic infection (following maternal amnionitis, perforation of bowel, etc.).

Predisposing conditions and bacteriologic hints can alert the physician, who may apply diagnostic procedures to ascertain the nature of the pathogens and the extent of the infection. Bacteriologic findings suggestive of anaerobic infection are[1]

1. Inability to grow, organisms seen on Gram stain in aerobic cultures.
2. Typical morphology on Gram stain.
3. Anaerobic growth on proper media containing antibiotics supressing aerobes.
4. Growth in anaerobic zone of fluid or agar media.
5. Gas, foul-smelling odor in specimen or bacterial culture.

6. Characteristic colonies on anaerobic plates.
7. Colonies of B. *melaninogenicus* may fluoresce red under ultraviolet light, and older colonies produce a typical dark pigment.

The classic diagnostic clinical signs and clues for the presence of anaerobic infections in adults were described first by Finegold.[1] These signs generally can be applied to pediatric patients; however, certain modifications of these clinical clues should be made when they are applied to children, in whom the infection may have unique features and predisposing conditions.

Almost all anaerobic infections originate from the patient's own microflora. Poor blood supply and tissue necrosis lower the oxidation-reduction potential and favor the growth of anaerobic bacteria. Any condition that lowers the blood supply to an affected area of the body can predispose to anaerobic infection. Therefore, trauma, foreign body, malignancy, surgery, edema, shock, colitis, and vascular disease may predispose to anaerobic infection. Prior infection with aerobic or facultative organisms also may make the local tissue conditions more favorable for the growth of anaerobic bacteria.

The human defense mechanisms also may be impaired by anaerobic conditions. The ability of polymorphonuclear leukocytes to kill *Clostridium perfringens* is lowered in anaerobic conditions[2]; however, another report demonstrated their ability to eliminate potential anaerobic pathogens even under anaerobic conditions.[3]

Association of Infections with Mucosal Surfaces

The source of bacteria involved in most of the anaerobic infections is the normal indigenous flora of an individual. The mucous surfaces of the child become colonized with aerobic and anaerobic flora within a short time after birth.[4,5] Anaerobic bacteria are the most common residents of the skin and mucous membrane surfaces[6] and outnumber aerobic bacteria in the normal oral cavity and gastrointestinal tract at a ratio of 10:1 and 1000:1, respectively.[7] Examples of these mucous and skin surfaces are the oral, nasal, and sinus cavities, the gastrointestinal lumen and the conjunctiva, the skin surfaces of different locations, and the sebaceous glands. It is not surprising, therefore, that a large proportion of anaerobes that are part of the normal mucous membrane flora can be recovered from infection in proximity to these sites.

The inoculum of organisms that may penetrate into an infectious site (such as human bite, or perforated gut) usually is complex and contains a mixture of aerobic or anaerobic flora. Although the inoculum of certain organisms that possess greater pathogenicity (such as *Bacteroides fragilis*) can be initially small, they may become the predominant isolates as the infection evolves.

Anaerobes belonging to the indigenous flora of the oral cavity can be recovered from various infections adjacent to that area, such as cervical lymphadenitis[8]; subcutaneous abscesses[9] and burns[10] in proximity to the oral cavity; human and animal bites[11]; paronychia[12]; tonsillar and retropharyngeal abscesses[13]; chronic sinusitis[14]; chronic otitis media[15]; periodontal abscess[16]; thyroiditis[17, 18]; aspiration pneumonia[19]; and bacteremia associated with one of the above infections.[20] The predominant anaerobes recovered in these infections are species of *Bacteroides* (including *Bacteroides malaninogenicus* and *Bacteroides oralis*), *Fusobacterium,* and Gram-positive anaerobic cocci (peptococci and peptostreptococci), which are all part of the normal flora of the mucous surfaces of the oral, pharyngeal, and sinus flora.

A similar correlation exists in infections associated with the gastrointestinal tract. Such infections include peritonitis following rupture of appendix,[21] liver abscess,[22] abscess[23] and burns[10] near the anus, and bacteremia associated with any of these infections.[20] The anaerobes that predominate in these infections are *Bacteroides* species (predominantly *B. fragilis* group), clostridia (including *C. perfringens*), and Gram-positive anaerobic cocci.

Another site with a correlation between the normal flora and the anaerobic bacteria recovered from infected sites is the genitourinary tract. The infections involved are amnionitis, septic abortion, and other pelvic inflammations.[23] The anaerobes usually recovered from these sites are species of *Bacteroides* and *Fusobacterium* and Gram-positive anaerobic cocci. Organisms belonging to the vaginal-cervical flora are also important pathogens of neonatal infections.

Foul-Smelling Specimen or Discharge from an Infected Area

The presence of putrid smell is believed to be due to products of metabolic end products of the anaerobic organisms, which are mostly organic acids. It must be remembered that absence of a foul-smelling discharge does not exclude anaerobic infection. Conversely, the presence of such an odor can occur in an infection caused only by aerobic organisms.

The Presence of Gangrenous Necrotic Tissue

The presence of anoxic conditions can result in the formation of gangrenous necrotic tissue. This anoxic condition predisposes for anaerobic infections, since anaerobes thrive under such conditions.

Free Gas in Tissues

The formation of gas is due to the metabolic end products released by the growing anaerobic organism and is enhanced by anoxic conditions. It is important to remember that some aerobic organisms (such as *Escherichia coli*) also can produce gas in infected tissues. The formation of gas can be detected by palpation or by radiographic examination of the involved area.

No Growth in Aerobic Cultures of Infected Areas

The lack of growth in aerobic cultures is of particular significance in putrid specimens obtained prior to administration of antimicrobial therapy. This can occur also in anaerobic bacteremia, in which aerobic blood cultures will not reveal the infecting organisms. An additional clue to the presence of anaerobes could be the presence of bacterial forms in properly performed Gram stain preparations in which the aerobic bacterial cultures show no growth. Many laboratories assume that failure to cultivate anaerobes in thioglycolate broth excludes anaerobes from the infection, but thioglycolate broth inoculated in room air would not provide adequate anaerobic conditions. Furthermore, overgrowth of rapid growing aerobic organisms, which often are present also in many mixed infections, may mask the presence of slower growing anaerobes.

Infection Persisting after Administration of Antibiotics

Most anaerobes are susceptible to penicillins, although many *Bacteroides* species are resistant to that drug.[24] Other commonly used antibiotics are the aminoglycosides, to which almost all anaerobes are resistant. Therefore, persistence or recurrence of an infection in the face of either of these, or other antimicrobial agents to which anaerobes are resistant, should arouse suspicion of the presence of anaerobic bacteria in the infection.

Clinical Situations Predisposing to Anaerobic Infection

Any exposure of the sterile body cavity to indigenous mucous surface flora will result in infection. This can occur in infections following gastrointestinal surgery, septic abortion, amnionitis, human or animal bites, penetrating wounds of the abdominal or oral cavity, or aspiration pneumonia.

The newborn, and especially those suffering from fetal distress or delivered following maternal amniotic infection, are prone to anaerobic infection. Examples of such infections are the occurrence of neonatal pneumonia after aspiration of infected amniotic fluid[25] or the introduction of anaerobic bacteria indigenous to the vaginal-cervical area into the insertion site of the fetal monitoring needle, an event that can cause scalp abscess and osteomyelitis.[26]

REFERENCES

1. Finegold, S. M. *Anaerobic bacteria in human disease.* New York: Academic Press, 1977, p. 42.

2. Keresch, G. G., and Douglas, S. O. Intraleukocytic survival of anaerobic bacteria. *Clin. Res.* 22:445A, 1974.

3. Mandell, G. L. Bacterial activity of aerobic and anaerobic polymorphonuclear neutrophils. *Infect. Immun.* 9:337, 1974.

4. Brook, I. et al. Aerobic and anaerobic flora of maternal cervix and newborn gastric fluid and conjunctiva: a prospective study. *Pediatrics* 63:451, 1979.

5. Long, S. S., and Swenson, R. M. Development of anaerobic fecal flora in healthy newborn infants. *J. Pediatr.* 91:298, 1977.

6. Gibbons, R. J. Aspects of the pathogenicity and ecology of the indigenous oral flora of man. In *Anaerobic bacteria; role in disease,* eds. A. Ballow et al. Springfield, Ill.: Charles C Thomas, 1974.

7. Gorbach, S. L. Intestinal microflora. *Gastroenterology* 60:1110, 1971.

8. Brook, I. Aerobic and anaerobic bacteriology of cervical adenitis in children. *Clin. Pediatr.* 19:693, 1980.

9. Brook, I., and Finegold, S. M. Aerobic and anaerobic bacteriology of cutaneous abscesses in children. *Pediatrics* 67:891, 1981.

10. Brook, I., and Randolph, J. G. Aerobic and anaerobic flora of burns in children. *J. Trauma* 21:313, 1981.

11. Goldstein, E. J. C. et al. Bacteriology of human and animal bite wounds. *J. Microbiol.* 8:667, 1978.

12. Brook, I. Bacteriology of paronychia in children. *Am. J. Surg.* 141:703, 1981.

13. Brook, I. Aerobic and anaerobic bacteriology of peritonsillar abscess in children. *Acta Paediatr. Scand.* 70:831, 1981.

14. Brook, I. Bacteriologic features of chronic sinusitis in children. *JAMA* 246:967, 1981.

15. Brook, I. Microbiology of chronic otitis media with perforation in children. *Am. J. Dis. Child.* 130:564, 1980.

16. Brook, I.; Grimm, S.; and Kielich, R. B. Bacteriology of acute periapical abscess in children. *Journal of Endodontics* 7:378, 1981.

17. Abe, K. et al. Recurrent acute suppurative thyroiditis. *Am. J. Dis. Child.* 132:990, 1978.

18. Bussman, Y. C. et al. Suppurative thyroiditis with gas formation due to mixed anaerobic infection. *J. Pediatr.* 90:321, 1977.

19. Brook, I., and Finegold, S. M. Bacteriology of aspiration pneumonia in children. *Pediatrics* 65:1115, 1980.

20. Brook, I. et al. Anerobic bacteremia in children. *Am. J. Dis. Child.* 134:1052, 1980.

21. Brook, I. Bacterial studies of peritoneal cavity and postoperative surgical wound drainage following perforated appendix in children. *Ann. Surg.* 192:208, 1980.

22. Sabbaj, J.; Sutter, V. L.; and Finegold, S. M. Anaerobic pyogenic liver abscess. *Ann. Intern. Med.* 77:629, 1972.

23. Ledger, W. J.; Sweet, R. L.; and Hendington, J. T. *Bacteroides* species as a cause of severe infections in obstetrics and gynecologic patients. *Surg. Gynecol. Obstet.* 133:837, 1971.

24. Sutter, V. L., and Finegold, S. M. Susceptibility of anaerobic bacteria to 23 antimicrobial agents. *Antimicrob. Agents Chemother.* 20:736, 1976.

25. Brook, I.; Martin, W. J.; and Finegold, S. M. Neonatal pneumonia caused by members of the *Bacteroides fragilis* group. *Clin. Pediatr.* 19:541, 1980.

26. Brook, I. Osteomylitis and bacteremia caused by *Bacteroides fragilis:* a complication of fetal monitoring. *Clin. Pediatr.* 19:639, 1980.

Anaerobes as Pathogens in Childhood

Anaerobic bacteria differ in their pathogenicity. Not all of them are believed to be clinically significant, while others are known to be highly pathogenic. Table 4.1 lists the major anaerobes that clinically are most frequently encountered. The species of anaerobes most frequently isolated from clinical infections are, in decreasing frequency: *Bacteroides*, *Clostridium*, anaerobic Gram-positive cocci, *Fusobacterium*, Gram-positive rods (*Eubacterium*, *Lactobacillus*, *Propionibacterium*, *Actinomyces*), *Bifidobacterium*, and Gram-negative cocci (*Veillonella* and *Acidaminococcus*).[1] About three-fourths of the anaerobes isolated from clinical infections are members of these genera. The remaining isolates belong to species not yet described, but these usually can be assigned to the appropriate genus on the basis of morphologic characteristics and fermentation products. This chapter provides a discussion of each of the important anaerobic species recovered from children and their role in infectious processes.

Gram-Positive Spore-Forming Bacilli

Anaerobic spore-forming bacilli belong to the genus *Clostridium*. Morphologically, the clostridia are highly pleomorphic, ranging from short, thick bacilli to long filamentous forms, and are either ramrod straight or slightly curved. The three clostridia found most frequently in clinical infections are *Clostridium perfringens*, *Clostridium ramosum* and *Clostridium innocuum*.

   C. perfringens is an inhabitant of soil and of intestinal contents of humans and animals. It is the most frequently encountered histotoxic clostridial species. This microorganism, which elaborates a number of necrotizing extracellular toxins, is easily isolated and identified in the clinical laboratory. *C. perfringens* seldom produces spores in vivo. It can be characterized in direct smears of a purulent exudate by the pres-

ence of stout Gram-variable rods of varying length, frequently surrounded by a capsule. *C. perfringens* can cause a devasta   illness with
high mortality. Clostridial bacteremia is associated with   isive tissue
necrosis, hemolytic anemia, and renal failure. The inci‹   of clostridial endometritis, a common event following septic ab   ιs, has decreased as medically supervised abortions have increase

Table 4.1. Anaerobic Bacteria Most Frequently Encountered
in Clinical Specimens from Children

Organism	Infectious Site
Gram-positive cocci	
Peptococcus sp.	Respiratory tract, intraabdominal and subcutaneous infections
Peptostreptococcus sp.	Respiratory tract, intraabdominal and subcutaneous infections
Microaerophilic streptococci*	Sinusitis, brain abscesses
Gram-positive bacilli	
Non-spore-forming	
Actinomyces sp.	Intracranial abscesses, chronic mastoiditis, aspiration pneumonia, head and neck infections
P. acnes	Shunt infections (cardiac, intracranial)
Bifidobacterium sp.	Chronic otitis media, cervical lymphadenitis
Spore-forming	
Clostridium sp.	
C. perfringens	Wounds and abscesses, sepsis
C. septicum	Sepsis
C. difficile	Diarrheal disease, colitis
C. botulinum	Infantile botulism
C. tetani	Tetanus
Gram-negative bacilli	
Bacteroides sp.	
B. fragilis group	Intraabdominal and female genital tract infections, sepsis, neonatal infection
(*B. fragilis, B. thetaiotaomicron*)	
B. melaninogenicus group	Orofacial infections, aspiration pneumonia, periodontitis
B. oralis	Orofacial infections
B. ruminicola	Orofacial infections, intraabdominal infections
Fusobacterium sp.	
F. nucleatum	Orofacial and respiratory tract infections, brain abscesses, bacteremia
F. necrophorum	Aspiration pneumonia, bacteremia

*Not obligate anaerobes.

Clostridium septicum, long known as an animal pathogen, has been found in humans within the last decade, often associated with malignancy. The intestinal tract is thought to be the source of the organism, and most of the isolates are recovered from blood.

Although *Clostridium botulinum* usually is associated with food poisoning, wound infections caused by this organism are being recognized with increasing frequency. Proteolytic strains of types A and B have been reported from wound infections. Disease caused by *C. botulinum* usually is an intoxication produced by ingestion of contaminated food (uncooked meat, poorly processed fish, improperly canned vegetables), containing a highly potent neurotoxin. Such food may not necessarily seem spoiled, nor may gas production be evident. The polypeptide neurotoxin is relatively heat labile, and food containing this toxin may be rendered innocuous by exposure to 100°C for 10 minutes. Infection of a wound with *C. botulinum* occurs rarely and can produce botulism.

C. botulinum has been associated with newborns presenting with hypotonia, respiratory arrest, areflexia, ptosis, and poorly responding pupils. Botulism in growing infants is caused by toxin from the germination of ingested spores and *C. botulinum* in the bowel lumen.

Clostridium butyricum recently was isolated from blood cultures obtained from 12 newborns with necrotizing enterocolitis; however, the exact clinical association of this organism with the disease has not been established.[2] *Clostridium difficile* has been incriminated as the causative agent of antibiotic-associated and spontaneous diarrhea and colitis.[3,4]

Clostridium tetani rarely is isolated from human feces. Infections caused by this bacillus are a result of contamination of wounds with soil containing *C. tetani* spores. The spores will germinate in devitalized tissue and produce the neurotoxin that is responsible for the clinical findings. *C. tetani* has been recovered from patients presenting with otogenous tetanus.[5,6] Clostridia strains (*C. perfringens, C. butyricum,* and *C. difficile*) have been recovered from blood and peritoneal cultures of necrotizing enterocolitis and from infants with sudden death syndrome.[7-9] Strains of *Clostridium* were recovered from children with bacteremia of gastrointestinal origin[10] and with sickle cell disease.[11] Clostridial strains have been recovered from specimens obtained from children with acute[12] and chronic[13] otitis media, chronic sinusitis and mastoiditis,[14,15] peritonsillar abscesses,[16] peritonitis,[17] and neonatal conjunctivitis.[18]

Gram-Positive Non-Spore-Forming Bacilli

Anaerobic, Gram-positive, non-spore-forming rods comprise part of the microflora of the gingival crevices, the gastrointestinal tract, the vagina, and the skin. Because many of them appear to be similar morphologically, they have been difficult to separate by the usual bacteriologic tests. Several distinct genera are recognized: *Arachnia,* *Bifidobacterium, Propionibacterium, Eubacterium, Lactobacillus,* and Actinomyces.

The *Actinomyces, Arachnia,* and *Bifidobacterium* of the family *Actinomycetaceae* are gram-positive, pleomorphic, anaerobic to microaerophilic bacilli.

Actinomyces israelii and *Actinomyces naeslundii* are normal inhabitants of the human mouth and throat (particularly gingival crypts, dental calculus, and tonsillar crypts) and are the most frequently isolated pathogenic actinomycetes. These organisms have been recovered from intracranial abscesses,[19] chronic mastoiditis,[14] aspiration pneumonia,[20] and peritonitis.[17] Although actinomycetes often are present in mixed culture, they are clearly pathogenic in their own right and may produce widespread devastating disease anywhere in the body.[21] The lesions of actinomycosis occur most commonly in the tissues of the face and neck, lungs, pleura, and ileocecal regions. Bone, pericardial, and anorectal lesions are less common, but virtually any tissue may be invaded; a disseminated, bacteremic form has been described.

Most organisms of the genus *Eubacterium* and anaerobic lactobacilli seem to be nonpathogenic. These organisms are almost invariably isolated as part of mixed flora in the oral, vaginal, and gastrointestinal areas.

Propionibacterium ordinarily is not a pathogen but can be found in association with implanted cardiac or neurogenic prostheses or as a cause of endocarditis on previously damaged valves. Many nonpathogenic organisms may be involved in infection under these circumstances. The two most common species, *Propionibacterium acnes* and *Propionibacterium granulosum,* may be isolated with relative frequency from blood cultures but are associated only rarely with bacteremia or endocarditis. Because these organisms are part of the normal skin flora, they are common laboratory contaminants or may grow in blood cultures from skin contamination if the skin surface has been improperly decontaminated before the blood sample is drawn. Therefore, interpretation of the significance of an isolate must be undertaken with caution. There are, however, several well-documented cases of infection. *P. acnes* can cause bacteremia, especially in association with shunt infections.[22] The possible role of *P. acnes* in the pathogenesis of acne vulgaris was suggested. The data that support this are based on the recovery of this organism in large numbers from sebaceous follicles, especially in patients with acne, on its ability to elaborate enzymes such as lipase, protease, and hyaluronidase, and on its ability to activate the complement system and enhance chemotactic activity of neutrophils.[23]

Gram-Negative Bacilli

Bacteroides Species

The anaerobic Gram-negative rods are differentiated into genera on the basis of the fermentation acids they produce. The family Bacteroidaceae contains two genera of medical importance: *Bacteroides* and *Fusobacterium*.

The species of Bacteroidaceae that occur with greatest frequency in clinical specimens belong to the *Bacteroides fragilis* group. These organisms are resistant to penicillin by virtue of production of beta-lactamase, and by other unknown factors.[24] This organism was formerly classified as five subspecies of *B. fragilis* (ss. *distasonis*, ss. *fragilis*, ss. *ovatus*, ss. *thetaiotaomicron*, and ss. *vulgatus*). They have been recently reclassified into distinct species on the basis of DNA homology studies.[25]

B. fragilis (formerly known as *B. fragilis* ss. *fragilis*, one of the five subspecies of *B. fragilis*) is the anaerobe most frequently isolated from infections. Although *B. fragilis* is the most common subspecies found in clinical specimens, it is the least common *Bacteroides* species present in fecal flora, comprising only 0.5% of the bacteria present in stool. The pathogenicity of this organism probably is due to its ability to produce capsular material, which is protective against phagocytosis.[26] Because of its presence in normal flora of the gastrointestinal tract this organism is predominant in bacteremia associated with intraabdominal infections,[1] peritonitis and abscesses following rupture of viscus,[17] and subcutaneous abscesses or burns near the anus.[27] Although *B. fragilis* is not generally found as part of the normal oral flora, it can colonize the oral cavity of patients with poor oral hygiene or of those who previously received antimicrobial therapy (especially penicillin). Following the colonization of the oropharyngeal cavity, this organism can be recovered also from pediatric infections that originate in this area, such as aspiration pneumonia,[20] lung abscesses,[28] chronic sinusitis,[15] chronic otitis media,[13] brain abscesses,[19] and subcutaneous abscesses or burns near the oral cavity.[27, 29]

B. fragilis can be recovered from infectious processes in the newborn. The newborn infant is at risk of developing these infections when born to a mother with amnionitis, premature rupture of membranes, or during the newborn's passage through the birth canal, where *B. fragilis* is part of the normal flora.[30] *B. fragilis* was recovered from newborns with aspiration pneumonia,[31] bacteremia,[10] omphalitis,[32] and subcutaneous abscesses and occipital osteomylitis following fetal monitoring.[33]

Bacteroides oralis is part of the normal flora of the mouth and vagina. Unlike *B. fragilis*, however, strains of *B. oralis* generally are susceptible to penicillin and the cephalosporins, although more strains of *B. oralis* have shown resistance to these drugs. *B. oralis* almost never is found in pure culture in clinical infection. This organism can possess a capsule. It has been recovered from almost all types of respiratory tract and subcutaneous infections in children, including aspiration pneumonia,[20] lung abscess,[29] chronic otitis media,[13] sinusitis,[15] and subcutaneous abscesses around the oral cavity.[27]

Bacteroides melaninogenicus requires the presence of both hemin and vitamin K_1 for growth. The requirement for vitamin K_1 in vivo often is met by coexistence with organisms that are capable of supplying this need of *B. melaninogenicus*. *B. melaninogenicus* is part of the normal oral and vaginal flora and has emerged as the predominant *Bacteroides* species isolated from respiratory infections. These include aspiration pneumonia,[20] lung abscess,[28] chronic otitis media, and chronic sinusitis.[13, 15] This organism has been recovered also from abscesses and burns around the oral cavity,[27] human bites, paronychia,[34] urinary tract infection,[35] and brain abscesses.[19] Also, it has been isolated from children with bacteremia associated with infections of the upper respiratory tract.[10] Organisms of the *B. melaninogenicus* group have been found to play a major role in the pathogenesis of periodontal disease[36] and periodontal abscesses in children.[37]

Of the three designated species belonging to the *B. melaninogenicus* group, *B. asaccharolyticus* is the most frequent clinical isolate. Species *B. intermedius* is identified somewhat less frequently, and *B. melaninogenicus* is the least common. The presence of capsular material suppresses phagocytosis and therefore is an important factor influencing the pathogenicity of the *B. melaninogenicus* group.[38]

Subcutaneous and intraperitoneal abscesses could be induced in mice by inoculation with each of the three *B. melaninogenicus* species alone. The ability of these species to cause an abscess was correlated with the presence of a capsule.[39] Exposure of mice to viable, nonviable, or capsular material of *Klebsiella pneumoniae* also enables the nonencapsulated *Bacteroides* populations to become encapsulated populations. This phenomena was limited not only to coinoculation of *B. melaninogenicus* group with *K. pneumoniae,* but was achieved by inoculation of *B. melaninogenicus* with nonviable or capsular material from encapsulated *Bacteroides* strains or with other aerobic organisms causing inflammation. The presence of capsular material in the inoculum probably was sufficient to prevent phagocytosis of the organisms, and the final outcome was the selection of the encapsulated strain. This concept is supported by the observation that a few encapsulated organisms were found among the initially nonencapsulated strains.

Mixed infections caused by numerous aerobic and anaerobic organisms are observed commonly in clinical situations.[20, 28] The selection of encapsulated *Bacteroides* species in mixed infections with other encapsulated anaerobic or anaerobic organisms may take place also in patients, and it may explain the conversion of nonpathogenic organisms that are part of normal host flora into pathogenic bacteria. This phenomenon may justify directing therapy in such infections against potential pathogens such as *B. melaninogenicus*. Detection of the presence of a capsule in a clinical isolate may add significance to its possible role as a pathogen in the infection.

Bacteroides corrodens characteristically forms small colonies with a zone around or under the colony that has been described as "pitting" of the agar: thus the name "corrodens." *B. corrodens* is part of the normal flora of the mouth and has been isolated from blood cultures shortly after dental surgery, periodontal abscesses,[37] aspiration pneumonia,[20] and lung abscesses.[29] *Bacteroides ruminicola* ss. *brevis* also has been recovered from these sites, [20, 29] as well as from peritonsillar abscesses,[16] chronic sinusitis,[15] mastoiditis,[14] and peritonitis.[17]

Fusobacterium Species

The species of *Fusobacterium* seen most often in clinical infections are *Fusobacterium nucleatum*, *Fusobacterium necrophorum*, and *Fusobacterium mortiferum*. *Fusobacterium nucleatum* is the predominant *Fusobacterium* from clinical specimens, often associated with infections of the mouth, lung,[20] and brain.[40] Because these organisms are part of the normal flora of the oral and gastrointestinal flora, they are found in almost all types of infections in children. These include bacteremia,[10] meningitis associated with otologic diseases,[40] peritonitis following rupture of viscus,[17] and subcutaneous abscesses and burns near the oral or anal orifices.[17, 29] Cells of *Fusobacterium* species are moderately long and thin, with tapered ends, and have typical fusiform morphology.

Gram-positive Cocci

Anaerobic cocci have been most often reported either as "anaerobic streptococci" or "anaerobic Gram-positive cocci." Those that occur in clinical specimens are speciated easily according to differences in fermentation products and a few biochemical reactions. The species most commonly isolated are *Peptococcus magnus*, *Peptostreptococcus anaerobius*, *Peptostreptococcus intermedius*, *Peptococcus asaccharolyticus*, and *Peptococcus prevotii*. These organisms are part of the normal flora of the mouth, upper respiratory tract, intestinal tract, vagina, and skin. They are divided as peptococci or peptostreptococci on the basis of cell arrangement (peptococci are the anaerobic equivalent of staphylococci and peptostreptococci are the anaerobic equivalent of streptococci) and to species primarily on the basis of their metabolic products. Their presence has been documented in adults in a variety of syndromes, including endocarditis, brain abscesses, puerperal sepsis, traumatic wounds, and postoperative necrotizing fasciitis. They have been recovered in pediatric infections in subcutaneous abscesses and burns around the oral and anal area, intraabdominal infections,[17] decubitus ulcers, and also have been isolated as causes of bacteremia[10] and brain abscesses.[19, 40] These organisms are predominant isolates also in all types of respiratory infections, including chronic sinusitis,[15] mastoiditis,[14] acute[42] and chronic otitis media,[13] aspiration pneumonia, and lung abscess.[20, 29] They generally are recovered mixed with other aerobic or anaerobic organisms, but in many cases they are the only pathogens recovered. This may be of particular significance in cases of bacteremia[10] or acute otitis media.[42] Microaerophilic streptococci are of particular importance in chronic sinusitis[15] and brain abscesses.[19 40]

Gram-negative Cocci

There are three species described as anaerobic Gram-negative cocci: *Veillonella, Acidaminococcus,* and *Megasphaera.* There are two described species of *Veillonella* and only one each of the other two genera. The veillonellae are the most frequently involved of the three species and are part of the normal flora of the mouth, vagina, and the small intestine of some persons. Although they rarely are isolated from clinical infections, these organisms have been recovered occasionally from almost every type of pediatric infection.[2] Their exact pathogenic role is unclear, however.

Conclusion

Many infectious diseases in children can be produced by anaerobic bacteria. Anaerobes of major clinical importance tend to follow certain predictable patterns according to anatomic sites and their virulence. In the upper respiratory passages and lung, the major anaerobic pathogens are *Peptostreptococcus* species, *B. melaninogenicus,* and *Fusobacterium* species. In intraabdominal infections and female genital infections, the most frequent isolates are of the *B. fragilis* group, followed by *Clostridium* species and anaerobic Gram-positive cocci.

Recognition of the pathogenic features of these organisms enables prompt identification and initiation of appropriate management of the infections that they cause.

REFERENCES

1. Finegold, S. M. Anaerobic bacteria in human disease. New York: Academic Press, 1977.
2. Brook, I. The role of anaerobic bacteria in pediatric infections. In *Advances in pediatrics*, vol. 21, ed. L. A. Barnes. Chicago: Year Book, 1980, p. 163.
3. Brook, I. Isolation of toxin producing *Clostridium difficile* from two children with oxacillin and dicloxacillin associated diarrhea. *Pediatrics* 65:1154, 1980.
4. Viscidi, R. P., and Bartlett, J. G. Antibiotic associated pseudomembraneous colitis in children. *Pediatrics* 67:381, 1981.
5. Nourmand, A. Clinical studies on tetanus: notes on 42 cures in southern Iran with special emphasis on portal of entry. *Clin. Pediatr.* 12:652, 1973.
6. Fischer, M. G. W.; Sunakorn, P.; and Duangman, C. Otogenous tetanus: a sequelae of chronic ear infections. *Am J. Dis. Child.* 131:445, 1977.
7. Cashore, W. J. et al. *Clostridium* colonization and clostidial toxin in neonatal necrotizing enterocolitis. *J. Pediatr.* 98:308, 1981.
8. Sturm, R. et al. Neonatal necrotizing enterocolitis associated with penicillin resistant *Clostridium butyricum*. *Pediatrics* 66:928, 1980.
9. Cooperstock, M. S. et al. *Clostridium difficile* in normal infants and sudden infant death syndrome: an association with infant formula feeding. *Pediatrics* 70:91, 1982.
10. Brook, I. et al. Anaerobic bacteremia in children. *Am. J. Dis. Child.* 134:1052, 1980.
11. Brook, I., and Gluck, R. S. *Clostridium paraputrificum* sepsis in sickle cell disease: a report of a case. *South. Med. J.* 73:1644, 1980.
12. Brook, I.; Schwartz, R. H.; and Controni, G. *Clostridium ramosum* isolation in acute otitis media. *Clin. Pediatr.* 18:699, 1979.
13. Brook, I. Microbiology of chronic otitis media with perforation in children. *Am. J. Dis. Child.* 130:564, 1980.
14. Brook, I. Aerobic and anaerobic bacteriology of chronic mastoiditis in children. *Am. J. Dis. Child.* 135, 1981.
15. Brook, I. Bacteriological features of chronic sinusitis in children. *JAMA* 246:967, 1981.
16. Brook, I. Aerobic and anaerobic bacteriology of peritonsillar abscess in children. *Acta Pediatr. Scand.* 70:831, 1981.
17. Brook, I. Bacterial studies of peritoneal cavity and postoperative surgical wound drainage following perforated appendix in children. *Ann. Surg.* 192:208, 1980.
18. Brook, I.; Martin, W. J.; and Finegold, S. M. Effect of silver nitrate application on the conjunctival flora of the newborn and the occurrence of clostridial conjunctivitis. *J. Pediatr. Ophthalmol. Strabismus* 15:173, 1978.
19. Brook, I. Bacteriology of intracranial abscess in children. *J. Neurosurg.* 54:484, 1981.
20. Brook, I., and Finegold, S. M. Bacteriology of aspiration pneumonia in children. *Pediatrics* 65:1115, 1980.
21. Drake, D. P., and Holt, R. J. Childhood actinomycosis: report of 3 recent cases. *Arch. Dis. Child.* 51:979, 1976.
22. Beeler, B. A. et al. *Propionibacterium acnes:* pathogen in central nervous system infection. *Am. J. Med.* 61:935, 1976.
23. Esterly, N. B., and Furey, M. L. Acne: current concepts. *Pediatrics* 62:1044, 1978.

24. Olson-Liljequest, B.; Dornbusch, K.; and Nord, C. E. Characterization of three different beta-lactamases from the *Bacteroides fragilis* group. *Antimicrob. Agents Chemother.* 18:220, 1980.

25. Cato, E. P., and Johnson, J. L. Reinstatement of species rank for *Bacteroides fragilis, B. ovalus, B. distasonis, B. thetaiotaomicron,* and *B. vulgatus:* designation of neotype strains for *Bacteroides fragilis* (Veillin and Zuber) Castellani and Chalmers and *Bacteroides thetaiotaomicron* (Distaso) Castellani and Chalmers. *Int. J. Syst. Bacteriol.* 26:230, 1976.

26. Sperry, J. F., and Adamu, S. A. Polymorphonuclear neutrophil chemotaxis induced and inhibited by *Bacteroides* spp. *Infect. Immun.* 33:806, 1981.

27. Brook, I., and Finegold, S. M. Aerobic and anaerobic bacteriology of cutaneous abscesses in children. *Pediatrics* 67:891, 1981.

28. Brook, I., and Finegold, S. M. The bacteriology and therapy of lung abscess in children. *J. Pediatr.* 94:10, 1979.

29. Brook, I., and Randolph, J. Aerobic and anaerobic flora of burns in children. *J. Trauma* 21:313, 1981.

30. Brook, I. et al. Aerobic and anaerobic flora of maternal cervix and newborn's conjunctiva and gastric fluid: a prospective study. *Pediatrics* 63:451, 1979.

31. Brook, I.; Martin, W. J.; and Finegold, S. M. Neonatal pneumonia caused by members of the *Bacteroides fragilis* group. *Clin. Pediatr.* 19:541, 1980.

32. Brook, I. Bacteriology of neonatal omphalitis. *J. Infect. Dis.* 5:127, 1982.

33. Brook, I. Osteomyelitis and bacteremia caused by *Bacteroides fragilis:* a complication of fetal monitoring. *Clin. Pediatr.* 19:639, 1980.

34. Brook, I. Bacteriology of paronychia in children. *Am. J. Surg.* 141:703, 1981.

35. Brook, I. Urinary tract infection caused by anaerobic bacteria in children. *Urology* 16:596, 1980.

36. Slots, J. The predominant cultivable organisms in juvenile periodontitis. *Scand. J. Dent. Res.* 85:114, 1977.

37. Brook, I.; Grimm, S.; and Kielich, R. B. Bacteriology of acute periapical abscess in children. *J. Endod.* 7:378, 1981.

38. Okuda, K., and Takazoe, I. Antiphagocytic effects of the capsular structure of a pathogenic strains of *Bacteroides melaninogenicus. Bull Tokyo Med. Dent. Univ.* 14:99, 1973.

39. Brook, I. et al. The role of capsular material of *Bacteroides melaninogenicus* in mixed infection (abstr.). In *Report of the 82nd Annual Meeting of the American Society for Microbiology,* Atlanta, 1982.

40. Brook, I. et al. Complications of sinusitis in children. *Pediatrics* 66:568, 1980.

41. Brook, I. Anaerobic and aerobic bacteriology of decubitus ulcers in children. *Am. J. Surg.* 46:624, 1980.

42. Brook, I., and Finegold, S. M. Bacteriology of chronic otitis media. *JAMA* 241:487, 1979.

PART II

Neonatal Infections

CHAPTER 5

Introduction to Neonatal Infections

The incidence of infection in the fetus and newborn infant is high. As many as 2% of fetuses are infected in utero and up to 10% of infants are infected during delivery or in the first few months of life. The predominant microorganisms known to cause these infections are cytomegalovirus, rubella virus, herpes simplex virus, *Toxoplasma gondii*, *Treponema pallidum*, chlamydia, group B *Streptococcus*, *Escherichia coli*, and anaerobic bacteria. All of these agents can colonize or infect the mother and infect the fetus or newborn either intrauterinely or during the passage through the birth canal. Several factors have been associated with acquisition of local or systemic infection in the newborn. Most of these factors are vague and difficult to define; however, most studies have described the presence of one or more risk factors in the pregnancy and delivery in these infants: premature and prolonged rupture of membranes (longer than 24 hours), maternal peripartum infection, premature delivery, low birth weight, depressed respiratory function of the infant at birth or fetal anoxia, and septic or traumatic delivery.[1-3]

Maternal infection at the time of delivery, especially of the urogenital tract, can be associated with the development of infection in the newborn. Transplacental hematogenous infection that can spread before or during delivery is another way in which the infant can be infected.[4] The acquisition of infection while the newborn passes through the birth canal is, however, the most frequent mode of transfer.

During pregnancy the fetus is shielded from the flora of the mother's genital tract. Potentially pathogenic bacteria are found in the amniotic fluid (AF) even when the membranes are intact. Prevedourakis, Papadimitriou, and Ioannidou[5] documented bacterial invasion of the intact amnion from nearly 8% of the pregnant women in their sample, but this was of no consequence to the mother or the newborn infant. It was suspected that the AF may have antibacterial properties, probably owing to lack of nutritional factors.[5, 6] Larson, Snyder, and Galask[7] demonstrated that the AF actively inhibited the growth of aerobic bacteria, an ability thought to be due to a phosphate-sensitive cationic protein whose antimicrobial properties were regulated by the availability of zinc.[7] Its activity was independent of the muramidase and peroxidases and spermine.

The antimicrobial properties of the AF also vary with the period of gestation; it was the least inhibitory against *E. coli* and *Bacteroides fragilis* during the first trimester and most inhibitory during the third trimester.[7, 8] The relative sparsity of the *B. fragilis* population in the cervix at term labor and the added inhibitory effect of the amniotic fluid at term may together explain the relatively low incidence of *B. fragilis* infections at full term as compared to postabortal sepsis.[9, 10]

Following the rupture of the membranes the colonization of the newborn is initiated[4] by further exposure to the flora during the infant's passage through the birth canal. When premature rupture of the membranes occurs, the ascending flora can cause infection of the amniotic fluid with involvement of the fetal membranes, placenta, and umbilical cord.[11] Aspiration of the infected amniotic fluid can cause aspiration pneumonia. Since anaerobic bacteria are the predominant organisms in the mother's genital flora,[12] they become major pathogens in infections that follow early exposure of the newborn to that flora.

Genetic factors may be responsible for the predominance of sepsis in the newborn male.[13] The immaturity of the immunologic system, which is manifested by decreased function of the phagocytes and decreased inflammatory reactions, may also contribute to the susceptibility of infants to microbial infection.[14, 15] The presence of anoxia and acidosis in the newborn may interfere also with the defense mechanisms.

The support systems and procedures used in regular nurseries and intensive care units can facilitate the acquisition of infections. Offending instruments include umbilical catheters, arterial lines, and intubation devices. Contamination of equipment such as humidifiers and supplies such as intravenous solutions and infant formulas and poor isolation techniques can result in outbreaks of bacterial or viral infections in nurseries. Such spread is thought to contribute to clustering of cases of necrotizing enterocolitis in newborns.

REFERENCES

1. Gluck, L.; Wood, H. F.; and Fousek, M. D. Septicemia of the newborn. *Pediatr. Clin. North Am.* 13:1131, 1966.

2. Buetow, K. C.; Klein, S. W.; and Lane, R. B. Septicemia in premature infants. *Am. J. Dis. Child.* 110:29, 1965.

3. Overall, J. C., Jr. Neonatal bacterial meningitis. *J. Pediatr.* 76:499, 1970.

4. Grossman, J., and Tompkins, R. L. Group B beta-hemolytic streptococcal meningitis in mother and infant. *N. Engl. J. Med.* 290:387, 1974.

5. Prevedourakis, C.; Papadimitriou, G.; and Ioannidou, A. Isolation of pathogenic bacteria in the amniotic fluid during pregnancy and labor. *Am. J. Obstet. Gynecol.* 106:400, 1970.

6. Prevedourakis, C. et al. *E. coli* growth inhibition by amniotic fluid. *Acta Obstet. Gynecol. Scand.* 55:245, 1976.

7. Larson, B.; Snyder, I. S.; and Galask, R. P. Bacterial growth inhibition by amniotic fluid. *Am. J. Obstet. Gynecol.* 119:492, 497, 1974.

8. Thadepalli, H.; Bach, V. T.; and Davidson, E. C., Jr. Antimicrobial effect of amniotic fluid. *Obstet. Gynecol.* 52:198, 1978.

9. Ledger, W. J.; Sucet, R. L.; and Headington, J. T. *Bacteroides* species as a cause of severe infections in obstetrics and gynaecologic patients. *Surg. Gynecol. Obstet.* 133:837, 1971.

10. Pearson, H. E., and Anderson, G. V. Perinatal deaths associated with *Bacteroides* infections. *Obstet. Gynecol.* 30:486, 1967.

11. Benirschke, K. Routes and types of infection in the fetus and newborn. *Am. J. Dis. Child.* 99:714, 1960.

12. Brook, I. et al. Aerobic and anaerobic flora of maternal cervix and newborn gastric fluid and conjunctiva: a prospective study. *Pediatrics* 63:451, 1979.

13. Washburn, T. C.; Medearis, D. N., Jr.; and Childs, B. Sex differences in susceptibility to infection. *Pediatrics* 35:57, 1965.

14. Miller, E. M., and Stiehm, E. R. Phagocytic opsonic and immunoglobulin studies in the newborns. *Calif. Med.* 119:43, 1972.

15. Coen, R.; Grush, O.; and Kander, E. Studies of bacterial activity and metabolism of the leukocyte in full term neonates. *J. Pediatr.* 75:400, 1969.

Colonization of Anaerobic Flora in Newborns

Colonization of the Mucous Membranes, Gastrointestinal Tract, and Skin in the Normal Infant

The developing fetus is protected from the bacterial flora of the maternal genital tract. Initial colonization of the newborn and of the placenta usually occurs after rupture of the maternal membranes. During a vaginal delivery the neonate is exposed to the cervical birth canal flora, which includes many aerobic and anaerobic bacteria.[1, 2]

When appropriate cervical cultures are taken, at least 15 different bacterial strains can be recovered from a culture.[3] The predominant aerobic bacteria present in this flora are staphylococci, diphtheroids, alpha-hemolytic streptococci, *Corynebacterium vaginale (Haemophilis vaginalis)*, lactobacilli, and *Escherichia coli*. The anaerobic organisms most frequently isolated are the *Bacteroides fragilis* group, *Proprionibacterium acnes*, peptococci, *Bacteroides melaninogenicus*, clostridia, and anaerobic lactobacilli.

The newborn is colonized initially on the skin and mucosa of the nasopharynx, oropharynx, conjunctivae, umbilical cord, and the external genitalia. In most infants, the organisms colonize these sites without causing any inflammatory changes.

The colonization of the gastrointestinal tract by bacteria begins immediately after delivery. A recent prospective study of 35 mothers and infants examined the colonization of newborns and correlated the newborns' gastric fluid and conjunctival flora with maternal vaginal flora.[4] This study demonstrated that gastric aspirates of vaginally delivered infants contain many aerobic and anaerobic bacteria that are identical to the maternal genital flora.

The bacteriologic findings in the newborn infant (conjunctival and gastric contents) and the obstetric and neonatal data showed certain significant associations. As the newborn infant's birth weight increased, more pathogenic aerobic bacteria (such as *E. coli* and *Staphylococcus aureus*) were acquired in gastric contents; also, prolongation of labor brought about increased numbers of pathogenic anaerobes (such as the *B. fragilis* group). A number of groups of bacteria were found with statistically significant greater frequency in gastric contents with increased duration of pregnancy. Although a variety of pathogenic and nonpathogenic bacteria were ingested by the normal newborns, no apparent infection developed in any of these infants. It seems, therefore, that when appropriate aerobic and anaerobic cultures are done, gastric aspirates yield multiple potentially pathogenic aerobic and anaerobic bacteria that have no correlation with the clinical course of the newborn infants. These organisms represent a transient load of bacteria acquired during delivery, as has been indicated by previous investigations.[5, 6]

The development of normal fecal flora was studied in 50 newborns.[7] The initially sterile meconium becomes colonized in most instances within 24 hours with aerobic and anaerobic bacteria, predominantly micrococci, *E. coli*, *Clostridium* species, and streptococci. Other studies[8, 9] demonstrated the presence of various types of clostridia at that age. A recent study[9] involving 190 healthy infants has shown that the isolation rates of *B. fragilis* and other anaerobic bacteria in the gastrointestinal tract of term babies approach that of adults within a week. The percentage of stools containing anaerobic bacteria increased with age so that by four to six days of age 96% of the infants were colonized with anaerobic bacteria, and 61% were colonized with *B. fragilis*. There were, however, some variations in the colonization pattern that were related to gestational age, mode of delivery, and type of feeding.

E. coli, *Klebsiella* species, *Enterobacter* species, and *Proteus* species were the most frequently isolated aerobic Gram-negative bacilli. Almost three-fourths of term infants delivered vaginally, whether formula-fed or breast-fed, were colonized with at least one of these strains by 48 hours of age. In contrast, isolation rates of these coliform bacilli before 48 hours was lower in term infants delivered by cesarean section and in premature infants delivered by the vaginal route. The predominant anaerobes recovered, except for the *B. fragilis* group, included species of *Clostridium, Bifidobacterium, Eubacterium, Fusobacterium, Propionibacterium, Lactobacillus, Peptococcus, Peptostreptococcus,* and *Veillonella*. Non-*Bacteroides* anaerobic isolates were equally represented among study groups and age groups except for species of *Bifidobacterium* and *Veillonella*. *Bifidobacterium* isolates were recovered more frequently from breast-fed infants, while *Veillonella* isolates were isolated more frequently from stools of infants delivered by cesarean section.

The influence of breast-feeding on the predominance of the *Bifidobacterium* in the newborn was studied recently.[10] Specific growth factors for this organism were found in human milk, while other milks,

including cow's milk, sheep's milk, and infant formulas, did not promote the growth of this species. The investigators believe that *Bifidobacterium* inhibits the growth of *E. coli*[11] by producing large amounts of
acetic acid. Furthermore, because of the small buffering capacity of
human milk, the patient is maintained at acid levels that inhibit the
growth of *Bacteroides, Clostridium* and *E. coli*. It is postulated that these
conditions grant the breast-fed infant a resistance to gastroenteritis.

Colonization of the Respiratory Tract in Intubated Newborns

Bacterial colonization of the tracheobronchial tree almost always follows tracheal intubation.[12] It is not only difficult to differentiate between colonization and clinical infection,[13] but also to try to assess the
various factors that may influence the acquisition of these bacteria.[14]

The newborn infant who presents with respiratory distress syndrome may require intubation for extended periods of time. Studies of
bacterial colonization in newborns who require intubation rarely have
been done,[15] and the role of anaerobic bacteria in this setting was not
investigated until recently.[16] In a recent prospective study we have
summarized data obtained from a study of intubated newborns. This
report of 127 newborns requiring intubation describes the mode of tracheal colonization of both aerobic and anaerobic bacteria and the effect
of antibiotics on the colonization. Specimens were obtained twice a
week as long as the 127 newborns were intubated. The specimens were
obtained through tracheal suction done routinely in the nursery. Each
newborn had between one and eight specimens taken (average 1.7). No
bacterial or fungal growth was obtained from 65 specimens, whereas
the remaining specimens (147) yielded 209 bacterial and fungal isolates, accounting for 1.4 isolates per specimen. The total isolates recovered were 168 aerobes, 36 anaerobes, and 5 *Candida albicans*. Of
this total, 70 specimens yielded one isolate, 48 two isolates, 6 three isolates, 5 four isolates, and one aspirate yielded five isolates.

Aerobic organisms most frequently isolated were *Staphylococcus epidermidis* (61 isolates), alpha-hemolytic streptococci (41), *S. aureus* (14),
Klebsiella pneumoniae (12), and group B beta-hemolytic streptococci (6).

The predominant anaerobic bacteria isolated were *Propionibacterium acnes* (18 isolates), *Bacteroides* species (6), *Peptococcus* species (5),
and *Clostridium perfringens* (5). Anaerobic bacteria accounted for 20% of
the bacterial isolate recovered from the first three specimens.

Seventy-eight newborns (61%) received antimicrobial therapy. A
higher incidence of positive cultures and the presence of more than
one organism per culture were found in those infants not receiving antibiotics. More isolates per specimen were noted with increasing time
of incubation. The rate of isolation of *S. aureus, Pseudomonas aeruginosa*,

and *K. pneumoniae* remained constant with increased length of intubation, while the rate of recovery of *Staphylococcus epidermidis*, alpha-hemolytic streptococci, and *P. acnes* increased, and the rate of isolation of *E. coli*, *Bacteroides* species, and anaerobic Gram-positive cocci decreased.

This study demonstrates the occurrence of microbial colonization immediately after intubation in 70% of newborns. The bacteria recovered from the first specimens, which were obtained immediately after intubation and usually within 24 hours after delivery, may reflect microbial contamination acquired upon passage through the birth canal. Organisms recovered at that time were primarily Gram-positive cocci and *Bacteroides* organisms. These bacteria acquired from the mother's cervical flora tend to decrease in number and are replaced by normal skin flora such as alpha-hemolytic streptococci, *S. epidermidis*, and *P. acnes*.

The use of systemic antibodies in newborns can alter the bacterial flora of their respiratory tract, which may result in an overgrowth of Gram-negative bacteria.[17, 18] Bacterial colonization and superinfection also are common in adults treated with antimicrobial agents for pneumonia.[19] It is of interest that organisms such as *S. aureus*, *P. aeruginosa*, and a variety of anaerobes tend to increase in numbers in chronically intubated adults[14] and older children.[20] These organisms did not predominate in the newborn population, however.[16] This observation could be due to a variety of factors, including the relatively shorter intubation period in the neonate (which usually does not exceed one week), the relatively low levels of colonization with resistant bacteria,[15] the relatively short courses of antimicrobial agents, and the occurrence of early infant death.

In another study of colonization of newborns, endotracheal suction of intubated infants did provide a reliable specimen source for determining the etiology of perinatal pneumonia.[21] Presence of polymorphonuclear leukocytes in the aspirate correlated well with infection. Anaerobic bacteria were found to play a role in three of the five cases of pneumonia. The anaerobic organisms were isolated, all mixed with facultatives. In two instances *Bacteroides distasonis* was recovered with alpha-hemolytic streptococci. In one of these, the organism was recovered also from the mother's blood and amniotic fluid (amnionitis was present). *Clostridium perfringens*, *Peptococcus variabilis*, *Haemophilus influenzae*, and *S. epidermidis* were obtained from the third case of pneumonia, which occurred in a newborn delivered by cesarean section with meconium-stained amniotic fluid and meconium aspiration.

The technique of tracheal apsiration culture plus the Wright's staining procedure was shown, therefore, to be effective in defining infective and noninfective conditions in newborns with respiratory distress. Moreover, it seemed to be effective in early recognition of perinatal pneumonia caused by both aerobic and anaerobic bacteria.

Although the technique of obtaining tracheal cultures by aspiration of material from an endotracheal tube used for ventilation is not ideal, it seemed to be a simple and safe procedure with almost no side effects or risk. It is clear that anaerobes, along with facultative and aerobic bacteria, may play a role in perinatal pneumonia. This must be considered in devising therapeutic regimens.

Routine cultures of the tracheal secretions of intubated newborns for surveillance of aerobic and anaerobic bacteria would enable the clinician to predict changes in the tracheal flora and facilitate the selection of appropriate antimicrobial therapy whenever the patient is infected. Repeated tracheal cultures for aerobic and anaerobic bacteria during the course of the pneumonia would allow for adjustment of the therapy if and when the bacteria present change or become resistant to the antibiotics used.

REFERENCES

1. Linder, J. G. E. M.; Plantema, F. H. A.; and Hoogkamp-Korstanje, J. A. A. Quantitative studies of the vaginal flora of healthy women and obstetric and gynaecologic patients. *J. Med. Microbiol.* 11:233, 1978.

2. Coplerud, C. P.; Ohm, M. J.; and Galask, R. P. Aerobic and anaerobic flora of the cervix during pregnancy and puerperium. *Am. J. Obstet. Gynecol.* 126:856, 1976.

3. Larsen, B.; and Galask, R. P. Vaginal microbial flora: practical and theoretic relevance. *Obstet. Gynecol.* 55 (suppl.):1005, 1980.

4. Brook, I. et al. Aerobic and anaerobic bacterial flora of the maternal cervix and newborn gastric fluid and conjunctiva: a prospective study. *Pediatrics* 63:451, 1979.

5. Mims, L. C. et al. Predicting neonatal infections by evaluation of the gastric aspirate: a study in 207 patients. *Am. J. Obstet. Gynecol.* 114:232, 1972.

6. Hosmer, M. E., and Sprunt, K. Screening method for identification of infected infant following premature rupture of maternal membranes. *Pediatrics* 49:283, 1972.

7. Hall, I. C., and O'Toole, E. Bacterial flora of first specimens of meconium passed by fifty newborn infants. *Am. J. Dis. Child.* 47:1279, 1934.

8. Hall, I. C., and Matsumura, K. Recovery of *Bacillus tertius* from stools of infants. *J. Infect. Dis.* 35:502, 1924.

9. Long, S. S., and Swenson, R. M. Development of anaerobic fecal flora in healthy newborn infants. *J. Pediatr.* 91:298, 1977.

10. Simhon, A. et al. Effect of feeding on infant's faecal flora. *Arch. Dis. Child.* 57:54, 1982.

11. Bullen, C. L.; Tearle, P. V.; and Stewart, M. G. The effect of "humanized" milks and supplemental breast feeding on the faecal flora of infants. *J. Med. Microbiol.* 10:603, 1977.

12. Aass, A. S. Complications to tracheostomy and long term intubation. A follow-up study. *Acta Anaesthesiol. Scand.* 19:127, 1975.

13. Gotsman, M. S., and Whiby, J. L. Respiratory infection following tracheostomy. *Thorax* 19:89, 1964.

14. Bryand, L. R. et al. Bacterial colonization profile with tracheal intubation and mechanical ventilation. *Arch. Surg.* 104:647, 1972.

15. Harris, H.; Wirtschafter, D.; and Cassady, G. Endotracheal intubation and its relationship to bacterial colonization and systemic infection of newborn infants. *Pediatrics* 56:816, 1976.

16. Brook, I., and Martin, W. J. Bacterial colonization in intubated newborns. *Respiration* 40:323, 1980.

17. Dalton, H. P. et al. Pulmonary infection due to disruption of the pharyngeal bacterial flora by antibiotics in hamsters. *Am. J. Pathol.* 76:469, 1974.

18. Farmer, K. The influence of hospital environment and antibiotics on the bacterial flora of the upper respiratory tract of the newborn. *NZ Med. J.* 67:541, 1968.

19. Tillotson, J. R., and Finland, M. Secondary pulmonary infections following antibiotic therapy for primary bacterial pneumonia. *Antimicrob. Agents Chemother.* 8:326, 1968.

20. Brook, I. Bacterial colonization, tracheobronchitis and pneumonia, following tracheostomy and long term intubation. *Chest* 76:420, 1979.

21. Brook, I.; Martin, W. J.; and Finegold, S. M. Bacteriology of tracheal aspirates in intubated newborn. *Chest* 78:875, 1980.

CHAPTER 7

Conjunctivitis

Conjunctivitis in the newborn infant usually is due to chemical and mechanical irritation caused by the instillation of silver nitrate drops or ointment into the eye in order to prevent gonorrheal ophthalmia. Chemical conjunctivitis differs from infective forms in that it becomes apparent almost immediately after the instillation. The most common causes of infectious conjunctivitis in descending order of frequency are *Neisseria gonorrhoeae*,[1] *Staphylococcus*,[2] inclusion conjunctivitis caused by *Chlamydia trachomatis*,[3] A and B *Streptococcus*,[4] *Streptococcus pneumoniae*, *Haemophilus influenzae*, *Pseudomonas aeruginosa*, *Escherichia coli*, *Neisseria catarrhalis*,[5] *Neisseria meningitidis*,[6] *Corynebacterium diphtheriae*,[7] herpes simplex virus, echoviruses, and *Mycoplasma hominis*.[8] Recent work also has implicated clostridia and peptostreptococci as probable causes of neonatal conjunctivitis.[9]

The classical ophthalmia neonatonia caused by *N. gonorrhoeae* is an acute purulent conjunctivitis that appears from two to five days after birth. If untreated, the infection progresses rapidly until the eye becomes puffy and the conjunctiva is intensely red and swollen. The subsequent outcome would be corneal ulceration. Ophthalmia caused by organisms other than gonococcus, including *Clostridium* species, occurs usually from 5 to 14 days following delivery, is indistinguishable clinically, and the conjunctival inflammatory reaction usually is milder than in ophthalmia caused by gonococci.

A recent study investigated the role of anaerobes in neonatal conjunctivitis.[10] Newborn conjunctival cultures were obtained from 35 babies prior to silver nitrate application and 48 hours later. On initial culture, 46 facultative bacteria and 27 anaerobes were recovered.

It is apparent, therefore, that the conjunctiva of the newborn acquires many facultative and anaerobic bacteria soon after birth. This is due primarily to the acquisition of bacteria from the mother's cervical flora during passage through the birth canal. The organisms isolated in almost all of these cases were present also in the mother's cervical cultures and in the baby's gastric aspirates, taken concomitantly.

Of considerable interest is the change in the conjunctival flora after 48 hours. It was shown that *Haemophilus vaginalis, Bacteroides* species, and the anaerobic cocci all but disappeared, whereas *Staphylococcus epidermidis, Micrococcus* organisms, and *Propionibacterium acnes* increased in numbers. It is obvious that the conjunctiva of the newborn is exposed to not only *N. gonorrhoeae,* but to other potentially pathogenic bacteria as well. Most of those organisms disappeared from the conjunctiva within 48 hours.

Clostridial species were the only isolates recovered from two infants who developed conjunctivitis.[9] *Clostridium perfringens* was recovered from one newborn, and *Clostridium bifermentans* with *Peptostreptococcus* organisms were recovered from the other infant. Similar organisms were recovered from the mother's cervix immediately after delivery. These infections were noted on the second and third day postdelivery. The conjunctivitis was characterized by a profuse yellow-green discharge that was noted in both eyes. The conjunctivae were injected and the eyelids were edematous. There was normal light reflex and pupillary reaction, and the fundi were normal. The infants' body temperatures were normal, and there were no other abnormal findings.

Local therapy was initiated with 2% penicillin eye drops (two drops every two hours). The conjunctivitis subsided within three days, and repeat cultures of the eyes after 10 days were sterile. The babies were followed for three months with no residual of infection noted.

Of interest is that the silver nitrate solution of 1% currently used in newborns was efficacious in preventing in vitro growth of clostridia. The common practice of rinsing the eyes with distilled water after the addition of silver nitrate to prevent chemical conjunctivitis may alter the ability of this solution to effectively inhibit certain strains of *Clostridium.*

Since anaerobic bacteria have been recovered recently from children[11] and adults[12, 13] suffering from bacterial conjunctivitis, their presence in neonatal conjunctivitis is not surprising. These organisms, however, certainly are not the most prevalent cause of inflammation of the eye in these age groups. Their presence should be suspected in children whose aerobic and chlamydial cultures are negative, in those who do not respond to conventional antimicrobial therapy, and in children at high risk of developing anaerobic infection (as from maternal amnionitis or premature rupture of membranes).

The experience acquired from the documented cases of anaerobic conjunctivitis indicates that local therapy with appropriate antimicrobial agents is generally adequate.

REFERENCES

1. Friendly, D. S. Gonococcal conjunctivitis of the newborn. *Clin. Proc. Childrens Hosp.* (Washington, D.C.) 25:1, 1969.

2. Kaivonen, M. Prophylaxis of ophthalmic neonatorum. *Acta Ophthalmol.* (Suppl.) 79:1, 1965.

3. Heggie, A. D. et al. Chlamydia trachomatis infection in mothers and infants: a prospective study. *Am. J. Dis. Child.* 135:507, 1981.

4. Howard, J. B., and McCracken, G. F., Jr. The spectrum of group B streptococcal infections in infancy. *Am. J. Dis. Child.* 128:815, 1974.

5. Armstrong, J. H.; Zacarias, F.; and Rein, M. F. Ophthalmia neonatorum: a chart review. *Pediatrics* 57:884, 1976.

6. Hansman, D. Neonatal meningococcal conjunctivitis (letter). *Br. Med. J.* 1:748, 1972.

7. Naiditch, M. J., and Bower, A. G. Diphtheria. A study of 1433 cases observed during a ten-year period at Los Angeles County Hospital. *Am. J. Med.* 17:229, 1954.

8. Moore, R. A., and Schmitt, B. D. Conjunctivitis in children. A refresher survey of diagnosis and contemporary treatment. *Clin. Pediatr.* 18:26, 1979.

9. Brook, I.; Martin, W. J.; and Finegold, S. M. Effect of silver nitrate application on the conjunctival flora of the newborn, and the occurrence of clostridial conjunctivitis. *J. Pediatr. Ophthalmol. Strabismus* 15:179, 1978.

10. Brook, I. et al. Aerobic and anaerobic bacterial flora of the maternal cervix and newborn gastric fluid and conjunctiva: a prospective study. *Pediatrics* 63:451, 1979.

11. Brook, I. Anaerobic and aerobic bacterial flora of acute conjunctivitis in children. *Arch. Ophthalmol.* 98:833, 1980.

12. Perkins, R. E. et al. Bacteriology of normal and infected conjunctiva. *J. Clin. Microbiol.* 1:147, 1975.

13. Brook, I. et al. Anaerobic and aerobic bacteriology of acute conjunctivitis. *Ann. Ophthalmol.* 11:389, 1979.

CHAPTER 8

Omphalitis

Exposure

The umbilical stump becomes colonized with bacteria soon after delivery.[1] The devitalized umbilical stump is an excellent medium that supports bacterial growth, and the umbilical vessels provide direct access to the blood stream. The colonizing bacteria may invade the wound and spread through the blood vessels or the connective tissues to cause phlebitis or arteritis. The infection may also spread into the thrombi within the lumen of the umbilical vessels, and from there into the peritoneum or by emboli to various organs.[2] Although infection of the cord stump is rare, its potential sequelae such as cellulitis, peritonitis, septicemia, multiple hepatic abscesses, or portal vein thrombosis may be fatal.

Omphalitis manifests itself by drainage from the umbilical stump or from its base at its point of attachment to the abdominal wall or from the navel after the cord has separated. Secretions may be thin and serous, sanguineous, or frankly purulent, and at times they are foul smelling. Infection may remain restricted to the cord or may spread to involve the surrounding skin.

Staphylococcus aureus, Escherichia coli, Klebsiella pneumoniae, and *Proteus mirabilis* have been the predominant isolates recovered from the inflamed umbilicus in newborns.[3, 4]

Although group B beta-hemolytic streptococci and anaerobic bacteria can colonize the skin and mucous surfaces[1, 5, 6] of the newborn and may be associated with infections in this age group, their role in neonatal omphalitis has only recently been reported.[7]

A recent study[7] demonstrated the polymicrobial aerobic and anaerobic etiology of neonatal omphalitis. Aerobic and anaerobic cultures were obtained from 23 newborns with omphalitis (table 8.1). Aerobes were isolated from 20 specimens (87%). In 6 cases (26%) they were mixed with anaerobes, and in 14 cases (61%) they were the only isolates. Anaerobes were recovered from 39% of the patients. Anaerobes alone were recovered in three instances (13%). There were 47 aerobic isolates (2.1 per specimen), including 11 group B beta-hemolytic streptococci, 9 of *E. coli*, 6 of *S. aureus*, 5 group D streptococci, and 4 of *Proteus mirabilis*. There were 22 anaerobic isolates (0.9 per specimen). They included 7 of the *Bacteroides fragilis* group, 4 anaerobic Gram-positive cocci, and 2 of *Clostridium perfringens*. Beta-lactamase production was detected in 13 isolates recovered from 12 patients.

Although anaerobic bacteria were reported as colonizers of uninfected ligated or nonligated umbilical cords,[8] only a few case reports described their isolation from cases of omphalitis.[9] The anaerobes recovered in these cases were *Fusobacterium* organisms, *Clostridium tertium*, *C. perfringens*, and *Clostridium sordellii*.[10] Neonatal tetanus caused by *Clostridium tetani* usually results from contamination of the umbilical cord during improperly managed deliveries outside a medical facility. The disease is now rare in the United States[11]; however, in developing countries, tetanus still is one of the most common causes of neonatal death.[12]

Table 8.1. Bacteria Isolated from 23 Newborns with Omphalitis

Aerobic and Facultative Isolates	No. of Isolates	Anaerobic Isolates	No. of Isolates
Gram-positive cocci		Anaerobic cocci	
Alpha-hemolytic streptococci	4	*Peptococcus* sp.	3
		Peptostreptococcus sp.	1
Gamma-hemolytic streptococci	2	*V. parvula*	1
Group B beta-hemolytic streptococci	11	Gram-positive bacilli	
		P. acnes	2
Group D streptococci	5	*P. avidum*	1
S. aureus	6	*C. perfringens*	2
S. epidermidis	3	Gram-negative bacilli	
Gram-negative bacilli		*F. nucleatum*	3
E. coli	9	*Bacteroides* sp.	2
K. oxytoca	2	*B. fragilis*	4
P. mirabilis	4	*B. thetaiotaomicron*	2
C. freundii	1	*B. vulgatus*	1
Total number of aerobes and facultatives	47	Total number of anaerobes	22

SOURCE: Brook, I. Bacteriology of neonatal omphalitis. *J. Infect.* 5:129, 1982.

The recovery of anaerobes from umbilical infection is not surprising since during vaginal delivery the neonate is exposed to the cervical canal flora, which includes anaerobic bacteria.[9] A recent study[6] demonstrated that almost every newborn delivered by the vaginal route becomes colonized with potentially pathogenic aerobic and anaerobic bacteria that can be recovered from gastric contents and conjunctiva.

The predominant anaerobic isolates recovered from patients studied belonged to the *Bacteroides fragilis* group (i.e., *B. fragilis*, *Bacteroides vulgatus*, and *Bacteroides thetaiotaomicron*). These organisms are part of the normal flora of the female genital tract[9] and are frequently involved in ascending infections of the uterus and septic complications of pregnancy such as amnionitis, endometritis, and septic abortion.[13] They were recovered also from newborns with neonatal pneumonia[14] and sepsis.[15] It is of interest that maternal amnionitis caused by *B. fragilis* developed in three of the newborns reported in this study.[7] Maternal infection could have led to the early exposure of the infants to this organism.

Treatment

Simple omphalitis, without evidence of periumbilical spread, responds readily to local application of alcohol and drying of the infected area. Sometimes antibiotic compresses or ointments are applied. Bacitracin and neomycin, or a combination of these, are the local antibiotics of choice.

Systemic antibiotic medication is indicated if the discharge is purulent of if any evidence of periumbilical spread appears. Such spread can cause generalized sepsis and metastatic infection. Final choice of antibiotic will depend upon culture and sensitivity tests. It must be remembered, however, that the rate of growth of anaerobic bacteria is slower than their aerobic counterparts in mixed infection, and sometimes they may be overgrown if there is delay in the inoculation of cultures.

It is recommended that specimens from umbilical infection be routinely cultured for anaerobic organisms. Although the rate of growth of most anaerobic bacteria, including the *B. fragilis* group, is relatively slow, recent development of immunofluorescent methodology[16] may facilitate the identification of these anaerobes. Until such methodology is available on a routine basis, proper antimicrobial therapy effective against these organisms should be considered in newborns with omphalitis. This is especially important in infants who are at a high risk for developing anaerobic infection, such as those whose mother had amnionitis or those who have a foul-smelling secretion from the amniotic cord stump.

A penicillin derivative and an aminoglycoside generally are administered to newborns for the treatment of serious amnionitis. While most anaerobic organisms are susceptible to penicillin G, members of the *B. fragilis* group and some strains of *Bacteroides melaninogenicus*[17] are known to be resistant to that agent. It is noteworthy that of the seven newborns studied from whom organisms belonging to *B. fragilis* were recovered, three received the conventional combination of ampicillin and gentamicin, which was inappropriate for treatment of their infection.

Our study[7] suggests that anaerobes play a role in neonatal omphalitis. Since *B. fragilis* was the predominant anaerobe recovered and is resistant to penicillin, other antimicrobial agents effective against this organism, such as clindamycin, chloramphenicol, cefoxitin, carbenicillin, ticarcillin, or metronidazole, should be considered for the treatment of this infection and its septic complications.

REFERENCES

1. Speck, W. T. et al. Staphylococcal and streptococcal colonization of the newborn infant. *Am. J. Dis. Child.* 131:1005, 1977.

2. Forshall, I. Septic umbilical arteritis. *Arch. Dis. Child.* 32:25, 1957.

3. McKenna, H., and Johnson, D. Bacteria in neonatal omphalitis. *Pathology* 9:111, 1977.

4. Mason, W.; Ros, L.; and Wright, H. T. Omphalitis: epidemiology and etiological agents and chemotherapy (abstr. 220). In *Proceedings of the 17th Interscience Conference on Antimicrobial Agents and Chemotherapy*, New York, 1977.

5. Eickoff, T. C. et al. Neonatal sepsis and other infections due to group B beta-hemolytic streptococci. *N. Engl. J. Med.* 272:1221, 1964.

6. Brook, I. et al. Aerobic and anaerobic flora of maternal cervix and newborn's conjunctiva and gastric fluid: a prospective study. *Pediatrics* 63:451, 1979.

7. Brook, I. Bacteriology of neonatal omphalitis. *J. Infect.* 5:127, 1982.

8. Bernstine, J. B.; Ludmir, A.; and Fritz, M. Bacteriological studies in ligated and nonligated umbilical cords. *Am. J. Obstet. Gynecol.* 78:69, 1959.

9. Finegold, S. M. *Anaerobic bacteria in human disease.* New York: Academic Press, 1977.

10. Scott, M. A.; Kauch, Y. C.; and Luscombe, H. A. Neonatal anaerobic (clostridial) cellulitis and omphalitis. *Arch. Dermatol.* 113:683, 1977.

11. Center for Disease Control. *Tetanus surveillance.* Report no. 4, 1970–1971. Atlanta: Center for Disease Control, 1974.

12. Pinheiro, D. Tetanus of the newborn infant. *Pediatrics* 34:32, 1964.

13. Pearson, H. E., and Anderson, G. V. *Bacteroides* infections and pregnancy. *Obstet. Gynecol.* 35:31, 1970.

14. Brook, I.; Martin, W. J.; and Finegold, S. M. Neonatal pneumonia caused by members of the *Bacteroides fragilis* group. Clin. Pediatr. 19:541, 1980.

15. Brook, I. et al. Anaerobic bacteremia in children. *Am. J. Dis. Child.* 134:1052, 1980.

16. Holland, J. W.; Stauffer, L. R.; and Altemeier, W. A. Fluorescent antibody test kit for rapid detection and identification of members of the *Bacteroides fragilis* and *Bacteroides melaninogenicus* groups in clinical specimens. *J. Clin. Microbiol.* 10:121, 1979.

17. Sutter, V. L., and Finegold, S. M. Susceptibility of anaerobic bacteria to 23 antimicrobial agents. *Antimicrob. Agents Chemother.* 10:736, 1976.

CHAPTER 9

Bacteremia and Septicemia

Because the newborn generally is less able to overcome infections than an older child, localized infection may enter the infant's blood stream. The septic infant manifests generally clinical signs and symptoms that distinguish him from infants with transient bacteremia. The incidence of sepsis neonatorum is approximately one to four cases per 1000 live births and varies between nurseries. Factors such as prematurity or obstetric complications can change these rates.

Incidence and Bacterial Etiology

Within the last three decades, changes have occurred in the bacterial etiology of neonatal bacterial septicemia. In the preantibiotic era before 1940, the predominant organism was group A beta-hemolytic streptococci. In the 1950s, *Staphylococcus aureus* became the major pathogen, to be replaced by *Escherichia coli* and group B streptococci. Since the beginning of the 1960s[1] the latter two pathogens have accounted for up to 70% bacteremia in the newborn. The role of anaerobic bacteria in neonatal bacteremia has not been studied adequately. The true incidence of neonatal anaerobic bacteremia is difficult to ascertain since anaerobic blood cultures were not employed in the reported major series of neonatal sepsis and still are not routinely performed in some medical centers. Furthermore, many medical centers do not employ appropriate culture media for recovery of anaerobes.

Tyler and Albers[2] obtained cultures from 319 newborns. These authors reported the recovery of anaerobes in four instances, which allowed them to predict an incidence of 12.5 cases per 1000 live births, and 13% of all cases of neonatal bacteremia.

A recent report described anaerobic bacteremia in 23 newborns. The yield of anaerobic bacteria in 23 newborns seen over a period of 3.5 years represented 1.8 cases per 1000 live births and accounted for 26% of all instances of neonatal bacteremia at that hospital.[3]

In the study of Salem and Thadepalli[4], 180 per 1000 live births had self-limiting transplacental bacteremia. Thirumoorthi, Keen, and Dajani[5] conducted a prospective survey of all neonate blood cultures that were specially processed for anaerobes and observed that anaer-. obes were isolated from only 1% of the 1599 blood cultures processed. It is difficult to generalize about the population of anaerobic bacteria in newborns in these studies, since cultures were obtained through the umbilical artery in many of the infants. The possibility of umbilical artery contamination occurring in some of these patients cannot be discounted.

The majority of cases for neonatal bacteremia reported in the literature were obtained, therefore, from selected case reports. Table 9.1 summarizes 126 cases of anaerobic neonatal bacteremia reported in the literature.[6-28] The predominant organisms are *Bacteroides* (53 cases). Of these, the *Bacteroides fragilis* is predominant. The other organisms, in descending order of frequency, are clostridia (33 instances), anaerobic Gram-positive cocci (32), *Propionibacterium acnes* (4), veillonellae (3), and fusobacteria (1).

Multiple organisms, aerobic and anaerobic, were isolated from eight patients reported in one study[3]: anaerobic coisolates from six (*Peptococcus* or *Peptostreptococcus*, five; *Veillonella parvula*, one) and aerobic coisolates from only two (*E. coli* and alpha-hemolytic streptococcus).

Simultaneous isolation of the anaerobes from other sites was reported by several authors.[3, 11-14, 28] This was especially common with *B. fragilis*.

Chow and co-workers[3] reported the simultaneous isolation of *Bacteroides* organisms from gastric aspirate in four instances, from the amniotic fluid or uterus at cesarean section in two cases, and from the maternal and fetal placental surfaces and the external auditory canal in one instance each.

Brook, Martin, and Finegold[14] reported the recovery of *B. fragilis* from lung aspirates of two patients with pneumonitis; Harrod and Sevens[17] recovered *B. fragilis* from the inflamed placenta; Dysant and associates[13] and Brook, Martin, and Finegold[14] recovered *B. fragilis* from the cerebrospinal fluid of two patients with meningitis.

Brook[12] recovered *B. fragilis* from an occipital abscess that developed following neonatal monitoring with scalp electrodes. Ahonkhai and colleagues[23] reported the concomitant isolation of *Clostridium perfringens* in the placenta of a newborn.

Diagnosis

The diagnosis of septicemia can be made only by recovery of the organism from blood cultures. Blood should be obtained from a peripheral vein rather than from the umbilical vessels, which frequently

Table 9.1. Literature Summary: Neonatal Bacteremia Due to Anaerobic Bacteria

Organism	No. of Patients (deaths)	Remarks	Reference
Bacteroides sp.	14 (14)		6
	5 (0)	Omphalitis	7
	2 (1)		8
	1 (0)		2
	1 (0)		9
	1 (0)		10
	15 (1)		3
	1 (0)	Adrenal abscess	11
	1 (0)	Neonatal scalp monitoring	12
	1 (0)	Meningitis	13
	5 (2)	Pneumonia, meningitis	14
	2 (0)		15
	3 (0)		16
	1 (1)	Pneumonia	17
Subtotal	53 (19)	*36% mortality*	
Anaerobic Gram-positive cocci	19 (0)		7
	3 (0)		2
	2 (1)		18
	7 (0)		3
	1 (0)		19
Subtotal	32 (1)	*3% mortality*	
Veillonella sp.	2 (0)		19
	1 (0)		3
Subtotal	3 (0)		
Fusobacterium sp.	1 (0)		7
Subtotal	1 (0)		
Clostridium sp.	1 (1)		20
	1 (1)		21
	1 (1)		22
	1 (0)		23
	1 (0)		3
	18 (0)		24
	9 (0)	Necrotizing enterocolitis	25
	1 (0)	Necrotizing enterocolitis	26
Subtotal	33 (3)	*10% mortality*	
P. acnes	1 (0)		27
	1 (0)	Periorbital cellulitis	28
	2 (0)		19
Subtotal	4 (0)		
Total	126 (23)	*18.3% mortality*	

are colonized by aerobic and anaerobic bacteria. Femoral vein aspiration may result in cultures contaminated with organisms from the perineum such as *Bacteroides* and coliforms. It is helpful to obtain cultures of other sites prior to initiating antimicrobial therapy.

This is of particular importance in relation to maternal amnionitis or septicemia. In many cases, organisms identical to those found in the newborn's blood can be recovered from the mother's blood or amniotic fluid.[14] The rate of growth of most anaerobic bacteria, including the *B. fragilis* group, is relatively slow, and it may take several days to identify them with culture. The recent development of immunofluorescent methodology[29] may facilitate the identification of these anaerobes. Examination of gastric aspirates generally is not helpful in the prediction of anaerobic sepsis, since the gastric fluid of the normal infants can contain many aerobic and anaerobic bacteria that were ingested during delivery.[30] Examination of the gastric aspirate for white blood cells may suggest the presence of maternal amnionitis.

None of the other blood tests can be helpful in the diagnosis of bacterial septicemia. The white blood count can be elevated above 20,000 cells/cu ml, but in some cases it may be below 10,000 cells/cu ml.

Predisposing Conditions

A number of factors have been shown to dispose to aerobic neonatal septicemia, including maternal age, quality of prenatal care, sex of the infant, gestational age, and associated congenital anomalies. Perinatal maternal complications such as abruptio placentae, placenta previa, maternal toxemia, premature rupture of the membranes, and chorioamnionitis all increase the incidence of neonatal septicemia. Congenital anomalies that cause a breakdown of anatomic barriers or of the immunologic system predispose to infection.

The factors predisposing for anaerobic bacteremia were found to be similar to predisposing factors for aerobic bacteremia. The frequency of various perinatal factors associated with anaerobic bacteremia in newborns was reported by Chow and associates.[3] Prolonged time after premature rupture of membranes and maternal amnionitis were the most commonly associated obstetric factors. The median duration of time after membrane rupture until delivery in the 15 mothers studied by these authors was 57 hours. Seven of 12 mothers who had evidence of intrapartum amnionitis were noted to have foul-smelling vaginal discharge, suggestive of an anaerobic infection. Other investigators[31-33] also had demonstrated a relationship between premature rupture of fetal membranes and neonatal bacteremia. Prolonged rupture of fetal membranes often is associated with amnionitis, and it is generally accepted that an important pathway for fetal infection is by an ascending route through the membranes from the cervix.[34, 35] Tyler and Albers[2] also found an increasing frequency of neonatal bacteremia directly related to the duration after membrane rupture; they further demonstrated a highly significant association of neonatal bacteremia with the presence of foul-smelling amniotic fluid.

Prematurity was reported in about a third of the newborns with anaerobic bacteremia, and a male to female ratio of 1.6:1, which is similar to the finding of increased male susceptibility to neonatal aerobic bacteremia,[36] also was reported in anaerobic bacteremia.[3] Of interest is the correlation between certain predisposing conditions and some bacterial isolates (table 4.1). Neonatal pneumonia and abscesses were reported in association with the recovery of *B. fragilis* and necrotizing enterocolitis with the recovery of clostridia. *Clostridium butyricum* recently was isolated from blood cultures obtained from 12 newborns with that disease.[25]

Pathogenesis

Studdiford and Douglas[37] demonstrated placental bacteremia caused by Gram-negative bacteria, with the fetal blood vessels distended. They considered this to be peculiar to neonatal deaths with vascular collapse. Mandsley and colleagues[38] examined at random the fetal adnexa in 494 patients and found evidence of inflammation in 34.2%. They found chorionitis in 21% and inflammation of the cord in 17%. They also have studied the bacteriology of the surface of the placenta and failed to correlate these findings with the histologic findings. They found deciduitis in 89.5%, suggesting that normal labor may not be that normal after all. Salem and Thadepalli[4] have examined the histology of the cord, placenta, and membranes and tried to correlate the cord blood cultures with the neonatal outcome in 50 consecutive births. Thirty percent of the cord blood cultures were positive for aerobic-anaerobic bacteria soon after birth. Anaerobes were found in cord cultures in nine samples (18%), anaerobic cocci dominating. Excellent correlation was found between the cord blood culture results and the morphotypes of the bacteria seen in the Gram-stained sections of the placenta, cord, and membranes. Inflammation as evidenced by leukocyte infiltration was rare, found in only one instance. It appears, therefore, that transplacental transmission of aerobic and anaerobic bacteria is a common, but fortunately benign, feature of normal labor. In most instances it results from the contamination of the amniotic fluid with the cervical flora, followed by the transplacental influx of microorganisms created by the intrauterine pressure changes during active labor.

Clinical Manifestations

The early signs and symptoms of septicemia are caused by aerobic bacteria, are nonspecific, and frequently are recognized by the mother or nurse. Temperature imbalance, tachypnea, apnea, tachycardia, lethargy, vomiting, or diarrhea may be noted. Jaundice, petechiae, seizures, and hepatosplenomegaly are late signs and usually denote a poor prognosis.

The relative frequency of various clinical manifestations of neonatal anaerobic bacteremia in newborns is not different from those seen in aerobic bacteremia.[3] Over half of the infants had evidence of fetal distress, and three-fourths had a low Apgar score. A positive correlation between the presence of foul-smelling discharge at birth and bacteremia caused by *Bacteroides* organisms was noted also.[3] About two-thirds of the infants may manifest respiratory distress, with tachypnea and/or cyanosis shortly after birth. Chest films may reveal pneumonitis, confirming a correlation between prenatal aspiration of infected amniotic fluid and subsequent development of pneumonia or sepsis in the newborn infant.

Other clinical manifestations of these infants were nonspecific, and included poor sucking and feeding activity, lethargy, hypotonia, irritability, and tonic-clonic seizures. In general, the clinical manifestations of neonatal anaerobic bacteremia are indistinguishable from other causes of neonatal sepsis.

Prognosis

The mortality following anaerobic bacteremia depends on such factors as age of the patient, underlying disease, nature of the organism, speed with which the diagnosis is made, and surgical or medical therapy instituted. The overall mortality from anaerobic bacteria in the 126 patients reported in the literature (table 9.1) is 18.3%. The highest mortality is observed in the *Bacteroides* group (36%), while the mortality from other organisms is generally below 10%.

In the series of Chow and colleagues[3] the patients with neonatal anaerobic bacteremia had better prognoses than did newborns with bacteremia caused by facultative bacteria. Only one patient of the 23 (4%) died; however, the mortality from the cases of anaerobic bacteremia reviewed from the literature prior to this study was 26%.

Although several authors reported spontaneous recovery from anaerobic bacteremia,[3, 16] most of the reports in the literature describe the need to treat patients with such infection adequately[28] and describe infants who were inappropriately treated and died.[14] Following appropriate therapy and in the absence of complicating factors such as other sites of infections (meningitis, abscesses), there generally is complete recovery.

Therapy

Antimicrobial therapy must be initiated as early as possible in infants suspected of bacteremia. This should be done in most cases prior to the recovery of organisms and before information about their susceptibility is available. The clinician cannot wait in most cases for this information because of the vulnerability of newborns to bacterial infection. The time needed for the recovery and performance of blood cultures for susceptibility of anaerobes generally is longer than the time needed for culture of aerobes, and delay in therapy may be deleterious.

In most instances, a penicillin derivative (ampicillin, carbenicillin) and an aminoglycoside are administered for treatment of newborns. While most anaerobic organisms are susceptible to penicillin G, members of the *B. fragilis* group, and some strains of *Bacteroides melaninogenicus*[40] are known to be resistant to that agent. In one series, two newborns died after receiving the conventional antimicrobial therapy of combination ampicillin and gentamicin, treatment inappropriate for their infection by *B. fragilis*.[14] The third newborn in that study, however, recovered following therapy with a broader treatment that included therapy with clindamycin, a drug known to be effective in the treatment of anaerobic infections in adults and children.[11] Clindamycin was used in the treatment of anaerobic bacteremia by other authors also.[17]

There is, however, only limited experience in the use of clindamycin in the newborn period, and exact recommendations for dosage and frequency of administration are not available. Since clindamycin does not penetrate the blood-brain barrier in sufficient quantities, it is not recommended for treatment of meningitis. Other antimicrobial agents such as chloramphenicol or metronidazole, which are known to penetrate to the central nervous system, should be administered in the presence of meningitis. Although the experience in newborns is limited, metronidazole has been used successfully in the treatment of neonatal bacteremia.[42]

The length of treatment time for anaerobic infections is not established. It is apparent from data derived from older children,[28] however, that prolonged therapy of at least 14 days is adequate in eliminating the infection.

Surgical drainage is essential when pus has collected. Organisms identical to those causing anaerobic bacteremia were recovered from other infected sites in many patients. No doubt these extravascular sites serve as a source of persistent bacteremia in some cases; however, the majority of patients will recover completely when prompt treatment with appropriate antimicrobial agents is instituted before any complications develop. The early recognition of anaerobic bacteremia and administration of appropriate antimicrobial and surgical therapy play a significant role in preventing mortality and morbidity in newborns.

REFERENCES

1. Vaugham, V. C., III; McKay, R. J.; and Behman, R. E. *Nelson's textbook of pediatrics,* 11th edition. Philadelphia: W. B. Saunders, 1979.

2. Tyler, C. W., and Albers, W. H. Obstetric factors related to bacteremia in the newborn infant. *Am. J. Obstet. Gynecol.* 94:970, 1966.

3. Chow, A. W. et al. The significance of anaerobes in neonatal bacteremia: analysis of 23 cases and review of the literature. *Pediatrics* 54:736, 1974.

4. Salem, F. A., and Thadepalli, H. Microbial invasion of the placenta, cord and membranes during normal labor. *Clin. Pediatr.* 18:50, 1978.

5. Thirumoorthi, M. C.; Keen, B. M.; and Dajani, A. S. Anaerobic infections in children: a prospective survey. *J. Clin. Microbiol.* 3:318, 1976.

6. Pearson, H. E., and Anderson, G. V. Perinatal deaths associated with *Bacteroides* infections. *Obstet. Gynecol.* 30:486, 1967.

7. Kelsall, G. R. H.; Barter, R. A.; and Manessis, C. Prospective bacteriological studies in inflammation of the placenta, cord and membranes. *Journal of Obstetrics and Gynaecology of the British Commonwealth* 74:401, 1967.

8. DuPont, H. L., and Spink, W. W. Infections due to gram-negative organisms: an analysis of 860 patients with bacteremia at the University of Minnesota Medical Center, 1958–1966. *Medicine* 48:307, 1969.

9. Tynes, B. S., and Frommeyer, W. B., Jr. *Bacteroides* septicemia: culture, clinical and therapeutic features in a series of twenty-five patients. *Ann. Intern. Med.* 56:12, 1962.

10. Lee, Y., and Berg, R. B. Cephalhematoma infected with *Bacteroides. Am. J. Dis. Child.* 121:77, 1971.

11. Ohtu, S. et al. Neonatal adrenal abscess due to *Bacteroides. J. Pediatr.* 93:1063, 1978.

12. Brook, I. Osteomyelitis and bacteremia caused by *Bacteroides fragilis. Clin. Pediatr.* 19:639, 1980.

13. Dysant, N. K. et al. Meningitis due to *Bacteroides fragilis* in a newborn. *J. Pediatr.* 89:509, 1970.

14. Brook, I.; Martin, W. J.; and Finegold, S. M. Neonatal pneumonia caused by members of the *Bacteroides fragilis* group. *Clin. Pediatr.* 19:591, 1980.

15. Maguire, G. C. et al. Infections acquired by young infants. *Am. J. Dis. Child.* 135:693, 1981.

16. Echeverria, P., and Smith, A. L. Anaerobic bacteremia observed in a children's hospital. *Clin. Pediatr.* 17:688, 1978.

17. Harrod, J. R., and Stevens, D. A. Anaerobic infections in the newborn infant. *J. Pediatr.* 85:399, 1974.

18. Robinson, S. C. et al. Significance of maternal bacterial infection with respect to infection and disease in the newborn. *Obstet. Gynecol.* 25:664, 1965.

19. Spector, S.; Tickner, W.; and Grossman, M. Studies of the usefulness of clinical and hematological findings in the diagnosis of neonatal bacteremia. *Clin. Pediatr.* 20:385, 1981.

20. Wilson, W. R. et al. Anaerobic bacteremia. *Mayo Clin. Proc.* 47:639, 1972.

21. Isenberg, A. N. *Clostridium welchii* infection: a clinical evaluation. *Arch. Surg.* 92:727, 1966.

22. Freedman, S., and Hollander, M. *Clostridium perfringens* septicemia as a postoperative complication of the newborn infant. *J. Pediatr.* 71:576, 1967.

23. Ahonkhai, V. I. et al. Perinatal *Clostridium perfringens* infection. *Clin. Pediatr.* 20:532, 1981.

24. Alpern, R. J., and Dowell, V. R., Jr. Nonhistotoxic clostridial bacteremia. *Am. J. Clin. Pathol.* 55:717, 1971.

25. Howard, M. F. et al. Outbreak of necrotizing enterocolitis caused by *Clostridium butyricum. Lancet* 2:1099, 1977.

26. Khegman, R. M. et al. Clostridia as pathogens in neonatal necrotizing enterocolitis. *J. Pediatr.* 95:287, 1979.

27. Dunkle, L. M.; Brotherton, M. S.; and Feigin, R. D. Anaerobic infections in children: a prospective study. *Pediatrics* 57:311, 1976.

28. Brook, I.; Controni, G.; and Rodrigiuz, W. J. Anaerobic bacteremia in children. *Am. J. Dis. Child.* 134:1052, 1980.

29. Holland, J. W.; Stauffer, L. R.; and Altemeier, W. A. Fluorescent antibody test kit for rapid detection and identification of members of the *Bacteroides fragilis* and *Bacteroides melaninogenicus* groups in clinical specimens. *J. Clin. Microbiol.* 10:121, 1973.

30. Brook, I. et al. Aerobic and anaerobic flora of maternal cervix and newborns' conjunctivae and gastric fluid: a prospective study. *Pediatrics* 63:451, 1979.

31. Pryles, C. V. et al. A controlled study of the influence on the newborn of prolonged premature rupture of the amniotic membranes and/or infection in the mother. *Pediatrics* 31:608, 1963.

32. Kobak, A. J. Fetal bacteremia: a contribution to mechanism of intrauterine infection and to the pathogenesis of placentitis. *Am. J. Obstet. Gynecol.* 19:299, 1930.

33. Wilson, M. G. et al. Prolonged rupture of fetal membranes: effect on the newborn infant. *Am. J. Dis. Child.* 107:74, 1964.

34. Benirschke, K. Routes and types of infection in the fetus and the newborn. *Am. J. Dis. Child.* 99:714, 1960.

35. Blanc, W. A. Pathways of fetal and early neonatal infection. *J. Pediatr.* 59:473, 1961.

36. Davis, P. A. Bacterial infection in the fetus and newborn. *Arch. Dis. Child.* 46:1, 1971.

37. Studdiford, W. E., and Douglas, G. W. Placental bacteremia: a significant finding in septic abortion accompanied by vascular collapse. *Am. J. Obstet. Gynecol.* 71:842, 1956.

38. Mandsley, R. F. et al. Placental inflammation and infection. *Am. J. Obstet. Gynecol.* 95:648, 1966.

39. Naeye, R. L., and Blanc, W. A. Relation of poverty and race to antenatal infection. *N. Engl. J. Med.* 283:555, 1970.

40. Sutter, V. L., and Finegold, S. M. Susceptibility of anaerobic bacteria to 23 antimicrobial agents. *Antimicrob. Agents Chemother.* 10:736, 1976.

41. Brook, I. Clindamycin in the treatment of aspiration pneumonia in children. *Antimicrob. Agents Chemother.* 15:342, 1979.

42. Rom, S.; Flynn, D.; and Noone, P. Anaerobic infection in a neonate: early detection by gas liquid chromatography and response to metronidazole. *Arch. Dis. Child.* 52:740, 1977.

CHAPTER 10

Pneumonia

Pneumonia in the newborn can be classified according to the mode of acquiring the infection and the time when the infection took place. The infection can be acquired in utero by transplacental route or following intrauterine infection. The pneumonia could be acquired during delivery by inhalation of bacteria that colonize the birth canal. The type of infection contracted after birth is acquired by contact with environmental objects (e.g., a tracheostomy tube) or by human contact.

Congenital and intrauterine pneumonia usually is caused by viruses such as herpes simplex, cytomegalovirus, or rubella, and can be caused also by intrauterine exposure to *Treponema pallidum, Mycobacterium tuberculosis,* or *Listeria monocytogenes.*

Extensive reviews of these infections can be found in other textbooks.[1, 2] This chapter describes bacterial pneumonias in which anaerobes can participate.

During vaginal delivery, the neonate is exposed to the cervical birth canal flora, which includes both aerobic and anaerobic bacteria.[3, 4] A recent study[5] demonstrated that almost every normal baby born by vaginal delivery swallows potentially pathogenic aerobic and anaerobic bacteria.[5] These bacteria can be cultured in the infant's gastric contents. Moreover, similar bacteria can be found in the newborn's conjunctiva and external ear. In a few instances, especially in high-risk infants, aspiration of, or exposure to, these organisms could lead to the development of infections. The diagnosis of bacterial pneumonia has usually been achieved by cultures of tracheal aspirate, pleural fluids, needle aspirates of the lungs, and blood cultures.

The role of Gram-negative organisms, predominantly *Escherichia coli,* in causing perinatal pneumonia has been stressed in previous reports.[6–9] Most of these reports, however, relied on bacteriologic studies done at autopsy and did not use optimal anaerobic procedures. In other studies, Gram-positive organisms were found as the major cause of perinatal pneumonia, with *Staphylococcus aureus*,[10] group B beta-hemolytic streptococci,[11] group D streptococci, and alpha-hemolytic streptococci[12] the most frequently isolated organisms at autopsy. In approximately 40% of the cases previously reported, no organisms were recovered at necropsy.[12] Although the role of anaerobes as a cause of pulmonary infection in adults is well established,[13, 14] only two reports[15, 16] described the isolation of anaerobic organisms, namely *Bacteroides fragilis* from children with perinatal pneumonia.

Harrod and Stevens[15] described two newborns who presented with neonatal aspirate pneumonia that developed following maternal amnionitis. *B. fragilis* was recovered from the blood of these children.

Brook, Martin, and Finegold[17] reported three newborns with neonatal pneumonia caused by organisms belonging to members of the *B. fragilis* group. The mothers of all three infants had premature rupture of their membranes and subsequent amnionitis. The maternal membranes ruptured more than 24 hours before delivery, and the amniotic fluid was foul smelling. Organisms identical to those recovered from the newborns were recovered from the amniotic fluid of two of the mothers. In all three instances, the organisms were recovered from tracheal aspirates and in two from blood cultures as well. Two of the newborns were treated with ampicillin and gentamicin but succumbed to their infections; one of these infants also had meningitis. The third baby, treated with clindamycin, recovered.

Bacteroides organisms are part of the normal flora of the female genital tract.[3, 4] These organisms are involved frequently in ascending infections of the uterus and have been recognized as pathogens in septic complications of pregnancy, such as amnionitis, endometritis, and septic abortion,[15–19] and from infection in other clinical settings.[4] Amnionitis developed prior to delivery in two of the newborns, resulting in an early exposure of the infant to the organism. The relative immaturity of the cellular and humoral systems of the newborn may permit localized infections to invade the blood stream.

In most instances, a penicillin derivative and one of the aminoglycosides are administered for treatment of infection or pneumonia in newborns. While most anaerobic organisms are susceptible to penicillin G, members of the *B. fragilis* group and some strains of *Bacteroides melaninogenicus*[20] are known to be resistant to that agent. The first two newborns, who died of their infections, received the conventional antimicrobial therapy of a combination of ampicillin and gentamicin that was inappropriate for their infection. The third newborn, however, received a broader coverage that included therapy with clindamycin, a drug shown to be effective in the treatment of anaerobic infections in adults[21] and children.[22] There is limited experience in the use of this drug in the newborn period,[15] and exact recommendations for dosage and frequency of administration are not available. Since clindamycin does not penetrate the blood-brain barrier in sufficient quantities, it is not recommended for treatment of meningitis, as in the second patient. Other antimicrobial agents with better penetration to the central nervous system, such as chloramphenicol or metronidazole, should be administered in the presence of meningitis.

Anaerobic infections tend to occur in association with aspiration, tissue anoxia, and trauma.[3, 4] Such circumstances usually are present in high-risk newborns, which make them more vulnerable to anaerobic pneumonia, especially in the presence of maternal amnionitis.

REFERENCES

1. Schaffer, A. J., and Avery, M. E. *Diseases of the newborn,* 4th edition. Philadelphia: W. B. Saunders, 1977.

2. Remington, J. S., and Klein, J. O. *Infectious diseases of the fetus and newborn infant.* Philadelphia: W. B. Saunders, 1976.

3. Gorbach, S. L., and Bartlett, J. G. Anaerobic infections. *N. Engl. J. Med.* 290:1117, 1237, 1289, 1974.

4. Finegold, S. M. *Anaerobic bacteria in human disease.* New York: Academic Press, 1977.

5. Brook, I. et al. Aerobic and anaerobic flora of maternal cervix and newborn's conjunctiva and gastric fluid: a prospective study. *Pediatrics* 63:451, 1979.

6. Barson, A. J. Fatal *Pseudomonas aeruginosa* bronchopneumonia in a children's hospital. *Arch. Dis. Child.* 46:55, 1971.

7. Bernstein, J., and Wang, J. The pathology of neonatal pneumonia. *Am. J. Dis. Child.* 101:350, 1961.

8. Hable, K. A. et al. *Klebsiella* type 33 septicemia in an infant intensive care unit. *J. Pediatr.* 80:920, 1972.

9. Thaler, M. M. *Klebsiella-Aerobacter* pneumonia in infants. a review of the literature and report of a case. *Pediatrics* 30:206, 1962.

10. Penner, D. W., and McInnis, A. C. Intrauterine and neonatal pneumonia. *Am. J. Obstet. Gynecol.* 69:147, 1955.

11. Eickhoff, T. C. et al. Neonatal sepsis and other infections due to group B betahemolytic streptococci. *N. Engl. J. Med.* 271:1221, 1964.

12. Smith, J. A. M.; Jennison, R. F.; and Langley, R. A. Perinatal infection and perinatal death: clinical aspects. *Lancet* 2:903, 1956.

13. Bartlett, J. C., and Finegold, S. M. Anaerobic infections of the lung and pleural space. *Am. Rev. Respir. Dis.* 110:56, 1974.

14. Bartlett, J. G., and Finegold, S. M. Anaerobic pleuropulmonary infections. *Medicine* 51:413, 1972.

15. Harrod, J. R., and Stevens, D. A. Anaerobic infections in the newborn infant. *J. Pediatr.* 85:399, 1974.

16. Chow, A. W. et al. The significance of anaerobes in neonatal bacteremia: analysis of 23 cases and review of the literature. *Pediatrics* 54:736, 1974.

17. Brook, I.; Martin, W. J.; and Finegold, S. M. Neonatal pneumonia caused by members of the *Bacteroides fragilis* group. *Clin. Pediatr.* 19:541, 1980.

18. Pearson, H. E., and Anderson, G. V. *Bacteroides* infections and pregnancy. *Obstet. Gynecol.* 35:31, 1970.

19. Rotheram, E. B., and Schick, S. F. Nonclostridial anaerobic bacteria in septic abortions. *Am. J. Med.* 46:80, 1969.

20. Sutter, V. L., and Finegold, S. M. Susceptibility of anaerobic bacteria to 23 antimicrobial agents. *Antimicrob. Agents Chemother.* 10:736, 1976.

21. Gorbach, S. L., and Thadepalli, H. Clindamycin in the treatment of pure and mixed anaerobic infections. *Arch. Intern. Med.* 134:87, 1974.

22. Brook, I. Clindamycin in the treatment of aspiration pneumonia in children. *Antimicrob. Agents Chemother.* 15:342, 1979.

CHAPTER 11

Necrotizing Enterocolitis

Necrotizing enterocolitis is a relatively common disease in the newborn. The term necrotizing enterocolitis (NEC) has been applied to a clinical syndrome that probably has multiple factors in its etiology. Various studies have suggested that type of feeding, prematurity, low birthweight, umbilical catheterization, hypoxemia, and other conditions inhibiting oxygen delivery to the gut may predispose the newborn to the development of NEC.[1, 2, 3] The role of bacteria in necrotizing enterocolitis has been previously suggested, since *Escherichia coli, Klebsiella pneumoniae,* and other organisms have been isolated in various epidemics[4, 5]; however, the role of anaerobic bacteria in necrotizing enterocolitis has been studied only recently.[6]

Epidemiology

Occurrence of NEC was sporadic until 1965,[7] although epidemics of the disease were reported on many occasions, starting in South Africa in 1972[8, 9] and then in India.[10] The first epidemic of NEC reported in the United States occurred in 1974 and 1975.[11, 12] Sporadic cases are recognized with increasing frequency.

Conservative reports estimate occurrence of NEC at 1% to 2% of all admissions to newborn intensive care units. The disease accounts for about 2% of deaths of premature infants.[13] Other studies suggest that NEC will develop in as many as 5% to 15% of stressed, high-risk, premature infants during their hospitalization.

Predisposing Conditions

Certain infants have been identified as being at high risk. These infants often are premature, and some are small for gestational age. The mean weight of infants in most large series of NEC is between 1200 and 2000 gm, and almost all have sustained a period of stress or hypoxemia. Hyaline membrane disease, sepsis, congenital heart disease, hypothermia, and hypoglycemia have all been associated with development of NEC. Approximately half of the infants have a low Apgar score, and almost all have had either an umbilical artery or umbilical venous catheter. Many of the infants have been fed prior to developing necrotizing enterocolitis, and of those fed, most have not had breast milk. The few that had been fed breast milk received it from a breast milk bank and were not nursed. Maternal complications associated with fetal distress and shock, such as prolonged rupture of membranes and maternal infection, frequently are observed in these infants.

Etiology

Two sequential conditions are significant in the development of NEC. In the first stage there is an injury to the intestinal mucosa caused by ischemia, which is followed by the detrimental activity of intestinal bacteria.

The damage to the intestinal mucosa can be due to various factors that are synergistic in many infants. In response to systemic shock and hypoxia there is a shunting of the blood to the heart and brain and reduction in the supply to the intestinal tract and kidney. This reflex has been observed in diving mammals and is refered to as a "diving reflex."[14] With prolonged intestinal ischemia permanent damage to the mucosa may occur, including initial thrombosis of the vascular canal and local infarction of the bowel.

Some supportive procedures have been postulated to cause ischemia and have been associated with NEC, including the use of umbilical and venous catheters. These are frequently used for monitoring the biochemistry and gas exchange of stressed newborns and are used also for exchange transfusion and for infusion of fluids. The possibility exists that interruption of portal venous flow during the use of the catheters may result in compromise of the gut mucosa.

The role of diet also has been associated with the etiology of mucosal damage. It was noted that NEC rarely occurs prior to feeding, and it is especially prevalent in infants fed with hyperosmolar formulas. It was hypothesized that premature infants are relatively unable to handle large water and electrolyte loads. When these solutions are given to an infant with immature gut mucosa, severe fluid loss with damage to the mucosa can occur. The intestinal bacteria exploit the break in the integrity of the mucosa. Adynamic ileus and stasis develop, and in the fed infant whose immunologic defenses are deficient, bacteria colonize and multiply. Strains of *E. coli*, *K. pneumoniae*, and *Staphylococcus aureus* can produce enterotoxins that cause further fluid loss. The predominantly gas-forming organisms that generate pneumatosis may accumulate and rupture the intestinal wall, producing pneumoperitoneum and peritonitis. Further invasion into the lumen occurs, and bacterial proliferation extends into the lymphatics and radicles of the portal circulation and reaches the liver. Finally, there is overwhelming sepsis and death.

Numerous reports have implied that the fecal microflora may contribute to the pathogenesis of NEC. A broad range of organisms generally found in the distal gastrointestinal tract have been recovered from the peritoneal cavity and blood of infants with NEC. Roback and co-workers[15] found that organisms cultured from the blood usually matched organisms found in the stool of those patients, but they were unable to demonstrate a preponderance of any specific microorganism. Most of these reports describe the predominant recovery of members of the Enterobacteriaceae family of organisms, including *E. coli*[5, 16, 17] and *K. pneumoniae,*[2, 16, 18] although other organisms normally found in the gastrointestinal tract also have been reported. Among the various organisms isolated from infants with NEC, and thus implicated in the etiology of NEC, are acknowledged enteric pathogens (salmonellae,[9] Coxsackie B$_2$ virus,[19] and members of the normal flora of the neonatal gut such as klebsiellae[2, 16, 18]) and nonenteropathogenic organisms (*E. coli*[5, 16, 17] and clostridia).

Clostridia recently have been implicated as pathogens in some infants with NEC. Pedersen and colleagues[6] cultured *Clostridium perfringens* from the peritoneal fluids of babies who died of NEC and observed Gram-positive bacilli resembling clostridia in necrotic portions of the gut in six of seven infants. Howard and associates[20] reported an outbreak of nonfatal NEC from *Clostridium butyricum.* Strum and co-workers[21] recovered *C. butyricum* from the peritoneal fluid and cerebrospinal fluid of a neonate with NEC. Brook, Avery, and Glasgow[22] recovered *Clostridium difficile* mixed with *K. pneumoniae* from the peritoneal fluid and blood of a patient with NEC. Kosloske and Ulrich[23] obtained cultures of blood and of peritoneal fluid. Of 17 operated infants, 16 had bacteria in their blood and/or peritoneal fluid. The majority of resected bowel specimens from these infants contained a confirmatory morphologic type of bacterium within the wall. The clinical course of eight infants with clostridia was compared to that of eight infants with Gram-negative enteric bacteria (klebsiellae, *E. coli,* or *Bacteroides fragilis*). The infants with clostridia were sicker; they had more extensive pneumatosis intestinalis, a higher incidence of portal venous gas, more rapid progression to gangrene, and more extensive gangrene. These authors concluded that among infants who develop intestinal gangrene, the clostridia appear to be more virulent than Gram-negative enteric bacteria. However, Kliegman and associates,[24] who isolated clostridia from seven infants with NEC, reported a similar mortality among clostridial and nonclostridial infections.

The toxin of *C. difficile* has not been implicated in the pathogenesis of NEC, although it has been identified in the stools of healthy infants. Kliegman and colleagues found that 17 of 121 stools (14%) from infants up to five months of age caused cytotoxicity in tissue culture that was consistent with the effect of *C. difficile* toxin.[24] No toxin was identified in stools from 24 patients with NEC examined by Bartlett and associates[25] or from 18 patients with NEC studied by Chang and Areson.[26]

Cashore and co-workers[27] found *C. difficile* toxin in five samples from 15 patients with confirmed or suspected NEC. In addition, these authors recovered clostridia in 8 of 11 confirmed NEC cases, in 7 of 9 suspected cases, and in 4 of 13 asymptomatic cases. The difference in clostridial colonization between symptomatic and asymptomatic infants was statistically significant.

Clostridia are implicated as a possible source of NEC by almost all of the studies noted above. However, their definite role in NEC awaits further studies and confirmation. The hypoxia and circulatory disturbances in small premature infants at risk for NEC may lead to ischemic segments of bowel, in which multiplication of clostridia and toxin production may result in bowel ulceration, infarction, pneumatosis, and the clinical picture of enterocolitis.

Previous investigations failed to identify clostridia in NEC probably because peritoneal fluid was seldom cultured for anaerobes. In addition, the technology for detection of the more fastidious anaerobes has not been available until recently in many clinical laboratories. Clostridia in the gastrointestinal tract do not cause illness unless they invade the tissues and/or produce exotoxins. A low oxidation-reduction potential, which occurs in the presence of devitalized tissue, is essential for toxin production. Those infants colonized by clostridia and who have an episode of intestinal ischemia prior to the onset of NEC may, therefore, be at serious risk of clostridial invasion of the devitalized portions of their own intestines.

The gas-forming capability of certain clostridia may explain the more extensive pneumatosis intestinalis and the higher incidence of portal venous gas among the infants with clostridia. The production of clostridial exotoxins, which cause cell lysis and tissue necrosis, may explain the more rapid progression to gangrene and more extensive gangrene among infants with clostridia.[23] The lower platelet counts in the infants with Gram-negative rods may be due to endotoxin production by these bacteria. Endotoxin, which has been detected both in blood and peritoneal fluid of infants with severe NEC,[28] produces thrombocytopenia by direct destruction of platelets.

The anaerobic bacteria, including clostridia, are considered to be members of the normal flora of infants of this age. An investigation by Long and Swenson[29] of 196 healthy infants showed that the majority were colonized by 10 days of age with aerobic Gram-negative rods (most frequently *E. coli* and *Klebsiella*), as well as by an anaerobic flora, including *B. fragilis*. Various species of clostridia were found in a third of the infants. Although the clostridia are normal inhabitants of the human intestinal tract, reported colonization rates among neonates vary from 7% to 70%.[30] The source of the neonatal intestinal flora is the unsterile environment met by the infant the moment he leaves the uterus. The normal flora of the cervix and vagina contains many anaerobes, including clostridia.[37] Differences among neonates in gestational age, route of delivery, and type of feeding are associated with different colonization patterns of aerobic and anaerobic bacteria.[20]

Clinical Manifestation

The onset of acute necrotizing enterocolitis generally occurs in the first week of life, but in some victims it may be delayed to the second or third week. The typical infant with necrotizing enterocolitis is premature and recovering from some form of stress, but is well enough to begin gavage feedings. He develops temperature instability, lethargy, and moderate abdominal distention. Stools checked for reducing substance at this stage are likely to show an increase over the normal 1- to 2-reading on a Clinitest tape. The stools will show traces of occult blood, and diarrhea may be present. As abdominal distention progresses, the gastric residuals rise, and within a short period the urine volume decreases and osmolarity rises. The gastric aspirate then becomes bile stained. At this stage, the child may have hypotension and may have gross blood in diarrheal stools. If undetected or untreated at this stage, the patient will progress to massive abdominal distention, acidosis, disseminated intravascular coagulation, peritonitis, and vasomotor collapse.

Diagnosis

Radiological Findings

The earliest radiographic findings in necrotizing enterocolitis may be dilation of the small bowel. The pattern will suggest mechanical or aganglionic obstruction, most frequently in the form of multiple dilated loops of small bowel, but sometimes as isolated loops. Air fluid levels often are observed in the erect position. Commonly, intestinal loops will appear separated because of the presence of mural edema or peritoneal fluid. This then progresses to pneumatosis intestinalis in about 30% of infants studied, and about one-third of those with pneumatosis intestinalis will also have gas within the portal venous system of the liver.

A common finding is thickened bowel wall, bubbly appearance of the intestinal contents, and loops of unequal size. Free air ultimately will be identified within the peritoneal cavity of all infants with necrotizing enterocolitis who are not successfully treated. The site of perforation often is walled off, and in some infants with gas under the diaphragm the intestinal wall may be intact.

Laboratory Findings

Routine antemortem stool and cultures are consistently negative, but blood cultures will yield organisms in about one-fourth of patients. In some infants the white blood count may be very low or very high and the platelet count usually will be diminished and falling rapidly. At least 50% of infants with necrotizing enterocolitis have platelet counts of 50,000 per mm or less.[32] Prothrombin time and partial thromboplastin times are elevated. Hyponatremia is common at the outset of necrotizing enterocolitis.

Management

Medical Management

The management consists of withholding oral feeding, placement of nasogastric tube for suction, vigorous intravenous hydration containing electrolytes and calories, support of the circulation with plasma blood or dextran, and administration of oral and systemic antibiotics for the prevention and treatment of sepsis. The antibiotics should be of broad spectrum appropriate for covering of *E. coli, K. pneumoniae,* and enterobacteria. The antibiotic coverage should be based on the sensitivities or the expected susceptibility of those pathogens prevalent in the nursery at the time of treatment.

Parenteral ampicillin and an aminoglycoside (gentamicin or kanamycin) should be given parenterally. Bell and colleagues[32] found improved survival after administration of gentamicin or kanamycin by nasogastric tube in a dose two to three times the systemic dose. Caution should be used, however, in administration of aminoglycosides through the oral route, since rapid absorption of these drugs from the intestinal tract can occur in newborns with impaired mucosa.

In a recent study by Bell and co-workers,[33] parenteral clindamycin and gentamicin and topical gentamicin were administered to newborns with NEC. A reduction in aerobic Gram-negative organisms occurred following the treatment. The number of the anaerobic isolates did not, however, show a decrease. This study demonstrates the safety of the use of clindamycin in this age group. Conclusive results as for the ability to reduce the number of anaerobes cannot be obtained from this study because of the lack of quantitative cultures, but since clindamycin as well as penicillin is effective against most clostridia, these drugs could be used in the treatment of complications caused by this organism.

Surgical Treatment

When necrotizing enterocolitis has been detected early and appropriate therapy instituted promptly, only a small percentage of infants will require surgical intervention. Since perforation is an ominous complication, however, a close watch by a surgeon is essential. Signs such as persistent acidosis, a fall in the platelets, perfusion and urinary output deterioration in the face of adequate therapy, or if there is free air within the abdomen and if the child shows sudden onset of abdominal tenderness, the child must be surgically explored promptly.

Prevention

Many investigators have documented a sharp decrease in the incidence of NEC when the flora of the infants in their nurseries changed from klebsiellae or *E. coli* to a more innocuous member of the family Enterobacteriaceae. Stanley, Null, and DeLemos[34] noted that when klebsiellae were supplanted by *Serratia marcescens,* the incidence of NEC fell from 5.4% to 2.8%. Bell and colleagues[35] noted that when *Klebsiella* organisms and *E. coli* disappeared and were replaced by *Proteus mirabilis* as the predominant organism in the nursery, NEC disappeared. Such observations support the use of aminoglycoside antibiotics, which are effective against the Enterobacteriaceae for the therapy of NEC.[33] Bell and co-workers[32] reported a reduced incidence of intestinal perforation in affected infants treated orally with kanamycin sulfate or gentamicin sulfate. Egan and associates[36] demonstrated a reduced number of NEC cases in high-risk infants treated with kanamycin. Some neonatologists have advocated further prophylactic oral aminoglycoside antibiotics in high-risk premature infants,[37] which theoretically might decrease the risk of NEC by decreasing the colonization rate by all Enterobacteriaceae, including the more pathogenic strains. Two recent studies, however, have shown both prophylactic oral kanamycin[38] and prophylactic oral gentamicin[39] to be ineffective in preventing NEC. Moreover, Nelson[40] and McCracken and Eitzman[41] have warned against the use of prophylactic oral aminoglycoside antibiotics because of lack of convincing efficacy, plus a risk of emergence of resistant strains of bacteria, including clostridia. These authors pointed out that the oral administration of antimicrobials that selectively suppress the coliform flora of the gut will promote growth of other bacteria, some of which may be deleterious. This is of particular importance since it has recently been shown, first in adults and then in children, that antibiotic-associated pseudomembranous colitis is most likely caused by proliferation of toxin-producing clostridial strains that are resistant to the ingested drugs.[42] This argument is bolstered by the recent description of colitis caused by *C. difficile* in a newborn.[43] This is important also because clostridia have been implicated in the etiology of NEC[6] or NEC-like illnesses,[20] and these organisms are resistant to the aminoglycosides and polymyxins.

REFERENCES

1. Santulli, T. V. et al. Acute necrotizing enterocolitis in infancy. A review of 64 cases. *Pediatrics* 55:376, 1975.
2. Frantz, I. D., III. et al. Necrotizing enterocolitis. *J. Pediatr.* 86:259, 1975.
3. Torma, M. J. et al. Necrotizing enterocolitis in infants. Analysis of forty-five consecutive cases. *Am. J. Surg.* 126:758, 1973.
4. Frantz, I. D., III. et al. Necrotizing enterocolitis. *J. Pediatr.* 86:259, 1975.
5. Speer, M. E. et al. Fulminant neonatal sepsis and necrotizing enterocolitis associated with a "nonenteropathogenic" strain of *Escherichia coli. J. Pediatr.* 89:91, 1976.
6. Pedersen, P. V. et al. Necrotizing enterocolitis of the newborn—is it gas-gangrene of the bowel? *Lancet* 2:715, 1976.
7. Mizrahi, A. et al. Necrotizing enterocolitis in premature infants. *J. Pediatr.* 66:697, 1965.
8. Chappel, J. C., and Dinner, M. Neonatal necrotizing enterocolitis. *S. Afr. J. Surg.* 10:215, 1972.
9. Stein, H. et al. Gastroenteritis with necrotizing enterocolitis in premature babies. *Br. Med. J.* 2:616, 1972.
10. Bhargava, S. K. et al. An outbreak of necrotizing enterocolitis in a special care newborn nursery. *Indian Pediatr.* 10:551, 1973.
11. Virnig, N. L., and Reynolds, J. W. Epidemiologic aspects of neonatal necrotizing enterocolitis. *Am. J. Dis. Child.* 128:186, 1974.
12. Desai, N. S.; Cunningham, M. D.; and Wilson, H. D. Nosocomial epidemics of neonatal necrotizing enterocolitis. *Pediatr. Res.* 9:296, 1975.
13. Fetterman, G. H. Neonatal necrotizing enterocolitis—old pitfalls or new problem. *Pediatrics* 48:345, 1971.
14. Lloyd, J. R. The etiology of gastrointestinal perforations in the newborn. *J. Pediatr. Surg.* 4:77, 1969.
15. Roback, S. et al. Necrotizing enterocolitis: an emerging entity in the regional infant intensive care facility. *Arch. Surg.* 109:314, 1974.
16. Bell, M. J. et al. Evaluation of gastrointestinal microflora in necrotizing enterocolitis. *J. Pediatr.* 92:589, 1978.
17. Yeager, A. S. et al. Cluster of cases of necrotizing enterocolitis (NEC) associated with *E. coli* 085. *Pediatr. Res.* 11:545, 1977.
18. Guinan, M. et al. Epidemic occurrence of neonatal necrotizing enterocolitis. *Am. J. Dis. Child.* 133:594, 1979.
19. Johnson, F. E. et al. Association of fatal Coxsackie B_2 infection and necrotizing enterocolitis. *Arch. Dis. Child.* 52:802, 1977.

20. Howard, F. M. et al. Outbreak of necrotising enterocolitis caused by *Clostridium butyricum. Lancet* 2:1099, 1977.

21. Strum, R. et al. Neonatal necrotizing enterocolitis associated with penicillin-resistant, toxigenic *Clostridium butyricum. Pediatrics* 66:928, 1980.

22. Brook, I.; Avery, G.; and Glasgow, A. *Clostridium difficile* in pediatric infection. *J. Infection* 5:127, 1982.

23. Kosloske, M. A., and Ulrich, J. A. A bacteriologic basis for the clinical presentation of necrotizing enterocolitis. *J. Pediatr. Surg.* 15:558, 1980.

24. Kliegman, R. M. et al. Clostridia as pathogens in neonatal necrotizing enterocolitis. *J. Pediatr.* 95:287, 1979.

25. Bartlett, J. G. et al. Role of *Clostridium difficile* in antibiotic-associated pseudomembranous colitis. *Gastroenterology* 75:778, 1978.

26. Chang, T. W., and Areson, P. Neonatal necrotizing enterocolitis: absence of enteric bacterial toxins. *N. Engl. J. Med.* 299:424, 1978.

27. Cashore, W. J. et al. Clostridia colonization and clostridial toxin in neonatal necrotizing entercolitis. *J. Pediatr.* 98:308, 1981.

28. Fumarola, D. Endotoxemia and neonatal necrotizing enterocolitis. *Infection* 5:202, 1977.

29. Long, S. S., and Swenson, R. M. Development of anaerobic fecal flora in healthy newborn infants. *J. Pediatr.* 91:298, 1977.

30. Kindley, A. D.; Riderts, P. J.; and Tulloch, W. H. Neonatal necrotising enterocolitis. *Lancet* 1:649, 1977.

31. Brook, I. et al. Aerobic and anaerobic flora of maternal cervix and newborn's conjunctiva and gastric fluid: a prospective study. *Pediatrics* 63:451, 1979.

32. Bell, M. J. et al. Neonatal necrotizing enterocolitis: prevention of perforation. *J. Pediatr. Surg.* 8:601, 1973.

33. Bell, M. J. et al. Alterations in gastrointestinal microflora during antimicrobial therapy for necrotizing enterocolitis. *Pediatrics* 63:425, 1979.

34. Stanley, M. D.; Null, D. M.; and DeLemos, R. A. Relationship between intestinal colonization with specific bacteria and the development of necrotizing enterocolitis. *Pediatr. Res.* 11:542, 1977.

35. Bell, M. J. et al. Epidemiologic and bacteriologic evaluation of neonatal necrotizing enterocolitis. *J. Pediatr. Surg.* 14:1, 1979.

36. Egan, E. A. et al. A prospective controlled trial of oral kanamycin in the prevention of neonatal necrotizing enterocolitis. *J. Pediatr.* 89:467, 1976.

37. Grylack, L. J., and Scanlon, J. W. Oral gentamicin therapy in the prevention of neonatal necrotizing enterocolitis: a controlled double-blind trial. *Am. J. Dis. Child.* 132:1192, 1978.

38. Boyle, R. et al. Alterations in stool flora resulting from oral kanamycin prophylaxis of necrotizing enterocolitis. *J. Pediatr.* 93:857, 1978.

39. Rowley, M. P., and Dahlenburg, G. W. Gentamicin in prophylaxis of neonatal necrotising enterocolitis. *Lancet* 2:532, 1978.

40. Nelson, J. D. Commentary. *J. Pediatr.* 89:471, 1976.

41. McCracken, G. H., and Eitzman, D. V. Necrotizing enterocolitis (editorial). *Am. J. Dis. Child.* 132:1167, 1978.

42. Bartlett, J. G. et al. Antibiotic-associated pseudomembranous colitis due to toxin-producing clostridia. *N. Engl. J. Med.* 298:531, 1978.

43. Adler, S. P.; Chandrika, T.; and Berman, W. F. *Clostridium difficile* associated with pseudomembranous colitis: occurrence in a 12-week-old infant without prior antibiotic therapy. *Am. J. Dis. Child.* 135:820, 1981.

CHAPTER 12

Ascending Cholangitis Following Porto-enterostomy

Atresias of the extrahepatic bile ducts are associated with an extremely poor prognosis; less than 5% are amenable to surgical repair. In 1959, Kasai and Suzuki[1, 2] devised a procedure that may improve this outlook, *hepatic porto-enterostomy.*

Infection of the biliary tract is a frequent complication following Kasai's procedure and, unfortunately, adequate anaerobic methodologies have not been applied to study of the bacteriology of cholangitis in patients who have had a porto-enterostomy.[3]

Previous bacterial studies of cholangitis following Kasai's procedure revealed coliform bacilli, *Proteus* species, and enterococci to be the predominant isolates recovered from these patients.[3, 4] Adequate culture methods for anaerobic bacteria were not performed in most of these studies, however. The largest study reporting the bacterial growth within the biliary tract following the Kasai operation was done by Hitch and Lilly,[3] who studied 19 patients over 23 months, obtaining 283 cultures. These investigators used methods for recovery of aerobic as well as anaerobic bacteria and reported the colonization of all the biloenteric conduits with colonic flora within the first postoperative month. *Escherichia coli, Klebsiella* species, group D streptococci, *Pseudomonas* species, *Proteus* species, and *Enterobacter* organisms were the predominant aerobic isolates. *Bacteroides* species, including *Bacteroides fragilis,* were recovered in 11% of the cultures. These authors report the recovery of similar organisms during episodes of cholangitis; however, no specific attention was given in that report to the role of anaerobes during cholangitis. Furthermore, the mode and speed of transportation of specimens to the laboratory and the methods of identification of anaerobes is not described. If the methodology was not strict it is possible that more anaerobes could have been recovered in that study.

Numerous studies in adults demonstrated that *E. coli,* klebsiellae, *Enterobacter* organisms, and enterococci are the typical isolates recovered from patients with biliary tract infection.[5] It has also been recognized for some time that *Clostridium perfringens* may occasionally be involved in serious complications of biliary tract infection, such as sepsis and emphysematous cholecystitis.[6] Several reports indicate that anaerobes, and especially *B. fragilis*, may be more common in biliary tract infections than had been appreciated,[5-7] and they may be recovered in up to 40% of such infections.

Based on the data obtained in adults with biliary tract infection, it is not surprising to find anaerobes as well as aerobes in children with cholangitis. The mechanism by which both aerobic and anaerobic bacteria reach the bile ducts in patients who had undergone Kasai's procedure is most probable by an ascending mode from the gastrointestinal tract.[4, 10] This mode of spread is favored by the surgical procedure that approximates a part of the jejunum to the bile system, by the lack of the normal choledochal sphincter action, and by the stasis that can develop after the surgery. Other mechanisms of development of cholangitis are transhepatic filtration of bacteria from the portal venous blood into the cholangiole[11] and periportal lymphatic infection.[12]

The authors recently have studied aspects of the bile duct system from six children with cholangitis following hepatic porto-enterostomy (Kasai's procedure).[13] All aspirates were cultured for aerobic and anaerobic bacteria. Aerobic bacteria were recovered from all six specimens, and anaerobic organisms were recovered from three. There were 17 isolates recovered, 14 aerobes and 3 anaerobes. The predominant aerobic organisms were *Klebsiella pneumoniae* (four isolates), *Enterococcus* organisms (three isolates), and *E. coli* (two isolates). The anaerobes recovered were *B. fragilis* (two isolates) and *C. perfringens* (one isolate). These findings demonstrate the role of anaerobic organisms in cholangitis following hepatic porto-enterostomy.

The anaerobes recovered in children with ascending cholangitis[3, 13] are part of the normal gastrointestinal flora in infants. The initial sterile meconium becomes colonized within 24 hours with aerobic and anaerobic bacteria, predominantly micrococci, *E. coli*, *Clostridium* species, *B. fragilis*, and streptococci.[14-16] The isolation rate of *B. fragilis* and other anaerobic bacteria in the gastrointestinal tract of term babies approaches that of adults within one week.[16]

Although the number of infants studied so far is small, the data suggest that anaerobes play a major role in cholangitis following Kasai's procedure, and that specimens obtained from these patients should be cultured routinely for anaerobic as well as aerobic bacteria. It is conceivable that some of the reported failures of conventional antimicrobial therapy to cure patients with postsurgical cholangitis[10, 17] could be due to failure to use antimicrobial agents effective against anaerobic bacteria, especially those belonging to the *B. fragilis* group.

While most anaerobic organisms are susceptible to penicillin G, members of the *B. fragilis* group are known to be resistant to that agent.[18] In administrating therapy to infected patients, consideration should be given to the possible presence of anaerobic organisms. It is reasonable, therefore, to treat children with this infection with antimicrobial agents effective also against *B. fragilis,* at least until results of cultures are known.

REFERENCES

1. Kasai, M., and Suzuki, S. A new operation for "non-correctable" biliary atresia: hepatic porto-enterostomy. *Shujutsu* 13:733, 1959.

2. Kasai, M. Treatment of biliary atresia with special reference to hepatic porto-enterostomy and its modification. *Prog. Pediatr. Surg.* 6:5, 1974.

3. Hitch, D. C., and Lilly, J. R. Identification, quantification and significance of bacterial growth within the biliary tract after Kasai's operation. *J. Pediatr. Surg.* 13:563, 1978.

4. Odièvre, M. et al. Hepatic porto-enterostomy or cholecystostomy in the treatment of extrahepatic biliary atresia: a study of 49 cases. *J. Pediatr.* 88:774, 1976.

5. Lykkegaard-Nielsen, M., and Justesen, T. Anaerobic and aerobic bacteriological studies in biliary tract disease. *Scand. J. Gastroenterol.* 11:437, 1976.

6. Finegold, S. M. *Anaerobic bacteria in human disease.* New York: Academic Press, 1977.

7. England, D. M., and Rosenblatt, J. E. Anaerobes in human biliary tracts. *J. Clin. Microbiol.* 6:494, 1977.

8. Shimada, K.; Inamatsu, T.; and Yamashiro, M. Anaerobic bacteria in biliary disease in elderly patients. *J. Infect. Dis.* 135:850, 1977.

9. Lykkegaard-Nielsen, M.; Asnaes, S.; and Justesen, T. Susceptibility of the liver and biliary tract to anaerobic infection in extrahepatic biliary tract obstruction: III. Possible synergistic effect between anaerobic and aerobic bacteria. An experimental study in rabbits. *Scand. J. Gastroenterol.* 11:263, 1976.

10. Kobayashi, A. et al. Ascending cholangitis after successful surgical repair of biliary atresia. *Arch. Dis. Child.* 48:697, 1973.

11. Danks, D. M., and Bishop, R. F. Bacterial antibodies in liver disease. *Lancet* 1:846, 1972.

12. Hirsig, J.; Kara, O.; and Rickham, P. P. Experimental investigations into the etiology of cholangitis following operation for biliary atresia. *J. Pediatr. Surg.* 13:55, 1978.

13. Brook, I., and Altman, P. Anaerobic in biliary tract infection in infants following Kasai's procedure, in press.

14. Hall, I. C., and O'Toole, E. Bacterial flora of the first specimens of meconium passed by fifty newborn infants. *Am. J. Dis. Child.* 47:1279, 1934.

15. Hall, I. C., and Matsumura, K. Recovery of *Bacillus tertius* from stools of infants. *J. Infect. Dis.* 35:502, 1924.

16. Long, S. S., and Swenson, R. M. Development of anaerobic fecal flora in healthy newborn infants. *J. Pediatr.* 91:298, 1977.

17. Chaudhary, S., and Turner, R. B. Trimethoprim-sulfamethoxazole for cholangitis following hepatic portoenterostomy for biliary atresia. *J. Pediatr.* 99:656, 1981.

18. Sutter, V. L., and Finegold, S. M. Susceptibility of anaerobic bacteria to 23 antimicrobial agents. *Antimicrob. Agents Chemother.* 10:736, 1976.

CHAPTER 13

Infections Following Intrauterine Fetal Monitoring

Fetal monitoring with scalp electrodes has gained wide acceptance in the last decade. The technique allows for close monitoring of the fetal heart beat, thus providing useful data for maternal obstetric management and the reduction of the risks to the infant. Intrauterine fetal monitoring (IFM) is considered safe and particularly beneficial to the fetus and is used routinely in some centers.[1] The benefits of IFM are well documented.

A number of fetal complications related to application of the scalp electrode have been observed, including minor ecchymoses and superficial lacerations, leakage of cerebrospinal fluid, osteomyelitis of the skull, sepsis, and scalp abscesses.[1-10]

Predisposing Factors

Several factors have been associated with predisposition of a monitored infant to scalp abscess. These include the duration of the monitoring and ruptured membranes, the presence of high-risk indications for monitoring, and the presence of amnionitis.[11, 12] It is thought that there is an ascending infection into the uterine cavity from organisms that are normal inhabitants of the female genital tract. These organisms can ascend into the uterine cavity when the membranes are ruptured. The introduction of the electrode into the scalp can permit the entrance of the vaginal flora into the subcutaneous tissues. The electrode is a nidus for infection, and the longer it is in place, the greater the possibility of infection. Although the membranes have not been shown to be a barrier against infection, recent data indicate that the amniotic fluid is bacteriostatic.[13] It is probable, therefore, that with prolonged duration of ruptured membranes, the fetal presenting part is less protected by amniotic fluid and more susceptible to invasion by normal vaginal flora.

The higher infection rate among infants with a high-risk indication for monitoring suggests that these fetuses may be somewhat compromised and therefore more susceptible to infection. Infants born of normal pregnancies and monitored electively are at a lower risk for developing a scalp abscess.

Incidence

The rate of scalp infection associated with fetal heart monitoring was estimated to be between 0.4% and 5.2%.[2, 3, 14] Osteomyelitis occurring with fetal monitoring has been described only in two infants[3, 10]; bacteremia has been reported in four instances.[3, 4, 8, 10]

The most recent study was done by Okada, Chow, and Bruce,[11] who observed that 4.5% of the newborn infants developed fetal scalp abscess. The incidence of scalp infections was not found to be related to the type of scalp electrode employed.[11]

Bacteriologic Etiology and Complications

The scalp abscesses may result from inadvertent bacterial inoculation of the fetus while placing the fetal scalp electrode. Bacteria that are present in the cervical canal as normal flora or as pathogens can, therefore, be introduced into the infant's scalp and cause local infections such as cellulitis, abscess and osteomyelitis, or systemic septicemia.

Several case reports describe the recovery of different pathogens from the infected infants. Thadepalli and colleagues,[15] Plavidol and Werch,[16] D'Aunia and co-workers,[17] and Brook and associates[18] have each described one infant who presented with *Neisseria gonorrhoeae* scalp abscesses. In one instance, the infant also presented with conjunctivits from this organism.[18] Solu and colleagues[19] reported a case of meningitis, ventriculitis, and hydrocephalus as a complication of IFM, in which *Escherichia coli* was recovered from all sites.

Overturf and Balfour[3] reported an infant with osteomyelitis from whom only *Staphylococcus epidermidis* was recovered and another infant whose skin and blood cultures yielded beta-hemolytic streptococci. Anaerobic cultures were not done in these two infants.

Brook[10] reported a neonate monitored with scalp electrodes who was delivered with a scalp abscess, osteomyelitis, and bacteremia. *Bacteroides fragilis* was recovered from the blood culture, and polymicrobial aerobic and anaerobic flora were isolated from the aspirated purulent material. Feder, MacLean, and Moxon[8] reported nine infants with scalp abscesses following IFM. In six of the nine infants the cultures were positive: five with a single organism (three with *Hemophilis influenzae* type B, one with beta-hemolytic streptococci group A, one with microaerophilic streptococci) and one with three organisms (beta-hemolytic streptococci group B and 2 anaerobes). In two infants an identical organism was cultured from blood and abscess (*H. influenzae* and beta-hemolytic streptococci group A).

In a recent study using techniques for cultivation of anaerobes, Okada, Chow, and Bruce[11] studied 42 infants who presented with scalp abscess following fetal monitoring. In all instances, bacteria were isolated from the lesion. These investigators have recovered anaerobic microorganisms mixed with aerobes in 58% of the children, aerobes alone in 33%, and anaerobes alone in 9%. The most common organisms in their experience were *Staphylococcus epidermidis, Streptococcus* (groups A and B), *Peptostreptococcus* and *Peptococcus* organisms, coliforms, and anaerobic Gram-positive rods.

Clinical Manifestations

Infants who are at high risk for developing a local or systemic infection following IFM usually develop a local lesion within two to three days[11] following delivery. The lesion usually is localized around the area where the electrode was installed. Sometimes the abscess can drain spontaneously, and in some cases osteomyelitis of the occipital bone can develop.[3, 10] If a cephalohematoma is present, it can become infected also. As the infection progresses the skin can become necrotic and sloughed. The infection can extend into the cerebrospinal fluid and cause meningitis and ventriculitis or spread systemically in the form of sepsis.[3, 10]

Diagnosis

Aspiration of the purulent fluid followed by inoculation of the aspirate into adequate aerobic and anaerobic culture is essential. Because the inoculum may contain mixed flora, adequate selective medium should be used. Blood cultures should be performed when indicated.

Cultures should also be obtained for other sites where an infection is suspected. These include the conjunctiva, bone, and spinal fluid.

Management

Local management of the abscess may require repeated aspiration or leaving a drain in place. For patients whose skin sloughed or became necrotic, extensive debridement may be required on several occasions, with subsequent covering of the wound site by skin graft.[10] For patients with small uncomplicated abscesses, local management of the abscess with adequate drainage of the abscess may be sufficient.

For patients whose abscess is large or in whom an extension of the infection is suspected, parenteral antimicrobial therapy should be initiated. The choice of the antimicrobial agents depends on the bacteria isolated. All antimicrobial agents should be administered parenterally. Where *N. gonorrhoeae* is recovered, penicillin therapy is adequate, but when aerobic Gram-negative enteric organisms are recovered, amino-glycosides should be administered. Penicillin usually is adequate for the treatment of most anaerobic organisms, except for the beta-lacta-mase-producing *Bacteroides* species. Since these organisms were re-covered from these infected sites, however, appropriate coverage with agents active also against these organisms should be used. These in-clude chloramphenicol, clindamycin, or metronidazole. When the ex-act identity of the organism is known, a narrower spectrum of therapy can be selected.

Prevention

Since the risk of developing an infection following IFM is about 1 in 20, caution should be used in selecting the infants for the procedure. IFM should be avoided in infants whose mothers are known to be in-fected with gonorrhoeae or who have amnionitis; however, when IFM is essential, the infants should be watched carefully for development of such a complication. Although no evidence exists to support the use of antimicrobial prophylaxis in infants at high risk of developing an in-fection, consideration and clinical judgement should be used in select-ing this procedure.

REFERENCES

1. Tutera, G. and Newman, R. L. Fetal monitoring: its effect on the perinatal mortality and cesarean section rates and its complications. *Am. J. Obstet. Gynecol.* 122:750, 1975.

2. Okada, D. M., and Chow, A. W. Neonatal scalp abscess following intrapartum fetal monitoring: prospective comparison of two spiral electrodes. *Am. J. Obstet. Gynecol.* 127:875, 1977.

3. Overturf, G. D., and Balfour, G. Osteomyelitis and sepsis: severe complications of fe-tal monitoring. *Pediatrics* 55:244, 1975.

4. Cordero, L., and Hon, E. H. Scalp abscess: a rare complication of fetal monitoring. *J. Pediatr.* 78:533, 1971.

5. Winkel, C. A.; Snyder, D. C.; and Schlaerth, J. B. Scalp abscess: a complication of the spiral fetal electrode. *Am. J. Obstet. Gynecol.* 126:720, 1976.

6. Turbeville, D. F. et al. Complications of fetal scalp electrodes: a case report. *Am. J. Obstet. Gynecol.* 122:530, 1975.

7. Plavidal, J. F., and Welch, A. Fetal scalp abscess secondary to intrauterine monitoring. *Am. J. Obstet. Gynecol.* 125:65, 1976.

8. Feder, H. M.; MacLean, W. C., Jr.; and Moxon, R. Scalp abscess secondary to fetal scalp electrode. *J. Pediatr.* 89:808, 1976.

9. Goodin, R., and Harrod, J. Complications of fetal spinal electrodes. *Lancet* 1:559, 1973.

10. Brook, I. Osteomyelitis and bacteremia caused by *Bacteroides fragilis*. A complication of fetal monitoring. *Clin. Pediatr.* 19:639, 1980.

11. Okada, D. M.; Chow, A. W.; and Bruce, V. T. Neonatal scalp abscess and fetal monitoring: factors associated with infection. *Am. J. Obstet. Gynecol.* 129:185, 1977.

12. Gunn, G. C.; Mishell, D. R., Jr.; and Morton, D. G. Premature rupture of the fetal membranes. *Am. J. Obstet. Gynecol.* 106:494, 1970.

13. Galask, R. P., and Snyder, I. S. Bacterial inhibition by amniotic fluid. *Am. J. Obstet. Gynecol.* 102:949, 1968.

14. Koh, K. S. et al: Experience with fetal monitoring in a university teaching hospital. *J. Calif. Med. Assoc.* 112:455, 1975.

15. Thadepalli, H. et al. Gonococcal sepsis secondary to fetal monitoring. *Am. J. Obstet. Gynecol.* 126:510, 1976.

16. Plavidol, F. J., and Werch, A. Gonococcal fetal scalp abscess: a case report. *Am. J. Obstet. Gynecol.* 127:437, 1977.

17. D'Aunia, A. et al. Gonococcal scalp wound infection. *Morbidity and Mortality Weekly Report,* March 28, 1975, p. 115.

18. Brook, I. et al. Gonococcal scalp abscess in newborn. *J. South. Med. Assoc.* 73:386, 1980.

19. Solu, A. et al. Meningitis, ventriculitis, and hydrocephalus: a complication of fetal monitoring. *Obstet. Gynecol.* 56:663, 1980.

CHAPTER 14

Infant
Botulism

Botulism is a neuroparalytic disease affecting humans and animals all over the world. The pathogenesis of botulism has been through intoxication by ingestion of the preformed toxin in an improperly preserved food, and rarely, in vivo toxin production resulting in illness from a wound infection. Young infants have been thought to be safe from this disease, mostly because of their inability to eat food that contains the toxin. In 1976, botulism in infants became appreciated as a clinical entity by Pickett and colleagues.[1] Laboratory and epidemiologic studies[2-5] have shown that infant botulism results from the ingestion of *Clostridium botulinum* organisms that colonize the intestine with subsequent multiplication and toxin production. Over 150 infants with this infectious disease have been diagnosed since the recognition of infant botulism as a distinct clinical entity.

Infant botulism is an age-limited neuromuscular disease caused by the bacterium *C. botulinum*. It is distinct from classic botulism in that the botulinal toxin is elaborated by the organism in the infant's intestinal lumen and is then absorbed. Botulinal toxin acts through inhibition of acetylcholine release from cholinergic nerve endings with resultant neuromuscular paralysis, the toxin producing weakness or paralysis by impairing release of acetylcholine from the terminal axon.

Epidemiology

C. Botulinum has been found in soil and dust all over the world, and the human susceptibility to certain botulinal toxins appears to be universal. In the United States, differences in the regional soil distribution of *C. botulinum* exist. Mainly type B spores are found east of the Mississippi River,[5] while type A spores predominate in the soils west of it. Similar distribution in the case of infant botulism was found; *C. botulinum* type A has been responsible for most of the cases of infant botulism west of the Mississippi and type B, east of the river.

Predisposing Conditions

Infant botulism is a restricted age-range disease. Ninety-five percent of all recognized cases have occurred in patients between three weeks and six months of age, and the oldest known case occurred in a nine-month-old child. The disease affects equally all major racial and ethnic groups and both sexes. Excretion of the organism has persisted for as long as 158 days after the onset of constipation, well after clinical recovery had occurred. The syndrome has occurred in both breast-fed and bottle-fed infants.[6] Preformed toxin has not been identified in food ingested by the infants, but the organism has been identified in honey, vacuum cleaner dust, and soil. *C. botulinum* organisms, but no preformed toxin, were identified in six different honey specimens fed to three California patients with infant botulism, as well as from 10% (9/90) of honey specimens studied.[6] By food exposure history, honey was significantly associated with type B infant botulism. In California, 30% of hospitalized patients had been fed honey prior to onset of constipation; worldwide, honey exposure occurred in 35% (28/75) of hospitalized cases. Of all food items tested, only honey contained *C. botulinum* organisms. The organism and its toxin have rarely been identified in the feces of normal infants.[3, 4, 7] A recent study reported the isolation of *C. botulinum* from the stools of three normal control infants and nine control infants who had neurologic diseases that clearly were not infant botulism. These infants were termed "asymptomatic carriers" of the organism. The occurrence of the asymptomatic carrier state suggests that a diagnosis of infant botulism cannot be made on a basis of culture results alone, but must rest in historical and physical confirmation of progressive bulbar and extremity weakness with ultimate complete resolution of symptoms and findings over a period of several months.

A distinct seasonal incidence to infant botulism was observed in one study done in Utah.[8] All the cases were reported between March and October with no reported cases during the winter months. The seasonal incidence suggests that the temperature and moisture factors that favor proliferation of *C. botulinum* in the soil could be of major importance.

A common set of environmental features was found to be characteristic of the home environment of children with infant botulism and asymptomatic carriers and includes nearby constructional or agricultural soil disruption, dusty and windy conditions, a high water table, and alkaline soil conditions.[8] These conditions of high soil water and alkaline content, which are favorable for the growth of *C. botulinum*,[5] were found near the homes of all affected infants. The dissemination of the organism appeared to be further enhanced by construction and agricultural soil disruption as well as windy conditions near the homes of most affected infants and asymptomatic carriers.

The ubiquitous distribution of *C. botulinum* spores[5] in nature allows for their ingestion by many infants. The fact that ingested spores can germinate in some, but not all, infants generally between one and six months old indicates that host factors unique to this age play a central role in pathogenesis. Host factors are of great importance, a point emphasized by the broad spectrum in the severity of disease.

Clinical Manifestation

The syndrome as initially described by Pickett and co-workers in 1976[1] is characterized by a history of constipation followed by a subacute progression of bulbar and extremity weakness (within four to five days) manifest in feeding difficulties, ptosis, hypotonia and, often, respiratory embarrassment. There is, however, a broad clinical spectrum of infant botulism. The mild end of the spectrum appears to be represented by infants who never require hospitalization but who have feeding difficulties, mild hypotonia, and failure to thrive, while the severe end of the spectrum may be characterized by a presentation resembling sudden infant death syndrome,[9] and these patients require hospitalization for treatment of their respiratory and feeding difficulties.

The main clinical feature of the syndrome is constipation. In one study by Johnson, Clay, and Arnon,[6] the age of onset of constipation ranges from 21 to 139 days (mean 56 days). The time between the onset of constipation and onset of weakness ranges from 0 to 24 days (mean 11 days). The infants also may manifest tachycardia, difficulty in sucking and swallowing, listlessness, weakening, hypotonia, general muscular weakness with a loss of head control, and pooling of oral secretion. These babies appear "floppy," and may manifest various neurologic signs such as ptosis, ophthalmoplegia, sluggish reaction of the pupils, dysphagia, weak gag reflex, and poor anal sphincter tone.[1-3, 10] In seriously ill babies respiratory arrest may occur.

The first signs noted in infant botulism are classically those of autonomic blockade. The parasympathetic nervous system is more vulnerable to cholinergic blockade by botulinum toxin than the sympathetic nervous system because the parasympathetic pre- and postsynaptic transmissions are affected. In infants with botulism, recognition of the signs and symptoms associated with parasympathetic blockade is important, since these findings precede generalized motor weakness and respiratory decompensation.[6, 11]

The orderly sequence of presentation and recovery of disease signs and symptoms in infant botulism generally follows the order of constipation and tachycardia, followed by loss of head control, difficulty in feeding, weakening, and depressed gag reflex, followed by peripheral motor weakness and subsequent diaphragmatic weakness.[12]

The resolution of disease signs and symptoms occurs in the inverse order of presentation, with autonomic findings the last to regress.

It is important to remember that at this stage of the disease, return of peripheral motor activity does not signify complete reversed cholinergic synapse. The infant is highly susceptible to events that will additionally stress or impair neuromuscular transmission. Such events may lead to sudden respiratory arrest or gradual respiratory failure. Two specific factors have been associated with respiratory decompensation in infant botulism: administration of aminoglycoside antibiotics and neck flexion during positioning for lumbar puncture or computerized axial tomography (CAT) scan.[13, 14]

Aminoglycoside antibiotics decrease acetylcholine release from nerve terminals innervating the diaphragm, leading to diaphragmatic weakness and respiratory failure.

Differential Diagnosis

The most frequent admission diagnoses of infants later found to have infant botulism include sepsis, viral syndrome, dehydration, failure to thrive, myasthenia gravis, poliomyelitis, Guillain-Barré syndrome, encephalitis, and meningitis. Several hereditary endocrine or metabolic disorders considered are amino acid metabolism disorder, hypothyroidation, myasthenia gravis, Werdnig-Hoffmann disease, and drug or toxin ingestion. Diagnoses less frequently considered include subdural effusion, infectious mononucleosis, brain stem encephalitis, animal bite or sting, organophosphate poisoning, carbon monoxide intoxication, methemoglobinemia, myoglobinuria, glycogen or lipid storage diseases, benign congenital hypotonia, congenital muscular dystrophy, myotonic dystrophy, atonic cerebral palsy, and diffuse cerebral degenerative disease.

Diagnosis

Routine laboratory tests such as blood chemistry, blood count, and urinalysis generally are normal. A few cases have shown slight elevation in the cerebrospinal fluid protein.[3, 10] The only procedure that consistently corroborated the clinical diagnosis of infant botulism was electromyography (EMG). The EMG shows a characteristic pattern of brief, small amplitude, abundant, motor-unit action potential (BSAP).[2] As clinical recovery occurs, normal motor-unit activity reappears.

EMG can provide rapid bedside substantiation of the clinical diagnosis of infant botulism. If the BSAP pattern is present,[2, 15] then many of the other diagnostic tests and procedures to which patients are subjected may be deferred while laboratory examination of fecal specimens for *C. botulinum* toxin and organisms proceeds.

Unfortunately, EMG is not in itself diagnostic. The BSAP pattern may be seen in diseases of the terminal motor nerve axons, the neuromuscular junction, or of muscle itself.[1, 16] Furthermore, failure to detect the BSAP pattern does not exclude the diagnosis of infant botulism. The EMG pattern of posttetanic facilitation, observed often in food-borne botulism, may be found in a variety of other disorders besides botulism.[1, 16]

The diagnosis of infant botulism is established unequivocally only when *C. botulinum* organisms are identified in a patient's feces, as *C. botulinum* is not part of the normal resident intestinal microflora of infants or adults.[2, 17–19] Confirmation of the clinical diagnosis requires the demonstration of botulinus toxin or *C. botulinum* in the feces of the infant. The mouse neutralization assay is used to test for the presence of toxin in feces or the serum. Therefore, serum and fecal specimens should be collected as soon as the diagnosis of botulism is suspected. Other specimens that are important for the epidemiologic investigation should be collected also, including suspected food, drug, and environmental samples. All specimens should be transported in insulated containers with cold packs and remain at temperatures of at least 4°C. Specimens for botulism investigation can be submitted to the Centers for Disease Control in Atlanta, Georgia.[10]

Management

Children with infant botulism presenting with mild symptoms require minimal care and can be managed as outpatients if careful follow-up examinations are arranged. Infants with severe infant botulism constitute a select group who are at risk for respiratory failure. These infants can be identified by their progressive sequential loss of neurologic functions.

Seriously ill patients require hospitalization for up to two months. Careful maintenance of adequate ventilation and caloric intake is of particular importance. The need for respiratory assistance, if any, generally occurs during the first week of hospitalization. Parenteral antibiotic therapy in an attempt to eradicate *C. botulinum* toxin and organisms from the intestinal tract usually is unsuccessful and should be reserved for cases with proved or suspected sepsis caused by other organisms.

When penicillin or its derivatives have been used,[6] neither oral nor parenteral administration succeeded in producing discernible clinical benefit or in eradicating either *C. botulinum* organisms or botulinus toxin from the intestine.[2] Another argument against the use of antimicrobial agents is that these agents may alter the intestinal microecology in an unpredictable manner and might actually permit intestinal overgrowth by *C. botulinum* by eliminating the normal flora.

Aminoglycosides may potentiate neuromuscular weakness caused by botulinus toxin. It is, therefore, suggested that these antibiotics should be used with caution in suspected cases of infant botulism. In large doses, gentamicin, along with other aminoglycosides, has been demonstrated to produce a nondepolarizing type of neuromuscular block.[20] As botulinus toxin is known to block the release of acetylcholine from cholinergic nerve endings,[21] gentamicin may potentiate sublethal concentrations of botulinus toxin and result in complete neuromuscular blockade and resultant paralysis. In recent reports, L'Hommedieu and co-workers[13] provide clinical data and Santos, Swenson, and Glasgow[22] provide animal data to support this hypothesis.

The present treatment of infant botulism consists of meticulous supportive care, with particular attention to nutrition and to pulmonary hygiene. Immediate access to an intensive care unit and to mechanical ventilation is especially important because aspiration or apnea may occur. Associated conditions such as dehydration, aspiration, pneumonia, and anemia should be treated also. The respiratory aspects of the patient should be addressed by performing frequent suctioning and stimulation, mechanical ventilation, and administration of oxygen. When infant botulism is suspected, monitoring for both apnea and bradycardia should be instituted; tracheostomy may be required in some cases. Monitoring should continue until sufficient breathing, coughing, and swallowing ability have returned so that apnea and aspiration are unlikely to occur. The need for nutritional support can require gavage feeding, intravenous glucose and electrolytes and sometimes hyperalimentation.

Tube feeding may stimulate peristalsis and has been used successfully in most patients. Patients should not be fed by mouth until they are able to gag and swallow. To reduce the quantity of *C. botulinum* organisms and toxin in the intestine, cathartic agents or bulk laxatives may be judiciously administered if adynamic ileus is absent, but rarely have these proved efficacious.

Since patients excrete *C. botulinum* toxin and organisms in their feces for weeks to months after they have returned home, it is important to adhere to careful handwashing and diaper disposal. The value of enemas and purgatives, clostridiocidal antibiotics, cholinomimetic drugs (i.e., guanidine, 4-aminopyridine),[23] and equine or human *C. botulinum* antitoxin[24] is unproved. Experience with patients treated with the antitoxin has indicated that antitoxin is not needed for complete recovery.[25–27]

Prevention

Since *C. botulinum* spores are heat resistant and may survive boiling for several hours,[1] home cooking of foods may not destroy *C. botulinum* spores. Washing and peeling raw foods before cooking may substantially reduce the number of spores, if present.

The single food fed to patients that has been identified as a source of *C. botulinum* spores, but not of preformed botulinus toxin, is honey.[2, 17, 28, 29] Furthermore, honey exposure has been implicated as a significant risk factor for type B infant botulism.[28] A survey of honey samples not associated with cases of infant botulism found that 7.5% contained *C. botulinum*, type A or type B or both. The honeys that contained *C. botulinum* originated in various parts of the United States.[29] Since honey is not essential for infant nutrition, it is recommended that honey not be fed to infants less than one year old.[29]

The full extent of infant morbidity and mortality that results from the intestinal production of botulinus toxin has not been determined. Because the disease may mimic many other disorders, it is possible that more cases of infant botulism may be recognized, and its role in sudden infant death syndrome will be elucidated.

REFERENCES

1. Pickett, J. et al. Syndrome of botulism in infancy: clinical and electrophysiologic study. *N. Engl. J. Med.* 295:770, 1976.

2. Arnon, S. S. et al. Infant botulism: epidemiological, clinical, and laboratory aspects. *JAMA* 237:1946, 1977.

3. Arnon, S. S., and Chin, J. The clinical spectrum of infant botulism. *Rev. Infect. Dis.* 1:614, 1979.

4. Midura, T. F. Laboratory aspects of infant botulism in California. *Rev. Infect. Dis.* 1:652, 1979.

5. Smith, L. The occurrence of *Clostridium botulinum* and *Clostridium tetani* in the soil of the United States. *Health Lab. Sci.* 15:74, 1978.

6. Johnson, R. O.; Clay, S. A.; and Arnon, S. S. Diagnosis and management of infant botulism. *Am. J. Dis. Child.* 133:586, 1979.

7. Chin, J.; Arnon, S. S.; and Midura, T. F. Food and environmental aspects of infant botulism in California. *Rev. Infect. Dis.* 1:693, 1979.

8. Thompson, J. A. et al. Infant botulism: clinical spectrum and epidemiology. *Pediatrics* 66:936, 1980.

9. Arnon, S. S. et al. Intestinal infection and toxin production by *Clostridium botulinum* as one cause of sudden infant death syndrome. *Lancet* 1:1273, 1978.

10. Gunn, R. A.; Dowell, V. R., Jr.; and Hatheway, C. L. *Infant botulism: clinical and laboratory aspects.* Atlanta: Center for Disease Control, 1978.

11. Brown, L. Commentary: infant botulism and the honey connection. *J. Pediatr.* 94:337, 1979.

12. L'Hommedieu, C., and Polin, R. A. Progression of clinical signs in severe infant botulism. *J. Pediatr.* 20:90, 1981.

13. L'Hommedieu, C. S. et al. Potentiation of neuromuscular weakness in infant botulism with aminoglycosides. *J. Pediatr.* 95:1065, 1979.

14. Paton, W. D. M., and Waud, D. R. The margin of safety of neuromuscular transmission. *J. Physiol.* 191:595, 1967.

15. Clay, S. A. et al. Acute infantile motor unit disorder: infantile botulism? *Arch. Neurol.* 34:236, 1977.

16. Berg, B. Commentary of syndrome of infant botulism. *Pediatrics* 59:321, 1977.

17. Midura, T. F., and Arnon, S. S. Infant botulism: identification of *Clostridium botulinum* and its toxins in feces. *Lancet* 2:934, 1976.

18. Arnon, S. S. et al. Intestinal infection and toxin production by *Clostridium botulinum* as one cause of sudden infant death syndrome. *Lancet* 1:1273, 1978.

19. Dowell, V. R., Jr. et al. Coproexamination for botulinal toxin and *Clostridium botulinum:* a new procedure for laboratory diagnosis of botulism. *JAMA* 238:1829, 1977.

20. Brazil, O. V., and Prado-Franceschi, J. The neuromuscular blocking action of gentamicin. *Arch. Int. Pharmacodyn. Ther.* 179:65, 1968.

21. Simpson, L. L. The action of botulinal toxin. *Rev. Infect. Dis.* 1:656, 1979.

22. Santos, J. I.; Swensen, P.; and Glasgow, L. A. Potentiation of *Clostridium botulinum* toxin by aminoglycoside antibiotics: clinical and laboratory observations. *Pediatrics* 68:50, 1981.

23. Cherington, M., and Ryan, D. W. Treatment of botulism with guanidine: early neurophysiologic studies. *N. Engl. J. Med.* 282:195, 1970.

24. Lewis, G. E., and Metzger, J. F. Botulism immune plasma (human). *Lancet* 2:634, 1978.

25. Black, R. E., and Arnon, S. S. Botulism in the United States, 1976. *J. Infect. Dis.* 135:829, 1977.

26. Fisher, C. J., Jr., and Woerner, S. J. Emergency case report: infantile botulism. *J. Am. Coll. Emerg. Phys.* 6:453, 1977.

27. Edmund, B. J. et al. Case of infant botulism in Texas. *Tex. Med.* 73:85, 1977.

28. Arnon, S. S. et al. Honey and other environmental risk factors for infant botulism. *J. Pediatr.* 94:331, 1979.

29. Midura, T. F. et al. Isolation of *Clostridium botulinum* from honey. *J. Clin. Microbiol.* 9:282, 1979.

PART III

Anaerobic Infections of Specific Organ Sites

CHAPTER 15

Central Nervous System Infections

Anaerobic bacteria frequently were found in central nervous system infections in the preantibiotic era.[1] Their main mode of spread was postulated to be contiguous by dissemination from chronic otitis media, mastoiditis, or sinusitis. Although anaerobic bacteria are found rarely in acute meningeal infection, they are the major cause of intracranial abscess.

Meningitis

Incidence

Anaerobic bacteria are recovered infrequently from patients with acute bacterial meningitis. Finegold[1] in a review of the literature cited only 125 well-documented cases and 73 other cases with details inadequate for complete analysis. Only a few case reports of children with meningitis caused by anaerobes are present in the literature.[2-5] Since anaerobic cultures of cerebrospinal fluid rarely are done on a routine basis, and specimens are infrequently submitted in transport media appropriate for anaerobes, the rate of anaerobic meningitis could be higher than the rate reported.

Bacterial Etiology and Pathogenesis

There have been a few reported cases[5, 6] of children in whom meningitis due to *Bacteroides* developed following upper respiratory infection; the oropharynx may be a frequent source of infection since it harbors large numbers of anaerobes. Bacteremia has been associated with meningitis in children in many instances.[7] It has been demonstrated in children with bacteremia caused by *Fusobacterium* organisms following pharyngitis, sinusitis, otitis media, and pulmonary infections.[5, 8] Meningitis due to *Bacteroides* also has been reported in infants and older children.[9, 10] Of the 13 cases reported in the literature, acute or chronic middle ear infection was associated with 6 of them.[9–14] This was noted particularly in infants six months or older. The other group of infants with meningitis due to *Bacteroides* generally were newborns. As a rule, these infants were born with delivery complicated by premature rupture of membranes, amnionitis, or fetal distress. The portals of entry of the *Bacteroides* species in neonatal infections were bacteremia following necrotizing enterocolitis,[15] gastric perforation and subsequent ileus followed by bacteremia,[16] aspiration pneumonitis and septicemia,[17, 18] infected ventriculo-peritoneal[19] or ventriculo-atrial shunt,[16] and complicating dermal sinus tract infections.[19] Ventriculitis and hydrocephalus were common sequelae in the survivors of that group. Bacteremia with identical organisms was present in all but one case. Of interest is the association of *Bacteroides* with pneumonitis[17, 20] or lung abscesses[9, 21] in several of these patients.

Compared with the multiple number of bacteria generally associated with brain abscesses, anaerobic meningitis is more apt to be a monomicrobial infection and less likely to be a mixed anaerobic-aerobic infection. Combined aerobic-anaerobic infection was reported recently in a one-year-old child whose cultures yielded *Haemophilus influenzae* mixed with *Clostridium perfringens*.[4]

It should be noted that anaerobic meningitis often is part of a more extensive intracranial infection. Concurrent brain abscess or extradural or subdural abscesses have been reported.[12]

Diagnosis

The clinical symptoms and signs associated with meningitis caused by anaerobic bacteria do not generally differ from those associated with other central nervous system infections occurring in pediatric age groups. Infants can present with lethargy, seizures, and bulging fontanels or papilledema. Older children can present with headache, vomiting, stiff neck, lethargy, or irritability and fever.

The cerebrospinal fluid findings are generally cloudy and contain more than 1000 neutrophils per cubic millimeter, the protein concentration generally is above 100 mg%, the glucose content is generally low (below 30 mg%), and the lactic acid concentration is elevated (above 35 mg%). In partially treated cases these values may vary, except for the lactic acid level, which generally remains elevated up to 72 hours following initiation of antimicrobial therapy.[22] Clues to the presence of meningitis caused by anaerobic bacteria are situations in which no bacterial growth or no bacterial antigens are present in a cerebrospinal fluid specimen that shows the presence of bacteria on Gram stain. Other clues to bacterial infection are indications in the cerebrospinal fluids of elevated neutrophil count, elevated protein concentration and lactic acid, and a reduced glucose concentration. Meningitis should be suspected if patients fit into this category, even if they have been partially treated with antibiotics. The presence of more than one bacterial strain in Gram stain and the ability to grow only one isolate is another indication. Patients who fail to respond to appropriate antimicrobial therapy should be examined for the presence of anaerobes because of the possibility of mixed aerobic and anaerobic infection.[4]

Meningitis caused by anaerobes should be suspected especially in clinical situations that facilitate their development, such as chronic otitis media, mastoiditis, dental abscesses, facial sinusitis, anaerobic bacteremia, or following perforation of an abdominal viscus. Special consideration should be given to newborns at high risk to develop anaerobic infection, especially those who were born to mothers with amnionitis.

Because of the association between subdural or epidural empyema and brain abscesses with meningitis, the presence of any of these intracranial abscesses in patients should warrant diagnostic workup to exclude possible concurrent meningitis.

Treatment

Most *Bacteroides* and *Fusobacterium* species are extremely susceptible to penicillin and its analogues. Some species, however, particularly *Bacteroides fragilis,* are usually resistant to these antibiotics, and therefore susceptibility testing is necessary to ensure proper therapy. The organism is reliably susceptible to only four agents: carbenicillin, clindamycin, chloramphenicol, and metronidazole. Clindamycin is not recommended in central nervous system infections because of its generally poor penetration into the cerebrospinal fluid.

Carbenicillin levels in the cerebrospinal fluid do not always exceed the usual high minimum inhibitory concentrations for this bacillus (up to 64 μg/ml).[23] Although most strains of *B. fragilis* are susceptible to clindamycin phosphate, its diffusion into the cerebrospinal fluid is almost nil.[24] Chloramphenicol reaches concentrations in the cerebrospinal fluid of 40% to 70% of serum levels, but because usual MICs for *B. fragilis* may be 4 to 6 μg/ml, administration of maximum doses of chloramphenicol are required and because of toxicity, *serum concentrations of drug must be measured.* Available schedules for chloramphenicol dosage for the neonate are more safe than effective. Concomitant administration of phenobarbital may decrease serum chloramphenicol concentrations by increasing hepatic metabolism of the drug. Ventricular instillation of chloramphenicol succinate or clindamycin phosphate may be ineffective since metabolic activation of both drugs is required.[16]

Metronidazole, a drug used effectively in the therapy of trichomoniasis and amebiasis, has been shown to be very active in vitro against *Bacteroides* and *Fusobacterium* species in addition to other anaerobes.[25, 26] Moreover, its clinical efficacy in anaerobic infections has been reported in several studies.[25, 27] High levels in cerebrospinal fluid were recorded in patients treated with this drug reported previously,[28, 29] and its bactericidal mode of action[26] could make it a promising agent for therapy of anaerobic infections of the central nervous system.

The length of time for administration of antimicrobial therapy depends on the patient's response and underlying illness. It should be given for at least 14 days, but the ultimate length has to be adjusted to the clinical condition.

In patients with mixed aerobic and anaerobic meningeal infection, antimicrobial coverage against all organisms present is of paramount importance. Since metronidazole is effective only against anaerobic organisms, additional coverage for the other organisms should be added in instances of mixed infection. Complete eradication of the organisms in the cerebrospinal fluid may be difficult when insufficient antimicrobial agents penetrate into the cerebrospinal fluid. Repeated spinal tap would ensure eradication of the organisms and would allow for measurement of concentration of the antimicrobial agents in the cerebrospinal fluid.

Elimination of associated foci of infection is crucial. Failure to drain inflamed foci adjacent to the cerebrospinal fluid such as purulent sinusitis or epidural or subdural abscesses can prevent complete cure of the infection.

Prognosis

The prognosis of anaerobic meningitis is usually grave, and the mortality rate in the newborn period and older child may reach 50%. Early recognition and adequate therapy may allow survival and recovery. Hydrocephalus and developmental delay following the infection has been reported.[15, 16]

Cerebrospinal Fluid Shunt Infections

Infections are a common and serious complication of cerebrospinal fluid shunts. A variety of species of microorganisms have been responsible for these infections, but *Staphylococcus epidermidis* has predominated by far.[30-33]

Infection of the shunt placed to control hydrocephalus occurs with an incidence ranging in various recent series from 15.7%[34] to 27%[35] and is a significant cause of mortality in these patients. Coagulase-negative staphylococci are the most common infecting organisms, infections with *Staphylococcus aureus* are the second most frequent.[35, 36] Other organisms, including rare pathogens such as *Bacillus cereus*, have also been reported.[37] These patients may present with sepsis, signs of increased intracranial pressure,[32] or nephrotic syndrome.[38]

Microbiology

Shunt infection with *Propionibacterium* species has been recently reported in a few cases, especially in association with ventriculo-auricular shunts, varying from asymptomatic colonization found at the time of elective removal of shunts and mixed infection with *S. epidermidis* to symptomatic disease.[30, 39, 40]

Multiple-organism meningitis was reported in two patients as a complication of ventriculo- and lumboperitoneal shunts. The distal portion of the shunts perforated the colon and recurrent meningitis developed with *B. fragilis*, peptostreptococci, *Escherichia coli*, and group D streptococci.[19]

Pathogenesis

Anaerobic diphtheroids, currently classified as *Propionibacterium* species, like *S. epidermidis*, are of low virulence and ubiquitous on the skin, where they outnumber the aerobes by 10- to 100-fold.[41] The organisms are most numerous in areas of the skin containing pilosebaceous glands, with the scalp being the most heavily colonized.[42] The exact pathogenesis of cerebrospinal fluid shunt infection has not been elucidated; many are thought to originate from colonization at the time of surgery.[43]

Although *Propionibacterium acnes* outnumber other aerobic organisms on the skin, they are unusual causes of shunt infections, accounting for only 1.4% of the cases.[44] The true rate of infection caused by this organism is unknown, however, because spinal fluids may not be cultured routinely in thioglycolate broth or anaerobically, cultures may not be held a sufficient length of time for growth, the isolation of the organism may be ignored as a contaminant by the clinician, or the physician may not recognize the organism as being a cause of central nervous system infections.

Of interest is a recent report that described *P. acnes* infections of a subdural hematoma that developed following a diagnostic tap.[45] Anaerobic meningitis caused by multiple organisms can develop as an unusual complication of ventriculoperitoneal and lumboperitoneal shunts. After placement in the peritoneal cavity, the distal end of the catheter penetrated the colon with retrograde contamination of the cerebrospinal fluid with enteric flora. In both cases reported in the literature[19] meningitis was caused by multiple microorganisms. The isolation of *E. coli* and *B. fragilis* (the most common enteric aerobic and anaerobic flora, respectively) were common to both cases. Similarly, in both patients, an interval of approximately six months elapsed following the placement of the shunt and the subsequent occurrence of meningitis. The isolation of *E. coli* and *B. fragilis* following shunt surgery is unusual and should alert the physician to the possibility of the penetration of the gastrointestinal tract by a peritoneal shunt.

Laboratory

Laboratory data generally show a mild peripheral leukocytosis, usually moderate pleocytosis of the cerebrospinal fluid, with a predominance of neutrophils and absence of profound hypoglycorrhachia. Gram stains when performed are frequently positive.

It is therefore imperative that spinal fluid specimens should have complete routine examination to include a Gram stain and be cultured aerobically and anaerobically, or at least in thioglycolate broth. Cultures should be held for a minimum of 14 days, since in many cases the cultures do not turn positive until 9 or 10 days of incubation.[46] Anaerobic diphtheroids are common contaminants, but in a patient with a ventricular shunt who has signs of infection and cerebrospinal fluid pleocytosis, the isolation of these organisms should not be ignored. In cases where clinical and laboratory findings of shunt infection are present but cultures are negative, special anaerobic culture methods must be used. This would include collection of spinal fluid in an anaerobic tube for transport to the laboratory and inoculation to prereduced media as well as thioglycolate broth.

Complications

Complications other than difficulty in eradicating the infection are few, providing the case was recognized as an anaerobic diphtheroid infection. Glomerulonephritis, a well-recognized complication of staphylococcal shunt infection,[38] has been reported following *P. acnes* infection.[47]

Therapy

P. acnes is universally sensitive in vitro to penicillin, chloramphenicol, clindamycin, and rifampin.[48] *P. acnes,* however, is generally resistant to metronidazole, which is very effective in the treatment of meningitis caused by other organisms.

The approach to the treatment of *P. acnes* shunt infection is generally identical to that outlined for *S. epidermidis* infection,[4] which includes antimicrobial therapy and removal of the shunt. In cases where multiple organisms are present due to perforation of the colon, surgical repair of the perforation as well as removal of the shunt may be necessary to eradicate infection.[19]

Intracranial Abscesses

Intracranial abscesses can be classified as brain abscesses or subdural or extradural empyema. They also can be classified according to their anatomic location or etiologic agent.

Microbiology

Previous studies of the bacteriology of intracranial abscess may be misleading for a number of reasons, including lack of appropriate sampling techniques to prevent contamination of specimens by normal flora and the failure to culture adequately for strict anaerobes.[1] Schwartz and Karchmer[49] found that streptococci, Enterobacteriaceae, and *S. aureus* were the most common isolates in 787 cases from the literature. Anaerobic streptococci or *Bacteroides* species were found in 37% of their most recently studied patients. Heineman and Braude[50] recovered anaerobes from 16 of 18 consecutive patients with brain abscesses, and aerobes from only six. Fourteen anaerobes were associated with chronic infection of the ear, sinus, or lung. Their most common isolates were anaerobic streptococci, *Bacteroides* species, veillonellae, fusobacteria, and actinomycetes. After summarizing the bacteriologic data available in the literature, Finegold[1] concluded that anaerobes are the major etiologic agents of brain abscess.

Various anaerobic and microaerophilic cocci and Gram-negative and Gram-positive anaerobic bacilli are the major causes of brain abscess. The predominant aerobic organisms are *S. aureus* and *Streptococcus pneumoniae,* group A streptococci, alpha-hemolytic streptococci.

Less common causes include *E. coli, Proteus* species, *Klebsiella* species, *Enterobacter* species, *Pseudomonas* species, *H. influenzae, Neisseria meningitidis, Nocardia asteroides,* mycobacteria, various fungi, and *Entamoeba histolytica.*

Only a few reports describe the microbiology of brain abscesses in children. Salibi[51] described the recovery of *Bacteroides funduliformis* from a frontal lobe brain abscess that developed two weeks after tonsillectomy and adenoidectomy. Khuri-Bulos[11] treated a posterior fossa brain abscess that developed following chronic otitis media. *Bacteroides fragilis,* bifidobacteria, anaerobic Gram-positive cocci, and *Proteus mirabilis* were recovered from the abscess. Idriss, Gutman, and Kronfol[52] described the recovery of 41 isolates from 34 children with brain abscesses. Seventeen of the 41 isolates (42%) were anaerobes, and they included 13 strains of anaerobic or microaerophilic streptococci, two *Bacteroides* species, and one *Actinomyces* species. In a retrospective review by Fisher, McLean, and Suzuki[53] of 94 episodes of brain abscess, 16 anaerobes were recovered. These included 11 isolates of Gram-positive anaerobic cocci, four *Bacteroides* species, and one *Clostridium* species.

Table 15.1. Clinical Characteristics of Patients with Intracranial Abscesses

	Brain Abscess	Subdural Empyema
Number of patients	9	10
Underlying conditions		
Sinusitis		
frontal	2	3*
sphenoid	1	3
maxillary	1	
mastoid	2†	2
Chronic otitis media	2†	
Dental abscess	1	1*
Meningitis		1
Head trauma		1
Congenital heart disease	2	
Site of abscess		
Frontal area	3	4
Temporal area	3	2
Parietal area	3	4

SOURCE: Brook, I. Bacteriology of intracranial abscess in children. *J. Neurosurg.* 54:485, 1981. Reprinted by permission.

*One patient with subdural empyema had two predisposing conditions (frontal sinusitis and a dental abscess).

†Two patients with brain abscess had two predisposing conditions (chronic otitis media and mastoiditis).

The bacteriologic and clinical findings in 19 pediatric patients with intracranial abscess was recently presented.[54] Ten children presented with subdural empyema and nine had brain abscess. Underlying conditions to abscess formation were present in all of the patients (table 15.1). Sinusitis was present in 14 children, and dental abscess in two. The abscess was located in the frontal and parietal area in seven instances each, and in the temporal area in five.

Anaerobic organisms alone were recovered from 12 (63%) of the patients (including eight with subdural empyema and four with brain abscess), aerobic bacteria alone were present in two children (11%), and mixed aerobic and anaerobic bacteria were present in five (26%) patients. There were 43 anaerobic isolates (2.3 per specimen). The predominant anaerobes were anaerobic Gram-positive cocci (16 isolates), *Bacteroides* species (10, including 2 *B. fragilis*); *Fusobacterium* species (9 isolates), and *Actinomyces* species (5 isolates). A total of eight isolates (0.4 per specimen), including five Gram-positive cocci and three *Haemophilus* species, were recovered (table 15.2).

These findings support the role of anaerobes in complications of sinusitis such as brain abscess and subdural empyema, as well as their pathogenic role in sinusitis itself.

Pathogenesis

Before the use of antibiotics, anaerobic bacteria were frequently found in intracranial infections.[1] It was thought that they spread from contiguous sites of existing infections, such as chronic otitis media, mastoiditis, or sinusitis. Intracranial extension is facilitated by the ability of the infectious organisms to cause tissue necrosis and invade blood vessels. This extension can result in epidural or cerebral abscesses, subdural empyema, or septic thrombophlebitis of the cortical veins or venous sinuses.[16]

Infection may enter the intracranial compartment by two routes. Direct extension may occur through necrotic areas of osteomyelitis in the posterior wall of the frontal sinus. This direct route of intracranial extension is more commonly associated with chronic otitic infection than with sinusitis.[1]

An alternative route of intracranial bacterial entry is provided by the valveless venous network that interconnects the intracranial venous system and the vasculature of the sinus mucosa. Thrombophlebitis originating in the mucosal veins progressively involves the emissary veins of the skull, the dural venous sinuses, the subdural veins, and finally the cerebral veins. By this mode of spread, the subdural space may be selectively infected without contamination of the intermediary structure; that is, a subdural empyema can exist without evidence of extradural pus or osteomyelitis. Intracranial extension of the infection

Table 15.2. Bacterial Isolates from Patients with Intracranial Abscess

	Brain Abscess	Subdural Empyema
Number of patients	9	10
Aerobic bacteria		
Gram-positive cocci		
Alpha-hemolytic streptococcus	1	
Group A beta-hemolytic streptococci	2	
Group F beta-hemolytic streptococci		1
Staphylococcus aureus	1	
Gram-negative bacilli		
Haemophilus aphrophilus	1	
Haemophilus parainfluenzae	1	
Haemophilus influenzae type B		1
Subtotal, Aerobes	6	2
Anaerobic bacteria		
Gram-positive cocci		
Peptococcus species	2	1
Peptococcus asaccharolyticus	2	
Peptococcus prevotii	1	
Peptostreptococcus magnus	1	
Peptostreptococcus intermedius	1	1
Peptococcus constellatus		1
Microaerophilic streptococci	2	4
Gram-negative cocci		
Veillonella parvula	1	2
Gram-positive bacilli		
Actinomyces odontolyticus	2	
Actinomyces species	3	
Gram-negative bacilli		
Fusobacterium species	1	1
Fusobacterium necrophorum		1
Fusobacterium nucleatum	3	2
Fusobacterium mortiferum		1
Bacteroides species	1	2
Bacteroides oralis		1
Bacteroides melaninogenicus	1	2
Bacteroides bivius		1
Bacteroides fragilis	1	1
Subtotal, Anaerobes	22	21
Total Number of Bacteria	28	23

Source: Brook, I. Bacteriology of intracranial abscess in children. *J. Neurosurg.* 54:485, 1981. Reprinted by permission.

by the venous route is common in paranasal sinus disease, especially in its acute exacerbation of chronic inflammation.

Contiguous spread could extend to the central nervous system, causing cavernous sinus thrombosis, retrograde meningitis, and epidural, subdural, and brain abscesses (fig. 15.1).[55]

Subdural empyema is a pyogenic infection that usually involves one cerebral hemisphere, but it may spread under the falx to the contralateral side. It frequently spreads from an inflamed frontal sinus, especially in young adult males.[56] In many cases, purulent drainage can be established from the infected sinus through the cribriform plates of the frontal bone into the subdural space.[56-58]

The site of the primary infection or the underlying condition is a determinant of the etiology of the brain abscess. *B. fragilis* is the most common anaerobic bacterium isolated in otogenic temporal lobe abscesses[1, 59]; however, streptococci (aerobic, microaerophilic, and anaerobic) and Enterobacteriaceae, especially *Proteus* species,[59] have also been found.[50, 60-62] Frederick and Braude[63] showed that over half of cultures obtained at surgery from 83 patients with chronic sinusitis yielded anaerobes; heavy growth of anaerobes in pure culture occurred in 23 patients. Brook[64] identified anaerobes from all 37 culture-positive specimens recovered from children with chronic sinusitis. Anaerobic streptococci and *Bacteroides* species predominated; *S. aureus* and *H. influenzae* were other notable isolates in these studies.[63, 64] There is excellent bacteriologic correlation with the anaerobic isolates from brain abscesses arising in the paranasal sinuses.[1, 59]

Abscesses spread by blood-borne bacteria usually originate in the lung. This source of infection is rare in children, however. Anaerobic and microaerophilic streptococci, as well as streptococci viridans, are common isolates in abscesses associated with congenital heart disease.[1, 61] A variety of Enterobacteriaceae and anaerobes may spread from intraabdominal or genitourinary sites.[1] *S. aureus* remains the most common isolate in brain abscess secondary to trauma[58, 65] and was recently reported as a major isolate recovered from children; however, the predisposing factors in these patients are not described. In children under five years of age,[66] subdural empyema almost invariably follows bacterial meningitis, and the causative organism is the same that causes the meningitis itself, usually *H. influenzae*, or, in neonates, Gram-negative bacilli.

Intracranial complications can develop secondary to periapical abscesses of the upper incisors.[67] In the children studied the infection spread to the central nervous system through the maxillary and frontal sinuses. Anaerobic bacteria were isolated from the infected subdural empyema. *Peptostreptococcus intermedius* and microaerophilic streptococci were recovered from one patient and fusobacteria from the other.

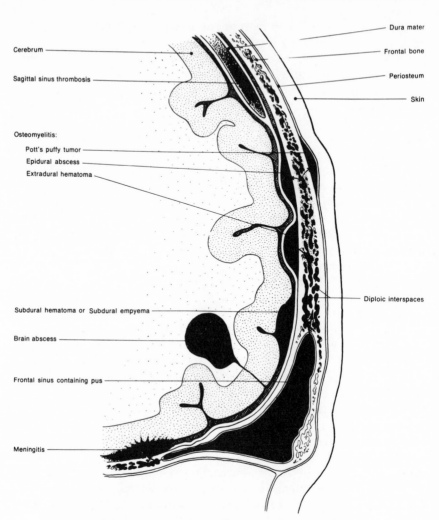

Figure 15.1. The brain membranes and the sites of intracranial abscesses. (Clairmont, A. A., and Per-Lee, J. H.
Complications of acute sinusitis. *Am. Fam. Physician* 11:80–
84, 1975. Reprinted by permission.)

   Anaerobic organisms were found to be the predominant isolate in
periodontal abscesses in children, outnumbering aerobes eight to
one.[68] This finding is important because of the association of anaerobes
with many examples of serious infections arising from dental foci, such
as bacteremia, endocarditis, sinusitis, meningitis, subdural empyema,
brain abscess, and pulmonary empyema.[1] Several reports[69] have demonstrated the spread of dental infections into the central nervous system, via the sinuses.

Clinical Manifestations

The clinical picture of brain abscess is usually manifested by symptoms of a space-occupying lesion. The symptoms include persistent headache that often is localized, drowsiness, confusion, and stupor, general or focal seizures, nausea and vomiting, and focal motor or sensory impairments. Localized neurologic signs are eventually found in most cases. In the initial stages of the infection, a brain abscess can present itself as a form of encephalitis accompanied by signs of increased intracranial pressure. Papilledema in the older child or bulging fontanels may be present in the younger infant.

A ruptured brain abscess may produce purulent meningitis associated with signs of neurologic damage.

Diagnosis

Aerobic, anaerobic, and acid-fast cultures and stain should be performed on all fluids. The opening pressure of the cerebrospinal fluid generally is elevated. If the diagnosis of intracranial suppuration is suspected from clinical examination, a lumbar puncture should be deferred to avoid brain herniation. The usual cerebrospinal fluid findings associated with subdural or parenchymal abscesses consist of an elevated protein, pleocytosis with a variable neutrophil count, a normal glucose, and sterile cultures.

The number of white blood cells is always very elevated and reaches 100,000 or more when a rupture of the abscess occurs into the cerebrospinal fluid. Many red blood cells generally are observed at that time, and the cerebrospinal fluid lactic acid is then elevated above 500 mg%.[22]

Skull films can be important in the diagnosis of sinusitis or the presence of free gas in the abscess cavity. Electroencephalogram occasionally can reveal a focus of high voltage with slow activity; however, this is the least accurate procedure in the diagnostic evaluation.[70, 71] Brain scan following the intravenous injection of radioisotopes is the most sensitive technique for the detection and localization of the brain abscess.[72] It is relatively noninvasive, is able to define even small purulent collections with exact localization, and minimizes the risk of missing a concomitant brain abscess or bilateral empyemas. Since brain abscess cannot always be differentiated from local cerebritis, other studies such as arteriogram or air encephalopathy may be needed. Computerized axial tomography also can be helpful in detecting the size and location of an abscess. Serial brain scans during the course of antimicrobial therapy are essential to monitor the patient's response.

Management

Before the abscess has become encapsulated and localized, antimicrobial therapy accompanied by measures to control the increase in the intracranial pressure are essential. Once an abscess has formed, surgical drainage is indicated. Some neurosurgeons advocate complete evacuation of the abscess, while others advocate repeated aspirations as indicated. In cases with multiple abscesses or in those with abscesses in essential brain areas, repeated aspirations are preferred to complete excision.

The antimicrobial treatment of the brain abscess is generally long because of the prolonged time needed for brain tissue to repair and close abscess space. Because of the difficulty involved in the penetration of venous antimicrobial agents through the blood-brain barrier, the choice of antibiotics is restricted.

With the exception of *B. fragilis* and some strains of *Bacteroides melaninogenicus,* most of the anaerobic pathogens isolated are sensitive to penicillin.[23] The recovery of these penicillin-resistant organisms requires antimicrobial agents that penetrate the blood-brain barrier, such as chloramphenicol, carbenicillin, or metronidazole. The administration of beta-lactamase-resistant penicillin for the treatment of *S. aureus* generally is recommended.

Injection of antibiotics into the cavity was advocated in the past in an effort to sterilize the area before operation; however, since chloramphenicol, penicillin, and methicillin penetrate brain abscess cavities fairly well, installation of antibiotics into the abscess after drainage is not needed.[73]

If not recognized early, both subdural empyema and brain abscess can be fatal. Although antibiotics have improved the outlook for children with these diseases, the mortality rate is about 40%.[1] Management of subdural empyema requires prompt surgical evacuation of the infected site and antimicrobial therapy. Failure to perform surgical drainage can lead to a higher mortality rate.[74] A recent report on four of eight children with subdural empyema noted that these patients did not respond to appropriate antimicrobial therapy and improved only after their empyemas were drained.[3]

Although it is important to emphasize the need for judicious selection of antimicrobial agents, it is essential to note that treatment of these infections frequently requires surgical drainage. This is of particular importance in patients with subdural or epidural empyema, for whom delay in surgical decompression has been associated with high mortality. There is growing evidence that brain abscess in the early phase of cerebritis may respond to treatment with antimicrobial agents without surgical intervention[75]; however, surgical drainage may be required in many instances to ensure adequate therapy.

REFERENCES

1. Finegold, S. M. Anaerobic bacteria in human diseases. New York: Academic Press, 1977.

2. Dysant, N. K. et al. Meningitis due to *Bacteroides fragilis* in a newborn infant. *J. Pediatr.* 89:509, 1976.

3. Brook, I. et al. Complications of sinusitis in children. *Pediatrics* 66:586, 1980.

4. Gehz, R. C. et al. Meningitis due to combined infections associated with *H. influenzae* type B and *Clostridium perfringens. Am. J. Dis. Child.* 130:877, 1976.

5. O'Grady, L. R., and Ralph, E. D. Anaerobic meningitis and bacteremia caused by *Fusobacterium* sp. *Am. J. Dis. Child.* 130:871, 1976.

6. Sanders, D. Y., and Stevenson, J. *Bacteroides* infections in children. *J. Pediatr.* 72:673, 1968.

7. Brook, I. et al. Anaerobic bacteremia in children. *Am. J. Dis. Child.* 134:1052, 1980.

8. Rubenstein, E.; Onderdank, A. B.; and Rahal, J. J. Peritonsillar infection and bacteremia caused by *Fusobacterium gonidiaformans. J. Pediatr.* 85:673, 1974.

9. Alston, J. M. Necrobacillus in Great Britain. *Br. Med. J.* 2:1524, 1955.

10. Ballenger, J. J.; Schall, L. A.; and Smith, W. E. *Bacteroides* meningitis: report of a case with recovery. *Ann. Otol. Rhinol. Laryngol.* 52:895, 1943.

11. Khuri-Bulos, N.; McIntosh, K.; and Ehret, J. *Bacteroides* brain abscess treated with clindamycin. *Am. J. Dis. Child.* 126:96, 1973.

12. Lifshitz, F.; Liu, C.; and Thurn, A. N. *Bacteroides* meningitis. *Am. J. Dis. Child.* 105:487, 1963.

13. McVay, L. V., Jr., and Sprunt, D. H. *Bacteroides* infections. *Ann. Intern. Med.* 36:56, 1963.

14. Rist, E. *Bacteroides* septicemia. *J. R. Coll. Surg. Edinb.* 2:41, 1956.

15. Berman, B. W. et al. *Bacteroides fragilis* meningitis in a neonate successfully treated with metronidazole. *J. Pediatr.* 93:793, 1978.

16. Feldman, W. E. *Bacteroides fragilis* ventriculitis and meningitis: report of two cases. *Am. J. Dis. Child.* 130:880, 1976.

17. Brook, I.; Martin, W.; and Finegold, S. M. Neonatal pneumonia caused by members of the *Bacteroides fragilis* group. *Clin. Pediatr.* 19:541, 1980.

18. Brook, I. et al. The recovery of anaerobic bacteria from pediatric patients: a one-year experience. *Am. J. Dis. Child.* 133:1020, 1979.

19. Brook, I. et al. Mixed bacterial meningitis: a complication of ventriculo and lumbo-peritoneal shunts. Report of two cases. *J. Neurosurg.* 47:961, 1977.

20. Tynes, B. S., and Frommeyer, W. B., Jr. *Bacteroides* septicemia: cultural, clinical and therapeutic features in a series of 25 patients. *Ann. Intern. Med.* 56:12, 1962.

21. Flamm, H., and Skala, O. Eitrige meningitis durch baccillus funduliformis bei einem kind. *Zentralbl. Allg. Pathol.* 96:157, 1957.

22. Brook, I. et al. Measurement of lactic acid in cerebrospinal fluid of patients with infections of the central nervous system. *J. Infect. Dis.* 137:384, 1978.

23. Sutter, V. L., and Finegold, S. M. Susceptibility of anaerobic bacteria to 23 antimicrobial agents. *Antimicrob. Agents Chemother.* 10:736, 1976.

24. Finegold, S. M. UCLA Conference: management of anaerobic infections. *Ann. Intern. Med.* 83:375, 1975.

25. Tally, F. P.; Sutter, V. L.; and Finegold, S. M. Metronidazole vs anaerobes: in vitro data and initial clinical observations. *Calif. Med.* 117:22, 1972.

26. Nastro, L. J., and Finegold, S. M. Bactericidal activity of five antibiotics against *Bacteroides fragilis. J. Infect. Dis.* 126:104, 1972.

27. Brook, I. Metronidazole for the treatment of anaerobic infections in children. In *First United States metronidazole conference,* ed. S. M. Finegold. New York: Biomedical Information Corporation, 1982, p. 319.

28. Ralph, E. D. et al. Pharmacokinetics of metronidazole as determined by bioassay. *Antimicrob. Agents Chemother.* 6:691, 1974.

29. Davies, A. H. Metronidazole in human infections with syphilis. *Br. J. Vener. Dis.* 43:197, 1967.

30. Bruce, A. M. et al. Persistent bacteremia following ventriculocaval shunt operations for hydrocephalus in infants. *Dev. Med. Child. Neurol.* 5:461, 1963.

31. Holt, R. The classification of staphylococci from colonized ventriculo-atrial shunts. *J. Clin. Pathol.* 22:475, 1969.

32. Nulsen, F. E., and Becker, D. P. Control of hydrocephalus by valve-regulated shunt: infections and their prevention. *Clin. Neurosurg.* 14:256, 1966.

33. Shurtleff, D. B. et al. Therapy of *Staphylococcus epidermidis:* infections associated with cerebrospinal fluid shunts. *Pediatrics* 53:55, 1974.

34. Shurtleff, D. B.; Christie, D.; and Foltz, E. L. Ventriculoauriculostomy-associated infection (a 12-year study). *J. Neurosurg.* 35:686, 1971.

35. Schoenbaum, S. C.; Gardner, P.; and Shillito, J. Infections of cerebrospinal fluid shunts. Epidemiology, clinical manifestations and therapy. *J. Infect. Dis.* 131:543, 1975.

36. McLaurin, R. L.; and Dodson, D. Infected ventriculo-atrial shunts. Some principles of treatment. *Dev. Med. Child. Neurol.* 13(suppl. 25):71, 1971.

37. Leffert, H. L.; Baptist, J. N.; and Gidez, L. Y. Meningitis and bacteremia after ventriculoatrial shunt revision. Isolation of a lecithinase producing *Bacillus cereus. J. Infect. Dis.* 122:547, 1970.

38. Black, J. A.; Challcombe, D. N.; and Ockenden, B. G. Nephrotic syndrome associated with bacteremia after shunt operations for hydrocephalus. *Lancet* 2:921, 1965.

39. Fokes, E. C., Jr. Occult infections of ventriculoatrial shunts. *J. Neurosurg.* 33:517, 1970.

40. Nastasi, G. et al. Colonization of Spitz-Holter valves by rare bacterial flora. *Acta Neurochir.* 26:173, 1972.

41. McGinley, K. J. et al. Regional variations in density of cutaneous *Propionibacterium:* correlation of *Propionibacterium acnes* populations with sebaceous secretion. *J. Clin. Microbiol.* 12:672, 1980.

42. Marples, R. R., and McGinley, K. J. *Corynebacterium acnes* and other anaerobic diphtheroids from human skin. *J. Med. Microbiol.* 7:349, 1974.

43. Schimke, R. T. et al. Indolent *Staphylococcus albus* or *aureus* bacteremia after ventriculoatriostomy. *N. Engl. J. Med.* 264:264, 1961.

44. Everett, E. D.; Eickhoff, T. C.; and Simon, R. H. Cerebrospinal fluid shunt infections with anaerobic diphtheroids (*Propionibacterium* species). *J. Neurosurg.* 44:580, 1976.

45. Cohle, S. D.; Hinds, D.; and Yawn, D. H. *Propionibacterium acnes* infection following subdural tap. *Am. J. Clin. Pathol.* 75:1430, 1981.

46. Beeler, B. A. et al. *Propionibacterium acnes:* pathogen in central nervous system shunt infection. *Am. J. Med.* 61:935, 1976.

47. Stauffer, U. G. "Shunt nephritis": diffuse glomerulonephritis complicating ventriculoatrial shunts. *Dev. Med. Child. Neurol.* 22(suppl.):161, 1970.

48. Martin, W. J.; Gardner, M.; and Washington, J. A. II. In vitro antimicrobial susceptibility of anaerobic bacteria isolated from clinical specimens. *Antimicrob. Agents Chemother.* 1:148, 1972.

49. Schwartz, M. N., and Karchmer, A. E. Infections of the central nervous system. In *Anaerobic bacteria: role in disease,* eds. A. Balows et al. Springfield, Ill.: Charles C Thomas, 1974, p. 309.

50. Heineman, H. S., and Braude, A. I. Anaerobic infection of the brain. Observations

on eighteen consecutive cases of brain abscess. *Am. J. Med.* 35:682, 1963.

51. Salibi, B. S. Bacteroides infection of the brain. *Arch. Neurol.* 10:629, 1964.

52. Idriss, Z. H.; Gutman, L. T.; and Kronfol, N. M. Brain abscess in infants and children. Current status of clinical findings, management, and prognosis. *Clin. Pediatr.* 17:738, 1978.

53. Fisher, E. G.; McLean, J. E.; and Suzuki, Y. Cerebral abscess in children. *Am. J. Dis. Child.* 135:746, 1981.

54. Brook, I. Bacteriology of intracranial abscess in children. *J. Neurosurg.* 54:484, 1981.

55. Blumenfeld, R. J., and Skolnik, E. M. Intracranial complications of sinus disease. *Trans. Am. Acad. Ophthalmol. Otolaryngol.* 70:899, 1966.

56. Galbraith, J. G., and Barr, V. W. Epidural abscess and subdural empyema. In *Infectious diseases of the central nervous system*, eds. R. A. Thompson and J. R. Green. *Adv. Neurol.*, vol. 6. New York: Raven Press, 1974, p. 257.

57. Hitchcock, E., and Andreadis, A. Subdural empyema: a review of 29 cases. *J. Neurol. Neurosurg. Psychiatry* 27:422, 1964.

58. Kubik, C. S., and Adams, R. D. Subdural empyema. *Brain* 66:18, 1943.

59. de Louvois, J.; Gortvai, P.; and Hurley, R. Bacteriology of abscesses of the central nervous system: a multicenter prospective study. *Br. Med. J.* 2:981, 1977.

60. Beller, A. J.; Sahar, A.; and Praiss, I. Brain abscess. Review of 89 cases over a period of 30 years. *J. Neurol. Neurosurg. Psychiatry* 36:757, 1973.

61. Brewer, N. S.; MacCarty, C. S.; and Wellman, W. E. Brain abscess: a review of recent experience. *Ann. Intern. Med.* 82:571, 1975.

62. O'Callaghan, C. H. et al. Novel method for detection of beta-lactamase by using a chromatogenic cephalosporin substrate. *Antimicrobiol. Agents Chemother.* 1:283, 1972.

63. Frederick, J., and Braude, A. I. Anaerobic infection of the paranasal sinuses. *N. Engl. J. Med.* 290:135, 1974.

64. Brook, I. Bacteriologic features of chronic sinusitis in children. *JAMA* 246:967, 1981.

65. Holdeman, L. V., and Moore, W. E. C. *Anaerobic laboratory manual*, 3rd edition. Blacksburg, Va.: Anaerobic Laboratory, Virginia Polytechnic Institute and State University, 1975.

66. Farmer, T. W., and Wise, G. R. Subdural empyema in infants, children, and adults. *Neurology* 23:254, 1973.

67. Brook, I. and Friedman, E. M. Intracranial complications of sinusitis in children. A sequela of periapical abscess. *Ann. Otol. Rhinol. Laryngol.* 91:41, 1982.

68. Brook, I.; Grimm, S.; and Keilich, R. B. Bacteriology of acute periapical abscess in children. *J. Endodontics* 7:378, 1981.

69. Hollin, S. A.; Hayashi, H.; and Gross, S. W. Intracranial abscesses of odontogenic origin. *Oral Surg. Oral Med. Oral Pathol.* 23:277, 1967.

70. Garfield, J. Management of supratentorial intracranial abscess. A review of 200 cases. *Br. Med. J.* 2:7, 1969.

71. Carey, M. E.; Chous, S. N.; and French, L. Experience with brain abscess. *J. Neurosurg.* 36:1, 1972.

72. Crocker, E. F. et al. Technetium brain scanning in the diagnosis and management of cerebral abscess. *Am. J. Med.* 56:192, 1974.

73. Black, P.; Graybill, J. R.; and Charache, P. Penetration of brain abscess by systemically administered antibiotics. *J. Neurosurg* 38:705, 1973.

74. Yoshikawa, T. T.; Chow, A. W.; and Guze, L. B. Role of anaerobic bacteria in subdural empyema. Report of four cases and review of 327 cases from the English literature. *Am. J. Med.* 58:99, 1975.

75. Berg, B. et al. Nonsurgical care of brain abscess. Early diagnosis and followup with computerized tomography. *Ann. Neurol.* 3:474, 1978.

CHAPTER 16

Eye Infections

Conjunctivitis

Conjunctivitis is defined as redness of the conjunctivae associated with hyperemia and congestion of the blood vessels, with varying severity of exudate. Preauricular adenopathy may be present.

Although many infective agents can cause conjunctivitis, recognition of acute bacterial conjunctivitis is of utmost importance because of the rapidity of its development and its potential to cause irreversible ocular damage. Viruses, chlamydiae, richettsiae, fungi, parasites, and numerous noninfectious agents and metabolic diseases may all cause conjunctivitis. It is, therefore, important to arrive at a specific diagnosis for selection of appropriate antimicrobial therapy.

Microbiologic Etiology

The most common aerobic bacteria causing conjunctivitis in children are *Streptococcus pneumoniae, Haemophilus influenzae,* group A streptococci, *Staphylococcus aureus,* and *Staphylococcus epidermidis.* Others include *Neisseria gonorrhoeae* and *meningitidis,* gram-negative rods such as *Pseudomonas* and *Proteus, Corynebacterium* species, and *Moraxella* species.[1-5] The pneumococci, *Pseudomonas* organisms, and anaerobic Gram-positive cocci (peptococci and peptostreptococci) have a high tendency for corneal ulceration.

Two recent studies[6, 7] described the recovery of Gram-positive anaerobic cocci (peptococci and peptostreptococci) in statistically significant higher numbers from inflamed conjunctivae of adults and children compared to recovery from uninflamed conjunctivae.

In the pediatric population that was studied,[7] aerobic and anaerobic cultures and clinical data were obtained from 126 patients with acute conjunctivitis. Similar cultures were obtained from 66 persons who did not have a conjunctival inflammation. Anaerobes were isolated from 47 patients (37.3%). From 26 patients (20.6%) they were in mixed cultures with aerobes, and from 21 patients (16.7%) they were the only isolates. Aerobes alone were recovered from 72 patients (57.1%). No bacterial growth was noted in seven patients (5.6%). The organisms recovered from eyes with conjunctivitis in statistically significant numbers were *S. aureus, S. pneumoniae, H. influenzae,* and anaerobic Gram-positive cocci (tables 16.1 and 16.2).

Other anaerobes occasionally found in the infected eyes were *Bacteroides fragilis* and *Bacteroides melaninogenicus,* fusobacteria, and bifidobacteria. Of special note is that 38% of inflamed conjunctivae contained more than one organism (table 16.1).

Pathogenesis

Most studies of the bacterial flora of acute conjunctivitis have failed to record the presence of anaerobic bacteria. Appropriate culture media and proper anaerobic techniques were not employed in these studies, although occasional reports document anaerobes as part of the normal flora in conjunctivitis, other minor eye infections, and in panophthalmitis.[8] Clostridia,[9-12] non-spore-forming anaerobic organisms,[13] *Actinomyces* species,[14] and anaerobic Gram-positive cocci were recovered from various infections of the eye.

Gram-positive anaerobic cocci are well-documented pathogens. They are commonly isolated from pulmonary infections,[15] infections of the female genital tract,[16] and soft-tissue infections.[17] Although the findings of increased numbers of Gram-positive anaerobic cocci in inflamed conjunctivae may be due to their active role in the inflammatory process, it also could be incidental, resulting from inflammation from other causes.

Studies conducted in adults[5, 6, 18] demonstrated the presence of *Propionibacterium acnes* in the conjunctival sac of uninflamed eyes and an increased rate of recovery of peptostreptococci from patients with conjunctivitis.[18] A statistically significant increase in the numbers of anaerobic Gram-positive cocci in inflamed eyes was demonstrated also in the pediatric study group.

The recovery of anaerobes in the normal flora of the conjunctival sac does not exclude their ability to become pathogenic under the right circumstances. This can occur when foreign bodies, injuries, and underlying noninfectious diseases favor the establishment of conjunctival infections, thus allowing for the resident organisms to become patho-

Table 16.1. Bacterial Cultures of 126 Children With Acute
Conjunctivitis

Patients with Aerobic Organisms Only	No. of Patients
S. aureus	12
S. epidermidis	1
Alpha-hemolytic streptococci	2
Group A beta-hemolytic streptococci	2
Group D streptococci	3
S. pneumoniae	13
H. influenzae	14
H. parainfluenzae	3
N. meningitidis	1
E. coli	4
P. aeruginosa	1
S. aureus + *S. pneumoniae*	4
S. aureus + alpha-hemolytic streptococci	3
S. aureus + Group A beta-hemolytic streptococci	1
S. aureus + Group D streptococci	1
S. aureus + *Micrococcus* sp.	2
S. epidermidis + *Micrococcus* sp.	2
S. epidermidis + *C. albicans*	1
Group A beta-hemolytic streptococci + alpha-hemolytic streptococci	1
H. parainfluenzae + *S. pneumoniae*	1
Subtotal	72

Patients with Anaerobic Organisms Only	No. of Patients
Peptococci	2
Peptostreptococci	5
P. acnes	6
Bifidobacteria	2
B. melaninogenicus	1
B. fragilis	1
F. varium	1
Peptococci + lactobacillis + *P. acnes*	1
Peptococci + *P. acnes*	2
Subtotal	21

genic. The anaerobes recovered from children with conjunctivitis are all part of the normal oral flora.

Children often introduce saliva and its oral flora into their conjunctival sac. This can be done inadvertently while rubbing the eyes or wetting contact lenses. It is conceivable that these anaerobes can become pathogenic.

Table 16.1 Continued

Patients with Mixed Aerobic and Anaerobic Organisms	No. of Patients
Peptococci + *S. epidermidis*	4
Peptococci + *S. aureus*	1
Peptococci + *Micrococcus* sp.	1
Peptococci + lactobacilli + alpha-hemolytic streptococci	1
Peptococci + *P. acnes* + *S. pneumoniae*	2
Peptococci + *S. aureus* + *H. influenzae*	1
Peptococci + *S. aureus* + *S. pneumoniae*	1
Peptostreptococci + *A. israelii* + *S. pneumoniae*	1
Peptostreptococci + *S. epidermidis*	1
P. acnes + *S. epidermidis*	3
P. acnes + *Corynebacterium* sp.	3
P. acnes + micrococci	1
P. acnes + *E. coli*	2
P. acnes + alpha-hemolytic streptococci + lactobacilli	2
P. acnes + *S. aureus* + Group A beta-hemolytic streptococci	1
B. melaninogenicus + Peptostreptococci + *K. pneumoniae*	$\frac{1}{26}$
Total of all patients with positive cultures	119
Patients with negative cultures	7

SOURCE: Brook, I. Anaerobic and aerobic bacterial flora of acute conjunctivitis in children. *Arch. Ophthalmol.* 98:833–834, 1980. Copyright 1980, American Medical Association. Reprinted by permission.

Diagnosis

A bacterial etiology is suspected when severe conjunctivitis is present, and many polymorphonuclear leukocytes are found in conjunctival swab specimens. Conjunctivitis associated with anaerobes is indistinguishable from inflammation caused by other bacteria. Gram stain and aerobic and anaerobic cultures are necessary for correct diagnosis. The presence of mononuclear cells suggests nonbacterial infection, eosinophils and basophils suggest an allergic etiology, and intranuclear inclusions implicate herpes or adenoviruses. Intracytoplasmic inclusions suggest chlamydial agents.

Table 16.2. Comparison of Aerobic and Anaerobic Bacteria Isolated from 119 Pediatric Patients with Inflamed Conjunctiva and 60 Normal Controls

Aerobes	Patients		Control	
	No. of Isolates	Percentage of Patients	No. of Isolates	Percentage of Control
S. aureus	26	21.8	3	5.0
S. epidermidis	12	10.1	28	46.7†
Micrococci	6	5.0		
Alpha-hemolytic streptococci	9	7.6	8	13.3
Group A beta-hemolytic streptococci	5	4.2		
Group D streptococci	4	3.4	2	3.3
S. pneumoniae	22	18.5*	1	1.6
H. influenzae	15	12.8*	1	1.6
H. parainfluenzae	4	3.4		
E. coli	6	5.0		
K. pneumoniae	1	0.8	1	1.6
P. aeruginosa	1	0.8	2	3.3
Acinetobacter sp.			1	1.6
Corynebacterium sp.	3	2.5	13	25.0
N. meningitidis	1	0.9		
Total number of aerobes	115		60	

Anaerobes	Patients		Control	
	No. of Isolates	Percentage of Patients	No. of Isolates	Percentage of Control
Peptococci	16	11.8†	3	0.5
Peptostreptococci	8	6.7†		
P. acnes	23	18.5	8	13.3
Lactobacilli	4	3.4		
A. israelii	1	0.8	2	3.3
Bifidobacteria	2	1.7		
B. melaninogenicus	2	1.7		
B. fragilis	1	0.8		
F. varium	1	0.8		
Total number of anaerobes	58		13	
Total number of bacteria isolated	173		73	

SOURCE: Brook, I. Anaerobic and aerobic bacterial flora of acute conjunctivitis in children. *Arch. Ophthalmol.* 98:833–834, 1980. Copyright 1980, American Medical Association. Reprinted by permission.

*P < 0.001.

†P < 0.05.

Management

Treatment of bacterial conjunctivitis includes application of proper topical antibiotics selected according to the antimicrobial susceptibility of the infecting organism. Anaerobic Gram-positive cocci are the anaerobes most frequently recovered from inflamed conjunctivae and are susceptible to penicillins, erythromycin, and chloramphenicol. The penicillins should not be used topically because they are highly sensitizing in the conjunctival sac. Chloramphenicol should be used cautiously because it is absorbed from the conjunctivae. The bacteria, however, may be relatively resistant to sulfonamide and aminoglyloside preparations that are commonly applied to inflamed conjunctiva. Since anaerobes may be involved in severe cases of conjunctivitis and especially with the most serious complications of bacterial conjunctivitis, such as a penetrating corneal ulcer or orbital cellulitis, special coverage for these organisms should be considered. In such instances administration of parenteral antimicrobial agents should supplement the frequent topical application of medications.

Orbital and Periorbital Cellulitis

Cellulitis of the orbital and periorbital tissues includes a spectrum of disorders of varying etiologies that are commonly encountered in pediatric practice. The extent of involvement ranges from simple periorbital inflammation to cavernous sinus thrombosis. In the preantibiotic era, 17% of patients with cellulitis of the orbit died from meningitis, and 20% of the survivors had permanent loss of vision.[19] These serious complications have been modified so favorably by antibiotic therapy that the disorder can have a relatively benign course.

Microbiology

When the child is between 6 and 30 months of age and shows no evidence of trauma or overt clinical findings of acute purulent sinusitis, *H. influenzae* type B is the most probable causative organism of periorbital cellulitis. If the cellulitis is related to trauma or to extension from a neighboring soft tissue area, group A beta-hemolytic streptococci and *S. aureus* are the most likely causative organisms, regardless of the patient's age.[20-23]

Clostridium perfringens was reported[21] in a patient with orbital cellulitis that developed following a penetrating wound and involved the presence of a foreign body. Anaerobic bacteria could be associated with cellulitis that develops following chronic sinusitis or following sinusitis associated with dental infection.[24] The authors recently reported eight children (6 to 15 years of age) who presented with periorbital cellulitis and other complications of sinusitis. Both ethmoid and maxillary sinusitis were present in four patients, frontal sinusitis in two, and ethmoid sinusitis and pansinusitis in one patient each. Subdural empyema occurred in four patients, in one case accompanied by cerebritis and brain abscess and in another by meningitis. Periorbital abscess was present in two children who had ethmoiditis. Alveolar abscess in the upper incisors was present in two children whose infection had spread to the maxillary and ethmoid sinuses. Anaerobic bacteria were isolated from the infected sinuses and aspirated pus of all the patients. There were seven isolates of *Bacteroides* organisms, four fusobacteria, three microaerophilic streptococci, three Gram-positive anaerobic cocci, and two veillonellae. There was only one aerobic isolate recovered, a group F beta-hemolytic *Streptococcus*.

Pathogenesis

Orbital cellulitis is the most frequent serious complication of acute sinusitis and, despite antimicrobial therapy, is a potentially life-threatening infection. The anatomy of the orbit makes it highly vulnerable to inflammation from the paranasal sinuses. The continuity of the orbital veins with the cavernous sinus and the veins of the face and nose and the lack of valves from the ophthalmic venous system results in extensive two-way communication between the face, nasal cavity, and paranasal sinuses. The perivascular spaces associated with orbital veins may act as lymphatics, but there are neither true lymphatic vessels nor lymph nodes in the orbit.[25]

Periorbital cellulitis in a child with paranasal sinusitis may represent reactive edema, probably caused by impedance of blood flow in the veins of the orbit into the ethmoid and maxillary vessels from pressure in the corresponding chambers.[19] The eyelids may become noticeably swollen but are not tender, and usually there is no evidence of globe involvement.

Orbital cellulitis is less common than periorbital cellulitis and involves the globe or orbit. There is diffuse edema of the orbital contents and actual infiltration of the adipose tissue with inflammatory cells and bacteria. This can be a result of an extension from sinus infection with spread along the venous system and from contiguous spread through the very thin walls of the paranasal sinuses.[26] The teeth may be the primary site of pathology in cases of maxillary sinusitis. Orbital infection may also arise as a metastatic focus of infection of a systemic illness or extension through the orbital septum or through facial veins from a neighboring inflamed soft tissue area. In some cases there is direct infection from a penetrating wound.

Diagnosis

The child who appears with a "swollen eye" presents a difficult problem in differential diagnosis. Sinus infection is a major predisposing cause of a swollen eye, but there are other entities to be considered. Infected periorbital lacerations, conjunctivitis, dacryocystitis, systemic or contact allergy, seborrheic or eczematoid dermatitis, and nasal vestibular infections may cause swelling about the eye. A last important category of infections are those cases of *H. influenzae* type B periorbital or so-called preseptal cellulitis.

Infection in and around the eye must initially be differentiated from trauma, malignancy, dysthyroid exophthalmos, orbital pseudotumor, or cavernous sinus thrombosis. If infection is present, determination of the site of infection is important.

In considering infections of the orbit and lids, it is important to distinguish between infections of the superficial layers and orbital infections. The critical tissue plane separating the two types of infections is a fascial layer termed the *orbital septum*. Infection anterior to the orbital septum is most properly described as preseptal cellulitis (periorbital cellulitis). It is characterized by edema, erythema, tenderness, and warmth of the lid. Drainage either from the wound or the conjunctivae may be present. The eye itself is not involved in preseptal cellulitis and, therefore, the conjunctivae and orbital tissues are not involved. Preauricular lymphadenopathy may be present. Vision, mobility of the globe, and intraocular pressure are normal.

Infection deep to the orbital septum, *orbital cellulitis,* is characterized by marked lid edema and erythema, proptosis, chemosis, reduction of vision, restriction of mobility of the eye globe in proportion to orbital edema, pain on movement of the globe, fever, and leukocytosis.[19, 27] The distinctions between preseptal and orbital cellulitis may be difficult to make in children with minor degrees of orbital involvement.

If the infection is allowed to progress, subperiosteal or orbital abscess and cavernous sinus thrombosis may develop. In young children, sinusitis may be difficult to diagnose because of the lack of classical clinical or roentgenographic findings. Thus, a purulent discharge from the sinus cavity found during physical examination probably is more reliable evidence for sinusitis. In older children without trauma, the absence of sinusitis should prompt a search for another focus of infection. Roentgenographic studies for evidence of sinusitis can suggest an etiologic relationship.

CAT scan can assist in determining the degree of orbital disease.[28] The CAT scan can confirm the presence and define the location of an orbital abscess, and is especially valuable for diagnosis in children in whom severe lid edema prevents adequate eye examination.

Gram stains and cultures should be obtained of any purulent material available, and blood cultures are imperative. Aspiration and culture of the advancing border of cellulitis may be helpful in establishing an etiologic diagnosis.

Bacterial diagnosis from direct needle aspirate to the leading edge of the periorbital cellulitis is rare. In patients with purulent sinusitis, direct aspiration of the sinus is a superior procedure that is likely to provide bacterial diagnosis of the pathogen.

Although cultures of purulent material exuding from the eye may be helpful and should be done, the bacteria recovered may have no relationship to the true cause of the disorder. Blood cultures are helpful, and positive cultures were obtained in 23% of children tested[20]; however, there was a high incidence (34%) of positive blood cultures in children in whom there was no trauma or external lesions. This contrasts with results from children with trauma or external lesions, of whom only 5% had a positive blood culture.

In the last group, attempts to recover the organisms from external lesions may be helpful. This can be done by aspiration of the inflamed area or collection of secretions from a draining wound.

Management

Hospitalization is essential because of the severity of complications and the need for intravenous antibiotics. In children 30 months or younger without evidence of trauma, *H. influenzae* is the primary pathogen. Because of the high incidence of *Haemophilus* bacteremia in this group and because of the recent appearance of ampicillin-resistant strains, chloramphenicol and ampicillin appear to be the best antibiotics to use initially until the results of the blood cultures and the sensitivity of the organism become known.

In patients suspected of *S. aureus* infection a penicillinase-resistant penicillin should be included in the initial therapy. In the cellulitis that follows trauma or extension of infection from a neighboring site where group A streptococci and *S. aureus* are suspected, therapy with a penicillinase-resistant penicillin appears most appropriate.

Anaerobic bacteria should be suspected in children with periorbital cellulitis associated with chronic sinusitis. Most of the anaerobic pathogens isolated from inflamed sinuses are sensitive to penicillin, but *B. fragilis* and some strains of *B. melaninogenicus* are resistant to penicillin compounds.[29] The recovery of these penicillin-resistant organisms requires administration of appropriate antimicrobial agents such as chloramphenicol, carbenicillin, clindamycin, or cefoxitin.[8] Because of the possible intracranial extension of the infection, caution should be used with clindamycin and cefoxitin; these agents penetrate poorly into the central nervous system.

Although the need for judicious selection of antimicrobial agents must be emphasized, it is essential to note that the treatment of the complications of sinusitis frequently requires surgical intervention. Surgical drainage is essential also in cases where localized pus is observed. The mortality is reduced when therapy includes surgical drainage. Surgical drainage in these patients is therefore an integral part of the management and is necessary if there is no response to adequate antibiotic therapy, particularly if visual acuity is decreased.

Complications

Orbital cellulitis may progress into local accumulation of pus—a subperiostal or orbital abscess. Periorbital and orbital infections pose the risk of serious complications resulting from extension of the infectious process to the central nervous system and involvement of the eye.[24, 30] Complications have become infrequent with the availability of antibiotics; when present, they are of grave and serious nature and include loss of vision owing to involvement of the optic nerve, progression to cavernous sinus thrombophlebitis, meningitis, subdural or cerebral abscess, and death.

REFERENCES

1. Cason, L., and Winkler, C. H. Bacteriology of the eye: normal flora. *Arch. Ophthalmol.* 51:196, 1954.

2. Locatcher-Khorazo, D., and Seegal, B. C., eds. *Microbiology of the eye.* St. Louis: C. V. Mosby, 1972.

3. Smith, C. H. Bacteriology of the healthy conjunctiva. *Br. J. Ophthalmol.* 38:719, 1954.

4. Soudakoff, P. S. Bacteriologic examination of the conjunctiva. *Am. J. Ophthalmol.* 38:374, 1954.

5. Matsuura, H. Anaerobes in the bacterial flora of the conjunctival sac. *Jpn. J. Ophthalmol.* 15:116, 1971.

6. Brook, I. et al. Anaerobic and aerobic bacteriology of acute conjunctivitis. *Ann. Ophthalmol.* 11:389, 1979.

7. Brook, I. Anaerobic and aerobic bacterial flora of acute conjunctivitis in children. *Arch. Ophthalmol.* 98:833, 1980.

8. Finegold, S. M. *Anaerobic bacteria in human disease.* New York: Academic Press, 1977.

9. Cross, A. G. Gas gangrene of the eye. *Lancet* 2:515, 1941.

10. Henkind, P., and Fedukowiz, H. *Clostridium welchii* conjunctivitis. *Arch. Ophthalmol.* 70:791, 1963.

11. Kurz, G. H., and Weiss, J. F. Gas gangrene panophthalmitis: report of a case. *Br. J. Ophthalmol.* 53:323, 1969.

12. Frantz, J. F. et al. Acute endogenous panophthalmitis caused by *Clostridium perfringens. Am. J. Ophthalmol.* 78:295, 1974.

13. Jones, D. B., and Robinson, N. M. Anaerobic ocular infections. *Trans. Am. Acad. Ophthalmol. Otolaryngol.* 83:309, 1977.

14. Pine, L. et al. Actinomycotic lacrimal canaliculitis: a report of two cases with a review of the characteristics which identify the causal organism, *Actinomyces israelii. Am. J. Ophthalmol.* 49:1278, 1960.

15. Bartlett, J. G., and Finegold, S. M. Anaerobic infections of the lung and pleural space. *Am. Rev. Respir. Dis.* 110:56, 1974.

16. Mead, P. B., and Louria, D. B. Antibiotics in pelvic infections. *Clin. Obstet. Gynecol.* 12:219, 1969.

17. Rea, W. J., and Wyrick, W. J., Jr. Necrotizing fasciitis. *Ann. Surg.* 172:957, 1970.

18. Perkins, R. E. et al. Bacteriology of normal and infected conjunctivitis. *J. Clin. Microbiol.* 1:147, 1975.

19. Chandler, J. R.; Laagenbrunner, D. J. and Stevens, E. R. The pathogenesis of orbital complications in acute sinusitis. *Laryngoscope* 80:1414, 1970.

20. Gellady, A. M.; Shulman, S. T.; and Ayoub, E. M. Periorbital and orbital cellulitis in children. *Pediatrics* 61:272, 1978.

21. Smith, T. F.; O'Day, D.; and Wright, P. F. Clinical implications of preseptal (periorbital) cellulitis in childhood. *Pediatrics* 62:1006, 1978.

22. Haynes, R. E., and Cramblett, H. G. Acute ethmoiditis. Its relationship to orbital cellulitis. *Am. J. Dis. Child.* 114:261, 1967.

23. Feingold, M., and Gellis, S. S. Cellulitis due to *Haemophilus influenzae* type B. *N. Engl. J. Med.* 272:788, 1965.

24. Brook, I. et al. Complications of sinusitis in children. *Pediatrics* 66:568, 1980.

25. Hawkins, D. B., and Clark, R. W. Orbital involvement in acute sinusitis. *Clin. Pediatr.* 16:464, 1977.

26. Jarret, W. H. II, and Gutman, F. A. Ocular complications of infection in the paranasal sinuses. *Arch Ophthalmol.* 81:683, 1969.

27. Smith, A. T., and Spencer, J. T. Orbital complications resulting from lesions of the sinuses. *Ann. Otol. Rhinol. Laryngol.* 57:5, 1948.

28. Goldberg, F.; Berne, A. S.; and Oski, F. A. Differentiation of orbital cellulitis from preseptal cellulitis by computed tomography. *Pediatrics* 62:1000, 1978.

29. Sutter, V. L., and Finegold, S. M. Susceptibility of anaerobic bacteria to 23 antimicrobial agents. *Antimicrob. Agents Chemother.* 10:736, 1976.

30. Shaw, R. E. Cavernous sinus thrombophlebitis: a review. *Br. J. Surg.* 40:40, 1952.

CHAPTER 17

Dental Infections

Anaerobic bacteria are part of the normal oral flora and outnumber aerobic organisms by a ratio of 1:10 at this site. It is, therefore, not surprising to find them predominant in dental infection. These infections can, in addition to the local damage they inflict to the oral or dental structures, extend locally or disseminate, causing serious infections elsewhere in the body.

Dental Caries

Several factors interact in the formation of dental caries. These include the presence of a susceptible tooth surface, the proper microflora, and a suitable substrate for the microflora. Several oral acidogenic aerobic and anaerobic microorganisms, including *Lactobacillus acidophilus, Streptococcus mutans,* and *Actinomyces viscosus,* are capable of initating the carious lesion. Some microorganisms also contribute through synthesis of extracellular polysaccharides that adhere to the tooth surface. Fermentable carbohydrates serve as substrates for the microbial enzyme systems that produce organic acids (primarily lactic acid); sucrose is the optimum substrate for extracellular polysaccharide synthesis. Besides providing a source of fermentable carbohydrate for conversion to acid, these extracellular polysaccharides greatly increase the bulk of the dental plaque and heighten its capacity as an area of bacterial proliferation.

Dietary carbohydrates play a major role. The types of carbohydrates and their frequency of ingestion are more important than the total quantity that is consumed. Frequent between-meal snacks, especially of sucrose-containing foods, enhance the carious process; sticky foods linger in the mouth and are potentially more harmful than non-sticky foods.

Although clinically or radiographically observable caries may be arrested, none of the destroyed tooth structure will regenerate. Treatment by removal of all affected tooth structure and proper replacement with a restorative material is the responsibility of a dentist. Prophylaxis of caries can be achieved by ingestion of proper amounts of fluoride (about 1 mg/day) or local application of fluoride compounds, by daily brushing and mechanical removal of plaque, and by adhering to proper diet that contains fewer sugars.

Pulpitis

Pulpitis, an inflammation of the dental pulp, may result from thermal, chemical, traumatic, or bacterial irritation. Inflammation and infection secondary to dental caries is the most frequent cause.

Microbiology

The bacteria usually recovered from an inflamed pulp and root canal are aerobic organisms. *Streptococcus salivarius* usually constitutes less than 8% of the microorganisms of the contaminated root canal. *Streptococcus faecalis*, an enterococci, has been reported in 10% to 30% of infected root canals. Other microorganisms, which may be difficult to eliminate from contaminated root canals even when antibiotics are used, are yeasts and Gram-negative bacteria, mostly neisseriae and Gram-negative rods, such as *Proteus vulgaris* and *Escherichia coli*.[1]

There have been a number of studies of the bacteriology of root canals in which anaerobes have been detected.[2] The quality of these studies varies considerably, however, and the anaerobic techniques generally are not optimal. Most of the studies do not avoid contamination of the root canal specimen by microorganisms of the oral flora. A variety of anaerobes have been isolated in these past studies, accounting for 25% to 30% of the root canal isolates. These include anaerobic streptococci, *Bacteroides* species, propionibacteria, veillonellae, and others.[1]

Pathogenesis

The pulp of the tooth normally is protected from infection by oral microorganisms by the enamel and dentin. This barrier may be breached to permit entrance of bacteria into the pulp or periapical areas. This can occur through a cavity caused by trauma, dental caries, or operative dental procedures, through the tubules of cut or carious dentin, in periodontal disease by way of the gingival crevice and by invasion along the periodontal membrane, by extension of periapical infection from adjacent teeth that are infected, or by way of the bloodstream during bacteremia.

Virulent bacteria can migrate from the root canal into the apical regions. Toxic products from the pulp also may have a pathogenic role in these responses. As the abscess progresses, more tissue may be involved, as well as adjacent teeth; the pressure of accumulated pus can produce a sinus tract to the surface of the skin or to the oral or nasal cavity.

The most important route by which bacteria invade the pulp is through the tubules of carious dentin. This may occur even before the pulp is exposed directly to the oral environment by cavitation. The bacteria that penetrate the dentin before cavitation has exposed the pulp include streptococci, staphylococci, lactobacilli, and filamentous microorganisms.[3] Of this group, streptococci are the predominant known cause of pulpitis.[4] Staphylococci and filamentous microorganisms also may cause pulpitis.

The primary microorganism causing pulpitis is difficult to determine because of the technical difficulties associated with obtaining valid samples for culturing, and because the exact time of the initial infection is difficult to ascertain. Many studies have reported the recovery of anaerobes in dental abscesses and phlegmons. Most of these are single reports, and some are series that show a relatively low incidence of anaerobes.[2]

Diagnosis

Acute suppurative pulpitis can cause low-grade fever, pain, soreness of the tooth, and swelling of the face. The pain usually is induced by hot liquids, a reaction apparently caused by expansion of gases produced by gas-forming bacteria trapped inside the root canal.

Intense pain may be difficult to localize. It may be referred to the opposite mandible or maxilla or to areas supplied by common branches of the fifth cranial nerve. X-rays, pulp testers, percussion, and palpation are aids in diagnosis.

Treatment

In early pulpitis, cleansing of the cavity to remove debris and packing the cavity with zinc oxide-eugenol cement usually will afford relief. Infected pulpal tissue should be removed and root canal therapy instituted, or the tooth should be extracted.

Antimicrobial therapy supplementing the dental care should be considered, especially when local or systemic spread of the infection is suspected. Penicillin generally is effective against most of the aerobic and anaerobic bacteria recovered. The patient whose oral cavity may harbor penicillin-resistant organisms should be considered for treatment with drugs effective against these organisms.

Periapical Abscess

The alveolar, or apical, abscess may be either acute or chronic. The acute alveolar abscess is the extension of necrotic or putrescent pulp into the periapical area, which causes necrosis of bone and tissue and the accumulation of pus. As the abscess progresses, more and more tissue may be involved, including adjacent teeth, and the pressure of accumulated pus may produce a fistula to the gingival surface or to the oral or nasal cavity.[5]

Microbiology

Anaerobes were isolated also from cases of periodontal abscesses.[2] Studies done at the turn of the century of acute and chronic alveolar abscesses described the isolation of predominantly aerobic streptococci; however, fusiform bacilli and *Bacteroides* species were found in some abscesses, sometimes in pure culture. More recent studies report the isolation of a variety of anaerobes in periodontal abscesses, including anaerobic cocci, anaerobic Gram-negative bacilli, and anaerobic Gram-positive bacilli.[2]

In a recent study of the bacteriology of periapical abscess in 12 children,[6] anaerobic organisms were found to be the predominant isolates in periodontal abscess, outnumbering aerobes eight to one (table 17.1). All aspirates yielded bacterial growth when cultured for aerobes and anaerobes. Anaerobes were isolated in all patients; in two-thirds of the patients, the anaerobes were the only organism isolated, and in the rest they were mixed with aerobes. There were 53 anaerobic isolates (4.4 per specimen), 20 *Bacteroides* species (including nine *Bacteroides melaninogenicus*, three *Bacteroides oralis*, and three *Bacteroides corrodens*), 17 anaerobic Gram-positive cocci, 5 fusobacteria, and 3 *Actinomyces* species. There were six aerobic isolates (0.5 per specimen), three *Streptococcus salivarius*, two alpha-hemolytic streptococci, and one gamma-hemolytic *Streptococcus*. Beta-lactamase production was noticed in four isolates recovered from four patients (33%); these were three of nine *B. melaninogenicus*, and one of three *B. oralis*.

Table 17.1. Bacteria Isolated from 12 Children with Periapical Abscess

Aerobic organisms	Number
S. *salivarius*	3
Alpha-hemolytic streptococci	2
Gamma-hemolytic streptococci	1
Total aerobes	6

Anaerobic organisms	Number
Gram-positive cocci	
Peptococci	2
P. *intermedius*	3
P. *micros*	4
S. *constellatus*	3
Microaerophilic streptococci	5
Gram-negative cocci	
V. *parvula*	4
Gram-positive bacilli	
Actinomyces sp.	3
Eubacterium sp.	1
Lactobacillus sp.	3
Gram-negative bacilli	
Fusobacterium sp.	2
F. *nucleatum*	3
Bacteroides sp.	3
B. *melaninogenicus*	4
B. *melaninogenicus* ss. *asaccharolyticus*	2
B. *melaninogenicus* ss. *intermedius*	1
B. *melaninogenicus* ss. *melaninogenicus*	2
B. *oralis*	3
B. *corrodens*	3
B. *ochraceus*	1
B. *bifitus*	1
Total anaerobes	53

SOURCE: Brook, I.; Grimm, S.; and Kielich, R. B. Bacteriology of acute periapical abscess in children. *J. Endodontics* 7:379, 1981. Copyright 1981, American Dental Association. Reprinted by permission.

Pathogenesis

The abscess generally is secondary to an extension of infection, usually from caries, of the dental pulp. It may occur after trauma to the teeth or from periapical localization of organisms.

Diagnosis

Pain from an acute abscess usually is intense and continuous. The involved tooth is painful when percussed. Hot or cold foods may increase the pain.

A chronic periapical abscess presents few clinical signs, since it is essentially a circumscribed area of mild infection that spreads slowly. In time, the infection may become granulomatous. Radiographic studies of the involved tooth can be helpful, and free air eventually can be observed in the tissues.

Complications

If treatment is delayed, the infection may spread through adjacent tissues, causing cellulitis, varying degrees of facial edema, and fever. The infection may extend into osseous tissues or into the soft tissues of the floor of the mouth. Local swelling and gingival fistulas may develop opposite the apex of the tooth, especially with deciduous teeth.

Serious complications from periapical infections are relatively rare considering the enormous numbers of infected teeth that occur in the population. Serious complications from periapical infection are not unknown, however. In some cases, the infection spreads to tissues in other portions of the oral cavity, causing submandibular or superficial sublingual abscesses; abscesses may be produced also in the submaxillary triangle or in the parapharyngeal or submasseteric space.[7]

In the maxilla, periapical infection may affect only the soft tissues of the face, where it is not so serious. It may extend, however, to the intratemporal space including the sinuses and then to the nervous system, where it can cause serious complications such as subdural empyema, brain abscess, or meningitis.[2, 8]

The finding of anaerobic bacteria in periodontal abscesses is of importance because of the association of anaerobes with many serious infections arising from dental foci, such as bacteremia, endocarditis, sinusitis, meningitis, subdural empyema, brain abscess, and pulmonary empyema.[2] Previous reports have demonstrated the spread of dental infections into the central nervous system via the sinuses.[2, 9]

Intracranial suppuration following tooth extraction or dental infection is an uncommon but extremely serious complication. Most intracranial infections of buccodental origin concern cavernous sinus thrombosis, at times associated with brain abscess or subdural empyema.[2, 10, 11] Isolated brain abscesses occur much less frequently, and subdural empyema of odontogenic origin is quite rare. Infections of the molar teeth are more likely to cause intracranial complications because pus arising in the back of the jaw tends to collect between the muscles of mastication and spread upward in the fascial planes, whereas infection arising in the front of the jaw has free access to the oral cavity.[12]

Management

Since extraction or root canal therapy usually is indicated, a dentist should be consulted. If high fever persists, antibiotics should be administered. Most of the aerobic and anaerobic pathogens isolated from the abscesses are sensitive to penicillin. Some strains of *B. melaninogenicus* and *B. oralis* recovered from patients with periodontal abscesses may be resistant to penicillin, however.[13] In seriously ill patients, the recovery of these penicillin-resistant organisms may require the administration of antimicrobial agents also effective against these organisms. These include clindamycin, chloramphenicol, carbenicillin, or cefoxitin.[14] Although the need for judicious selection of antimicrobial agents must be emphasized, it is essential to note that the treatment of periapical abscess may require surgical intervention and that surgical drainage of these cases is, therefore, an integral part of the management.

Gingivitis and Periodontitis

Periodontal disease most commonly begins as a gingivitis and progresses to periodontitis. Periodontal disease may be complicated by purulent gingival pockets or gingival abscesses. Gingivitis is an inflammation of the gingivae, characterized by swelling, redness, change of normal contours, and bleeding. Swelling deepens the crevice between the gingivae and the teeth, forming gingival pockets. Gingivitis may be acute, or may be chronic with remissions and exacerbations. Periodontitis is due to the progression of gingivitis to the point that loss of supporting bone has begun.

Aspiration pneumonia and lung abscess can complicate gingival disease, especially in children who have poor dental hygiene. This has been noted especially in neurologically-impaired children who constantly aspirate their oral secretions and in children with gingivitis associated with Dilantin therapy.[15]

Recent observations suggest that specificity exists in the bacterial etiology of various forms of periodontal disease.[16] *Bacteroides asaccharolyticus* is a predominant isolate from some advancing lesions of adult periodontitis in humans[17, 18] and from experimental periodontitis lesions in monkeys. Localized juvenile periodontitis is associated with a predominance of *Actinobacillus actinomycetem-comitans*[18, 19] and *Capnocytophaga* species.[20]

The role of anaerobic organisms in this infection is strengthened by the finding of elevated levels of serum IgG antibodies specific for oral *B. asaccharolyticus* in children with periodontitis.[21] This immuno-serologic observation is strongly supportive of several bacteriologic studies[17, 18] that have indicated that *B. asaccharolyticus* is a predominant isolate from advancing chronic periodontitis lesions.

Vincent's Infection

This infection, sometimes called trench mouth, Vincent's infection, or acute necrotizing ulcerative gingivitis, occurs at the gingival papillae between the teeth. Although most cases occur in adults, the disease has been described also in young children.[22]

Microbiology

It is known to be caused by synergistic infection between unusually large spirochetes and fusobacteria,[22, 23] which are part of the normal oropharyngeal flora.

Pathogenesis

Poor oral hygiene, physical or emotional stress, nutritional deficiencies, blood dyscrasias, debilitating diseases, and insufficient rest may predispose to this disease.

Symptoms

Onset, usually abrupt, may be accompanied by malaise. The patients generally manifest bleeding of the gums, blunting and cratering of the interdental papillae, fetid breath, pain, and numbness. The ulcerations are usually limited to the marginal gingivae and interdental papillae. They have a characteristic punched-out appearance, are covered by a grayish membrane, and bleed on slight pressure or irritation. Swallowing and talking may be painful. Regional lymphadenopathy often is present. Lesions on the buccal mucosa are rare but may appear as diffuse ulcerations covered with an easily removed pseudomembrane. Rarely, lesions may occur on the tonsils, pharynx, bronchi, rectum, or vagina.

Diagnosis

The punched-out appearance of the interdental papillae, the interdental grayish membrane, spontaneous bleeding, and pain are pathognomonic. The presence of overwhelming numbers of fusospirochetal forms in stained smears from the lesions confirms the diagnosis. Early differentiation from diphtheria or agranulocytosis is essential when the tonsillar or pharyngeal tissues are involved. Streptococcal or staphylococcal pharyngitis and herpetic stomatitis must be considered in the differential diagnosis.

Management

Gentle debridement by a dentist, the establishment of good oral hygiene, adequate nutrition, and rest are essential. Rinsing the mouth with warm normal saline or 3% peroxide solution may be helpful for the first few days.[24] Analgesics may be required during the first 24 hours after initial debridement. Therapeutically, the various drugs that are active against anaerobes in general, including penicillin G, are effective in the management of Vincent's angina. Other antimicrobial agents used successfully in the treatment of this infection include metronidazole and erythromycin.[25]

REFERENCES

1. Burnett, G. W., and Schuster, G. S. *Oral microbiology and infectious diseases.* Baltimore: Williams & Wilkins, 1978, p. 244.

2. Finegold, S. M. *Anaerobic bacteria in human disease.* New York: Academic Press, 1977, p. 78.

3. Sabiston, C. B., Jr.; Grigsby, W. R.; and Segerstron, N. Bacterial study of pyogenic infections of dental origin. *Oral Surg.* 41(4):430, 1976.

4. Akpata, E. S. Total viable count of microorganisms in the infected dental pulp. *J. Dent. Res.* 53(6):1330, 1974.

5. Gorlin, R. J., and Goman, H. M., eds. *Thoma's oral pathology,* 6th edition. St. Louis: C. V. Mosby, 1970.

6. Brook, I.; Grimm, S.; and Kielich, R. B. Bacteriology of acute periapical abscess in children. *J. Endodontics* 7:378, 1981.

7. Rogers, A. H. The oral cavity as a source of potential pathogens in focal infection. *Oral Surg.* 42:245, 1976.

8. Brook, I. et al. Complications of sinusitis in children. *Pedriatrics* 66(4):568, 1980.

9. Hollin, S. A.; Hayashi, H.; and Gross, S. W. Intracranial abscesses of odontogenic origin. *Oral Surg.* 23:277, 1967.

10. Dixon, O. J. Dental infection as a cause of cavernous sinus thrombosis. *Dental Cosmos* 71:121, 1929.

11. Koeph, S. W.; Rosedale, S. R.; and Learn, G. E. Infection of gasserian ganglion following tooth extraction. *J. Am. Dent. Assoc.* 24:1813, 1937.

12. Haymaker, W. Fatal infections of the central nervous system and meninges after tooth extraction with an analysis of 28 cases. *Am. J. Orthodontics Oral Surg.* 31:117, 1945.

13. Brook, I.; Calhoun, L.; and Yocum, P. Beta lactamase producing isolates of *Bacteroides* species for children. *Antimicrob. Agents Chemother.* 18(1):164, 1980.

14. Sutter, V. L., and Finegold, S. M. Susceptibility of anaerobic bacteria to 23 antimicrobial agents. *Antimicrob. Agents Chemother.* 10(4):736, 1980.

15. Brook, I., and Finegold, S. M. Bacteriology of aspiration pneumonia in children. *Pediatrics* 65:1115, 1980.

16. Socransky, S. S. Microbiology and periodontal disease—present status and future considerations. *J. Periodontol.* 48:497, 1977.

17. Slots, J. The predominant cultivable microflora of advanced periodontitis. *Scand. J. Dent. Res.* 85:114, 1977.

18. Tanner, A. C. et al. A study of the bacteria associated with advancing periodontitis in man. *J. Clin. Periodontol.* 6:278, 1979.

19. Newman, M. G. et al. Studies on the microbiology of periodontosis. *J. Periodontol.* 47:373, 1976.

20. Newman, M. G., and Socransky, S. S. Predominant cultivable microbiota in periodontosis. *J. Periodontal Res.* 12:120, 1977.

21. Mouton, C. et al. Serum antibodies to oral *Bacteroides asaccharolyticus (Bacteroides gingivalis)*: relationship to age and periodontal disease. *Infect. Immun.* 31:182, 1981.

22. Stammers, A. F. Vincent's infection: observations and conclusions regarding the aetiology and treatment of 1017 civilian cases. *Br. Dent. J.* 76:147, 1944.

23. Listgarten, M. A., and Lewis, D. W. The distribution of spirochetes in the lesion of acute necrotizing ulcerative gingivitis. An electron microscopic and statistical survey. *J. Periodontol.* 38:379, 1967.

24. Wade, A. B., and Mirza, V. B. The relative effectiveness of sodium peroxyborate and hydrogen peroxide in treating acute ulcerative gingivitis (Vincent's type). *Br. Dent. J.* 115:372, 1963.

25. Davis, A. H.; McFadzean, J. A.; and Squires, S. Treatment of Vincent's angina with metronidiazole. *Br. Med. J.* 1:1149, 1964.

CHAPTER 18

Ear, Nose, and Throat Infections

Acute Otitis Media

Otitis media is one of the most common diseases of early childhood. Mawson believed that 5% of children will have an attack of acute otitis media during the first ten years of life, and one of these five will have a second attack.[1] Two-thirds of children experience at least one episode of otitis media by their second birthday, and one in seven children have more than six episodes by that time.[2] In a prospective study, 60% of children had at least one episode of otitis media, and 20% of children had three or more by their first birthday.[3]

Acute and chronic otitis media with effusion are frequent, and their complications and sequelae are significant health hazards in children. Otitis media is the result of an inflammatory reaction of the mucous membrane lining the middle ear cleft in its entirety, or part of its extent from the Eustachian tube to the mastoid antrum and air cells. The classification of the disease is based on the extent and degree of inflammatory reaction, with or without formation of pus. If there is pus in the middle ear cavity it is called *suppurative otitis media;* it is termed *nonsuppurative otitis media* if there is no pus in the middle ear cleft. A nonsuppurative condition may proceed to a suppurative one, however.

Acute otitis media usually is thought of as being suppurative or purulent, but serous effusions may also have an acute onset. There are many terms for chronic otitis media with effusion: serous, secretory, catarrhal, mucoid, nonsuppurative, or allergic otitis media. It is often difficult to determine the specific variety without a diagnostic aspiration of the middle ear effusion to determine if the fluid is serous, mucoid, or purulent in character, and whether bacteria are present.

Microbiology

Many studies[4-8] have established that two organisms, *Streptococcus pneumoniae* and *Haemophilus influenzae*, are the principal etiologic agents in acute bacterial otitis media. Of the two, *S. pneumoniae* has consistently been found more commonly, irrespective of age group, but its predominance has tended to increase with increasing age. *H. influenzae* previously was thought to be an infrequent cause of otitis media in older children, leading to the suggestion that penicillin alone is adequate therapy for otitis media in this age group. Several reports have documented the continued importance of this pathogen in older children.[8]

Of special concern is the increased rate of isolation of ampicillin-resistant strains from infected ears. The incidence of such strains may reach 30% in some areas.

Other organisms that less frequently cause acute otitis media include group A beta-hemolytic streptococci (GABHS), *Neisseria catarrhalis*, *Staphylococcus aureus*, and various Gram-negative bacilli,[9] including *Escherichia coli*, *Klebsiella pneumoniae*, *Pseudomonas aeruginosa*, and various *Proteus* species. Gram-negative bacilli and staphylococci are implicated as dominant etiologic agents in a study in otitis media of the neonate. Recent studies, however, have established that even among very young infants, *S. pneumoniae* and *H. influenzae* constitute the most common etiologic agents.

Despite confirmatory evidence for bacterial etiology in approximately 65% of episodes of acute otitis media, the remaining third of these middle ear cultures failed to grow definite pathogenic bacteria, using aerobic culture methods. Anaerobic bacteria have only recently been sought in these acute infections.[10,11]

Tympanocentesis with aerobic and anaerobic cultivation of middle ear fluid was performed through one or both tympanic membranes of 186 children with acute otitis media. A simplified method for performing myringotomy and tympanocentesis that avoids the use of complicated equipment and prevents contamination of the specimen was used in this study. This technique also allows for less exposure to oxygen in an effort to identify anaerobic as well as aerobic bacteria.[12] Aerobic bacteria alone, predominantly pneumococci and *H. influenzae*, were isolated from 118 (63.4%) patients. Anaerobic organisms alone, most commonly peptococci, were isolated from 24 (12.9%) patients. Twenty-six (14%) patients yielded mixtures of aerobes and anaerobes, and several had multiple aerobic or anaerobic agents. No bacterial growth was noted in 18 (9.7%) patients. Thus the addition of anaerobic methodology to the processing of specimens obtained from ear aspirates allowed isolation of bacteria from 90% of the patients studied. This rate is higher than that obtained in past studies in which anaerobic techniques were not used.

S. pneumoniae (table 18.1) was isolated from 62 patients (36.9%). In 44 cases, pneumococci were recovered in pure culture, in nine instances with *H. influenzae,* and from nine patients they were mixed with other aerobes or anaerobes. *H. influenzae* was isolated from 52 patients (30.1%) and *Haemophilus parainfluenzae* from two patients. *Staphylococcus epidermidis* was recovered in nine instances. *S. aureus* was isolated in pure culture from 5 patients, and from 10 patients they were mixed with other aerobic and anaerobic bacteria. *P. aeruginosa* was isolated in pure culture from three patients, and one of these had recurrent otitis media.

Anaerobic organisms were isolated from 50 patients (26.9%) (table 18.2). Gram-positive anaerobic cocci were identified in 39 instances (21%); eight of these were identified as *Peptostreptococcus* organisms. Gram-positive anaerobic cocci alone were recovered from 15 patients, and the rest of the isolates were mixed with other aerobic and anaerobic bacteria (table 18.2). *Propionibacterium* species were identified in 12 (7.1%) patients, in pure culture in 5 and in mixed culture in 7 patients. All of these isolates were identified as *Propionibacterium acnes* except

Table 18.1. Bacteria Isolated from 186 Cases of Acute Otitis Media

Isolates	No. of Isolates	Percent of Patients with Positive Cultures
Aerobic Bacteria		
S. pneumoniae	62	37
H. influenzae	52	30
S. aureus	15	9
Group A, beta-hemolytic streptococci	9	5
P. aeruginosa	3	2
Group D streptococci	3	2
Others	12	7
Total number of aerobic bacteria	156	
Anaerobic Bacteria		
Peptococci	31	17
Peptostreptococci	8	4
Propionibacterium sp.	12	7
Others	5	3
Total number anaerobic bacteria	56	
Total number of aerobic and anaerobic bacteria	212	

SOURCE: Brook, I. Otitis media in children: a prospective study of aerobic and anaerobic bacteriology. *Laryngoscope* 89:995, 1979. Reprinted by permission.

one, which was identified as *Propionibacterium avidum*. There were other anaerobic organisms identified: one each of *Veillonella* species, *Bifido-bacterium* species, *Eubacterium* species, *Clostridium ramosum*, and microaerophilic streptococci (table 18.1).

When anaerobes were recovered in pure culture, similar organisms were often seen in direct Gram stains of the aspirated effusions.

Although anaerobes were isolated in that study from 25% of children with acute otitis media, instillation of an antiseptic solution into the external auditory canal prior to tympanocentesis was not employed. Isolation of some of the anaerobic species may have represented contamination of the middle ear aspirate by the flora normally present on the canal walls and surface of the tympanic membrane.

Table 18.2. Bacterial Cultures of 186 Children with Acute Otitis Media

	Patients	
	No.	**%**
Patients with Aerobic Organisms Only		
S. pneumoniae	44	24
H. influenzae	32	18
S. pneumoniae + H. influenzae	9	5
Group A streptococci	9	5
S. aureus	5	3
Others	19	8
Subtotal	118	63
Patients with Anaerobic Organisms Only		
Anaerobic cocci	15	8
P. acnes	5	3
Others	4	2
Subtotal	24	13
Patients with Mixed Aerobic and Anaerobic Organisms		
Anaerobic cocci + H. influenzae	3	2
Anaerobic cocci + S. pneumoniae	2	1
Anaerobic cocci + S. aureus	7	4
Anaerobic cocci + H. influenzae + S. pneumoniae	3	2
Other combinations	11	5
Subtotal	26	14.0
Total of all patients with positive cultures	168	90.3
No growth	18	9.7

SOURCE: Brook, I. Otitis media in children: a prospective study of aerobic and anaerobic bacteriology. *Laryngoscope* 89:994, 1979. Reprinted by permission.

In another study[13] employing techniques for cultivation of anaerobes, there was an attempt to sterilize the external ear canal and surface of the tympanic membrane using povidone iodine. Three anaerobes were recovered from the 28 infants included in this study: two isolates of *Clostridium* organisms and one isolate of *Peptococcus magnus*.

The isolation of anaerobic bacteria from the middle ear even after antisepsis of the external auditory canal suggests that these bacteria may occasionally play a direct or ancillary role in the pathogenesis of acute otitis media in infants and young children.

Additional support for the role of anaerobic bacteria, and especially Gram-positive cocci, came from a study of the bacterial flora of the external auditory canal.[14] Seventy-two healthy children were included in the study. The most common aerobic isolates were *S. epidermidis* (56 isolates), alpha-hemolytic streptococci, and *P. aeruginosa*. The two anaerobic organisms recovered were *P. acnes* (13 isolates) and peptococci (two isolates).

It should be noted that peptococci were recovered from 17% of inner ear aspirates obtained from children with acute otitis media but were recovered from only 3% of external ear canal specimens obtained in this study. The differences in the isolation rate of this organism from the external ear canal and from the inner ear further supports its possible role in acute and chronic otitis media.

P. acnes, on the other hand, is a component of the skin flora and is rarely a pathogen.[15, 16] The rate of isolation of this organism from the external ear canal was 18%, which is higher than its recovery rate from inner ear aspirates in infected patients (7% in acute and 6% in chronic otitis media).

Pathogenesis

There are many factors in the etiology of otitis media. The Eustachian tubes have essential roles in protecting the middle ear from nasopharyngeal secretions. The tube provides drainage into the nasopharynx of secretions produced within the middle ear and permits equilibration of air pressure with atmospheric pressure in the middle ear, with replenishment of the oxygen that has been absorbed. Mechanical or functional obstruction of the Eustachian tube can result in middle ear effusion. Functional obstruction is common in infants and younger children since the amount and stiffness of the cartilage support of the tube is less than in older children and adults.

The horizontally placed Eustachian tube, which opens at a lower level in the infant's nasopharynx than in that of the child or adult, may allow easy access to infection through the medium of regurgitated milk or vomitus. The infant has a poorly developed immunity to upper respiratory infections of viral origin or bacterial sequela, and the infant's lymphoid tissue in the pharynx, and especially in nasopharynx, is in a state of active growth and is prone to infection. The middle ear content of mesenchyme forms a favorable medium for pathogenic growth.

Obstruction of the tube can result in formation of negative pressure in the middle ear and subsequent formation of a transudate in that space. This space can become contaminated through reflux of mucus from the nasopharynx, causing contamination of the middle ear space. This mode of infection can explain the route by which aerobic and anaerobic bacteria that are part of the oral flora gain access to the middle ear.

The anaerobic organisms that were recovered from the middle ear of infected children were isolated from serious pleuropulmonary infections and are part of the normal oropharyngeal flora.[17, 18] The isolation of anaerobes, all known pathogens of the upper and lower respiratory tracts, suggests a primary or ancillary role for these bacteria in the etiology of acute otitis media.

Diagnosis

The child may present with irritability and restless sleep. These may be the only signs in an infant, or the infant may rub or pull at the ear. Older children will complain of pain, dizziness, and headache. Fever in infants may be very high, sometimes with convulsions, or it may be absent. Symptoms of an upper respiratory tract infection usually are present. Vomiting or diarrhea, or both, may be prominent.

Examination of the ear may reveal distortion or absence of light reflex, impaired mobility of the drum, flaming and diffusely red drum rather than the normal pearl-gray, and the drum may bulge. If the tympanic membrane has ruptured, an opening may be seen as discharging pus or serous fluid. A conductive-type hearing loss is always present. It should be noted that mild redness of the drum in the presence of high fever is often entirely nonspecific and related only to the fever. Hyperemia of the drum may occur with crying.

Under certain circumstances, tympanocentesis or myringotomy should be performed. This procedure could be beneficial for some patients for whom determination of the etiology of the acute otitis media and relief of pain and acute symptoms is especially important. A simplified technique, using a modified Medicut (Aloe Medical, St. Louis, Mo.), can prevent gross contamination of the specimen (fig. 18.1).[10]

Management

Supportive therapy, including analgesics, antipyretics, and local heat, can be helpful. Although an oral decongestant may relieve some nasal congestion, and antihistamines may help patients with known or sus-

Figure 18.1. Intravenous cannula set used for tympanocentesis after the needle has been bent.

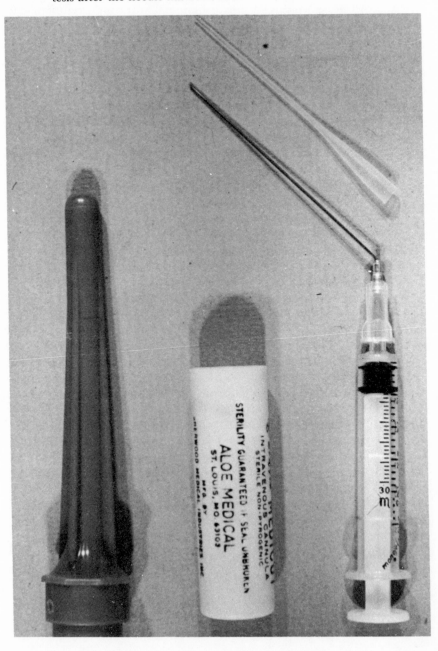

pected nasal allergy, their efficacy in the treatment of acute otitis media has not been proved.

Antimicrobial therapy is of utmost importance, and the selection of the agents used should depend on the bacterial cause of the infection. Since the common offending microbiological agents are *S. pneumoniae* and *H. influenzae,* most of the patients respond favorably to ampicillin or amoxicillin in appropriate dosage in divided doses for 10 days. In patients who are allergic to penicillin, erythromycin and/or sulfa drugs may be prescribed.[19]

Although cephalosporins have a limited role in the treatment of otitis media, the new cephalosporin, cefactor, has shown promise in the treatment of this disease.[20] This cephalexin analogue has enhanced anti-*Haemophilus* activity and is not inactivated by beta-lactamase-producing ampicillin-resistant bacteria. Combination antibacterial drug therapy also has gained in popularity in recent years, mostly because of the growing problem of ampicillin-resistant *H. influenzae.* The combinations successfully used are penicillin and sulfonilamide,[21] trimethoprim-sulfamethoxazole,[22] and erythromycin-sulphonamide.[23]

Since the anaerobes recovered in acute otitis media are susceptible to penicillins and other antibiotics commonly used to treat acute otitis media, no change in the recommended therapy is advocated. The recently licensed trimethoprim-sulfamethoxazole combination is effective against only 50% of anaerobic Gram-positive cocci isolates, the major anaerobe isolated in acute otitis media.

Complications

Perforation of drum, resulting in chronic otitis media, hearing loss, acquired cholesteatoma, mastoiditis, and occasionally meningitis, brain abscess, and chronic serous otitis (glue ear) are some of the complications of acute otitis media. Fortunately, the intracranial suppurative complications are uncommon in recent years. These complications usually occur following chronic otitis media or mastoiditis through direct extension or by vascular channels.

Facial paralysis secondary to involvement of facial nerves may occur during an episode of acute otitis media with effusion.

Suppurative labyrinthitis may occur during an episode of acute otitis media with effusion from the direct invasion of bacteria through the round or oval windows.

Secretory (Serous) Otitis Media

This is a common cause of mild hearing loss in children, most often between the ages of two and seven years. The middle ear contains fluid that varies from a thin transudate to a very thick consistency (glue ear). Eustachian tube obstruction usually is due to primary congenital tube dysfunction. Other possible contributing factors are allergic rhinitis, adenoidal hyperplasia, supine feeding position, or a submucous cleft. Middle ear effusion (MEE) was found to persist for at least one month in up to 40% of children who had suffered from acute otitis media, and for at least three months in 10% of afflicted children.[24]

Microbiology

Persistent or chronic MEEs usually have been assumed to be sterile because several reports had described unsuccessful attempts to culture bacteria from them.[25, 26] In 1958, however, Senturia and co-workers[27] examined 130 patients with chronic otitis media with effusion, using smears and cultures, and identified bacteria in 33% of ears with serous effusions, in 25% of ears with mucoid effusions, in 51% of ears with mucopurulent effusions, and in 29% of ears with purulent effusions. They acknowledged that the number of positive cultures may have been unduly high because bacteria from the unsterilized external canal may have contaminated the effusions. They did not use chocolate agar plates when culturing and, therefore, *H. influenzae* might not have grown except for satellite colonies around other organisms. Kokko[28] in 1974 cultured bacteria in 22% of ear effusions studied. Healy and Teele[29] attempted to sterilize the external canal with alcohol. They then investigated 57 children with chronic OME and reported that 35 of 96 specimens (36%) had positive cultures. The bacterial flora closely resembled those of acute OME. Riding and colleagues[30] studied the ear aspirates of 274 children with recurrent and chronic MEE after sterilizing the external canal with alcohol. They found that 45% contained bacteria, and 11% contained bacteria that were probable pathogens (*S. pneumoniae, H. influenzae,* and *Streptococcus pyogenes*).

In 1976, Liu and associates[31] examined 102 ears with chronic OME. They found organisms in 66% of ears with serous effusions, in 36% of ears with mucoid effusions, and in 80% of ears with leukocytic (purulent) effusions. Fifty-two percent of all effusions contained bacteria. The external canal was not sterilized in these studies, however, and the effusion cultures may have been contaminated. Diphtheroids and *S. epidermidis,* the two organisms thought to be contaminants, occurred most commonly. These authors cultured the ear canal in 30 patients, and although they did not report the organisms from the ear canal, they felt that types of bacteria recovered from the ear canal differed considerably from those recovered from the middle ear effusions.

Two authors have recently described the presence of antibody-coated bacteria (*S. epidermidis, Corynebacterium* species) in the sediments of middle ear effusions. Antibody titers against these bacteria are sometimes higher in the middle ear effusions than in the corresponding sera.[16, 17] These two studies may suggest that these organisms are not contaminants, but their role in the pathogenesis of otitis media cannot be determined at present.

Viral infections have not been ruled out as a major cause of middle ear effusions. Adlington and Davies[32] reviewed the literature on viruses and otitis media and concluded that there is little evidence for either viral growth in middle ear effusions or cytotoxic changes in the mucosa that would be characteristic of viral infection. Klein and Teele,[33] however, isolated viruses in 29 of 663 patients (4.4%), and respiratory syncytial virus was isolated most frequently (22 patients). Only one mycoplasma, *Mycoplasma pneumoniae*, was recovered.

Giebink and associates[34] recently studied 144 serous and mucoid effusions for aerobic and anaerobic bacteria, *M. pneumoniae,* and virus. Thirty percent of the effusions yielded aerobic bacteria. Although serous effusions were culture-positive as often as mucoid effusions, *H. influenzae* was isolated predominantly from serous effusions and *S. epidermidis* predominantly from mucoid samples. Only one effusion yielded a viral isolate *(Herpesvirus hominis),* and only one effusion yielded an anaerobe (*Propionibacterium* organisms). The anaerobic techniques used by these authors, however, were not appropriate for fastidious organisms, and the investigators used only liquid medium for the initial culturing of anaerobes.

In a recent study, Brook and co-workers[35] were able to recover bacteria from 23 of 57 (41%) of the patients studied. Anaerobes were present as the only isolates in 17% of the culture-positive aspirates, and in an additional 26% they were present mixed with aerobes.

Aerobic organisms only were recovered from 13 aspirates (57% of the culture-positive aspirates), anaerobic bacteria from 4 (17%), and mixed aerobic and anaerobic bacteria were recovered from 6 (26%). A total of 45 bacterial isolates were recovered, accounting for 2.0 isolates per specimen (1.4 aerobes and 0.6 anaerobes) (table 18.3). There were a total of 31 aerobic isolates, including *S. aureus* and *S. pneumoniae* (five of each), and *S. epidermidis* and alpha-hemolytic streptococci (four of each). A total of 14 anaerobes were recovered, including anaerobic Gram-positive cocci (six isolates), *B. melaninogenicus* and *P. acnes* (five and three isolates, respectively).

The anaerobes recovered from these patients are similar to anaerobic organisms previously recovered by these investigators from children with acute[10, 11] and chronic[36] otitis media.

Pathogenesis

Eustachian tube dysfunction is the primary cause of otitis media with effusion. All such patients have poor tubal function. Bluestone and co-workers[37] have suggested that there are two types of Eustachian tube obstruction that can result in middle ear effusion, mechanical and functional. Mechanical obstruction results from inflammation by bacteria or viruses, allergy, hypertrophic adenoids, or tumors of the nasopharynx. Functional obstruction results from persistent collapse of the cartilaginous tube. This collapse may be due to increased tubal compliance, an inadequate opening mechanism, or both. Evidence regarding the role of bacteria, viruses, and mycoplasmae in the etiology and pathogenesis of acute inflammatory disease in the middle ear is conflicting. The bacteria associated with acute suppurative otitis media in young children are *S. pneumoniae, H. influenzae,* and *S. pyogenes.*[4-8]

Table 18.3. Bacteria Isolated from 23 Culture-positive Serous Effusions*

Isolates	Number of Isolates
Aerobic Bacteria	
S. pneumoniae	5
Group D streptococci	1
Alpha-hemolytic streptococci	4
Gamma-hemolytic streptococci	1
S. aureus	5(5*)
S. epidermidis	4
Diphtheroids	2
H. influenzae	8(1*)
E. coli	1
Subtotal aerobes	31
Anaerobic Bacteria	
P. asaccharolyticus	3
P. micros	1
S. constellatus	1
V. alcalescens	1
P. acnes	3
B. melaninogenicus ss. *melaninogenicus*	3(2*)
B. melaninogenicus ss. *intermedius*	2(1*)
Subtotal anaerobes	14
Total bacteria	45

*Number of beta-lactamase-producing strains.

While there is general agreement that otitis media with a purulent effusion is usually a bacterial infection, there is no uniformity of opinion on the role of bacteria in the serous, seromucinous, and mucoid otitis media with effusion.

The presence of aerobic and anaerobic bacteria in some nonsuppurative effusions suggests that both are involved in the pathogenesis of serous otitis media.

Diagnosis

Onset is usually sudden, with a slight conductive hearing loss. Symptoms may include slight earache, a feeling of watery bubbles in the ear, or a sensation that the head is full. If the ear is not completely filled with fluid, there may be air bubbles or a meniscus visible through the tympanic membrane. The eardrum shows a loss of translucency, may be retracted, have diminished movement, and exhibit a change in color from the normal gray to a more pale or even bluish hue.

Management

The role of bacteria in the pathogenesis of this ear disease is not yet clear; however, antimicrobial agents often are used in an attempt to clear the ear effusion of bacteria. The presence of anaerobic bacteria as well as aerobic in the serous ear aspirate raises the question of whether the antimicrobial agents currently used are adequate and whether antibiotics effective also against some of the beta-lactamase producing organisms should be used. Additional controlled studies are needed to define the value of antimicrobial treatment in children with serous otitis media and to clarify the role of bacteria in the pathogenesis of serous otitis media.

The efficacy of antibiotics, decongestants, antihistamines, and corticosteroids has not been currently established. In most children the effusions are self-limited. If, however, the effusions persist for at least eight weeks or if there have been frequent episodes of acute otitis media, the patient requires evaluation for allergy, adenoid tissue obstruction, immunologic competence, and local malformations or abnormalities that may block the tubes.

In cases that fail to respond to medical management surgical intervention may be indicated. This includes myringotomy, suctioning, and the insertion of plastic ventilation tubes. Selected cases sometimes are referred for adenoidectomy. The efficacy of all of these procedures alone or in combination is debatable and awaits further study.

Chronic Otitis Media and Cholesteatoma

Chronic otitis media in children can be insidious, persistent, and very often destructive, with sometimes irreversible sequelae, such as hearing deficit and subsequent learning disabilities. In many patients with chronic otitis media a cholesteatoma may develop; a *cholesteatoma* is a pocket of skin that invades the middle ear and mastoid spaces from the edge of a perforation.

Chronic otitis media and cholesteatoma tends to be persistent and progressive and very often causes destructive irreversible changes in the bony structure of the ear. In many cases, the perforation of the tympanic membrane that occurs during acute otitis media persists into the chronic stage.

Microbiology

Although past studies reported the recovery of anaerobic organisms from many cases of chronic otitis media, aerobic organisms, mainly *S. aureus* and Gram-negative enteric bacilli, were considered to be the major pathogens.[18] Several recent studies reaffirmed the role of anaerobes in chronic otitis media.[36, 38, 39] Fulghum, Daniel, and Yarborough[38] recovered *Peptostreptococcus intermedius* and *P. acnes* in mixed cultures from four of ten cases of chronic serous otitis media. In another report, Jokipii and colleagues[39] recovered anaerobes from one-third of 70 patients. *Bacteroides* species accounted for 50% of the anaerobes (22 isolates), and anaerobic cocci for about 25% (13 isolates).

In a study of pediatric patients suffering from chronic otitis media,[38] anaerobic bacteria were isolated from 56% of ear aspirates (table 18.4). The majority of the anaerobic organisms isolated were Gram-positive anaerobic cocci, *Bacteroides* species (including the *Bacteroides fragilis* group), and *Fusobacterium nucleatum*. The predominant aerobic bacteria isolated were enteric Gram-negative rods (mostly *P. aeruginosa*) and *S. aureus*. Anaerobic isolates usually were mixed with other anaerobic or aerobic bacteria, and the number of isolates ranged between two and four per specimen, thereby demonstrating the polymicrobial etiology of chronic otitis media.

Only half of the bacteria recovered from the middle ear were also present in the external auditory canal.[40] Furthermore, external ear canal culture in many cases yielded bacteria that were not present in the middle ear. These findings demonstrate that cultures collected from the external auditory canal prior to its sterilization can be misleading. This is particularly important in the case of *P. aeruginosa*, which is more frequently recovered from the external auditory canal than from the middle ear. Although this organism is a common inhabitant of the external auditory canal, it can be recovered also from the middle ear, where it may participate in the inflammatory process. Direct middle-ear aspirations through the perforation in the eardrum are therefore more reliable in establishing the bacteriology of chronic otitis media and can assist in the selection of proper antimicrobial therapy.

The role of anaerobic bacteria in this infection is suggested also by their higher recovery rate from the middle ear only, compared with their recovery from the external canal. This is more apparent when *P. acnes* isolates are deleted from the total number of isolates. Thirty-eight anaerobic strains were recovered from the middle ear only, compared with seven from the external canal.

In a recent study, cholesteatoma specimens were obtained from 28 patients undergoing surgery for chronic otitis media and cholesteatoma.[41] All specimens were cultured for aerobic and anaerobic organisms. Bacterial growth was present in specimens of 24 of the 28 pa-

Table 18.4. Bacterial Isolates in 50 Patients with Chronic Otitis Media

Isolates	Patients
Aerobes and facultatives	
Gram-positive cocci (total)	18
S. aureus	6
Gram-negative bacilli (total)	50
Proteus sp.	7
P. aeruginosa	36
Total aerobes	68
Anaerobes	
Gram-positive cocci	24
Gram-positive bacilli	6
Gram-negative bacilli	
F. nucleatum	2
Bacteroides sp.	3
B. melaninogenicus group	6
B. fragilis group	7
Total anaerobes	48
Total number of bacteria	116

SOURCE: Modified from Brook, I., and Finegold, S. M. Bacteriology of chronic otitis media. *JAMA* 241:488, 1979. Copyright 1979, American Medical Association. Reprinted by permission.

NOTE: Only the important pathogens are listed in detail. The total number of the groups of organisms is represented.

Table 18.5. Bacterial Isolates Obtained from Surgical Specimens in 24 Patients with Cholesteatoma

	Concentrations of bacteria		Total No. of Isolates
	$10^6 >$ CFU/gm	$10^6 <$ CFU/gm	
Aerobes and facultatives			
Gram-positive cocci	2		2
Alpha-hemolytic streptococci			
Group A, beta-hemolytic streptococci		1	1
S. aureus	1	4	5
S. epidermidis	2	1	3
Gram-negative bacilli	2	3	5
P. mirabilis			
P. rettgeri		2	2
P. aeruginosa	2	7	9
K. pneumoniae		5	5
E. coli	1	3	4
S. marcescens	2		2
Providencia sp.	1		1
C. diversus		1	1
Total number of aerobes	13	27	40
Anaerobes			
Anaerobic Gram-positive cocci			
Peptostreptococcus sp.	1	3	4
Peptococcus sp.	2	6	8
Anaerobic Gram-positive bacilli			
Bifidobacterium sp.	2	1	3
P. acnes	2		2
Clostridium sp.	1	2	3
Gram-negative bacilli			
F. nucleatum		2	2
B. melaninogenicus		3	3
B. fragilis group		2	2
B. distasonis group	1	2	3
B. corrodens	1		1
B. oralis		1	1
Bacteroides sp.	1	1	2
Total number of anaerobes	11	23	34
Total number of bacteria	24	50	74

SOURCE: Brook, I. Aerobic and anaerobic bacteriology of cholesteatoma. *Laryngoscope* 91:251, 1981. Reprinted by permission.

NOTE: CFU = colony forming units.

tients. A total of 74 bacterial isolates were present (40 aerobes and 34 anaerobes) (table 18.5). Aerobes alone were isolated from 8 (33.3%) of culture-positive patients, 4 (26.7%) patients yielded only anaerobes, and 12 (50%) had both aerobic and anaerobic bacteria. Fifty isolates (27 aerobes and 23 anaerobes) were present in a concentration greater than 10^6 CFU/gm. The most commonly isolated aerobic organisms were *P. aeruginosa* (9), *Proteus* species (7), *K. pneumoniae* (5), *S. aureus* (5), and *E. coli* (4). The anaerobic bacteria most commonly isolated were Gram-positive anaerobic cocci (12). *Bacteroides* species (12 including 5 *B. fragilis* group), *Clostridium* species (3), and *Bifidobacterium* species (3). These findings indicate the polymicrobial aerobic and anaerobic bacteriology of cholesteatoma.

All cultures in the present study were obtained from surgical specimens, excluding any possibility of contamination of the specimen by skin flora. The results demonstrate the polymicrobial bacteriology of cultures obtained from patients presenting with chronic otitis media and cholesteatoma. They concur with data obtained in other recent studies of the bacteriology of chronic otitis media.[36, 38, 40] The bacterial isolates obtained in this study are similar to those obtained from pus aspirated from the inner ear in cases of chronic otitis media.

Pathogenesis

The absence of anaerobic methods may account for the relatively high rate of negative cultures of middle-ear effusions in certain studies. In one of these studies,[42] bacteria were shown on direct smears in 80% of middle ear effusions obtained from patients with chronic otitis media, while only 40% of the effusions yielded positive bacterial cultures. The presence of foul-smelling pus originating from the middle ear suggests the presence of anaerobic bacteria in many of the patients.

Cholesteatoma that accompanies chronic otitis media is known to induce the absorption of the bone underlying it, but the mechanism by which this occurs is not well understood. Various theories attempt to explain the possible role of different factors in the process of expansion of the cholesteatoma and the collagen degradation that occurs in its vicinity.[43, 44] A possible role of anaerobic and aerobic bacteria in the destructive process is suggested, and further study to ascertain their affects on the surrounding bone and collagen is warranted.

It is also clear that a cholesteatoma contains bacteria similar to that recovered from aspirates of chronically infected ears. It seems reasonable that the cholesteatoma present in a chronically infected ear serves as a nidus of chronic infection.

Diagnosis

The common symptom is the presence of recurrent or persistent ear drainage. Chronic otitis media may be painless and free of fever in the intervals between acute exacerbations.

The eardrum can be perforated and foul-smelling pus may be present. Peripheral perforations provide a greater risk of cholesteatoma formation. Mastoid tenderness may be present.

Radiographic studies for evidence of mastoid involvement may reveal pathologic organisms. Aerobic and anaerobic bacteriologic cultures are imperative. Specific etiologic diagnosis must be made by culture of drainage fluid. Secondary invaders following perforations are frequent causes of chronic drainage and are much more resistant to therapy.

Management

Attempts to treat chronic otitis media using parenteral antimicrobial therapy have not been successful.[45] The organisms usually treated were the aerobic isolates, mainly *S. aureus* and Gram-negative enteric bacilli. Brook[46] has used parenteral carbenicillin or clindamycin to treat chronic otitis media. Combined therapy with gentamicin was used when aerobic Gram-negative rods were present in the aspirate. Response to therapy was good in more than half of the patients. This study demonstrates that antimicrobial therapy directed against the aerobic and anaerobic bacteria isolated from patients' effusions could in many instances eradicate the infections in children with chronic otitis media. Since this study did not include a control group, more studies are warranted to evaluate further the role of antimicrobial therapy alone or in combination with surgery.

Instillation of appropriate antibiotic drops sometimes are recommended. Myringoplasty or tympanoplasty is done at about age 10 or older. Cholesteatoma should be treated surgically when diagnosed.

Complications

Mastoiditis or inflammation of the mastoid air cell system frequently accompanies chronic otitis media with effusion.

The intracranial complications of chronic otitis media are meningitis, focal encephalitis, intracranial abscesses (brain abscess, extradural abscess, subdural abscess), and otitic hydrocephalus.[18]

A patient with chronic otitis media who develops signs of intracranial complications should be treated rapidly and thoroughly. Intracranial involvement is signalled by severe earache, constant and persistent headache, nausea and vomiting, seizures, fever, or localized neurologic findings.

Sinusitis

Sinusitis is defined as an inflammation of the mucous membrane lining the paranasal sinuses (fig. 18.2). Acute purulent sinusitis can be defined as pus in a sinus cavity. Chronic sinusitis is best defined as a presumptive diagnosis based on radiologic evidence of mucosal thickening. The maxillary antrums and the anterior and posterior ethmoid cells are present at birth and usually are of sufficient size to harbor infection. The frontal sinuses rarely become infected before six years of age.

Sinuses are involved in most cases of upper respiratory tract infection, but sinus infection usually does not persist after the nasal infection has subsided.

Figure 18.2. Diagram of the skull; *shaded areas* indicate frontal, ethmoid, and maxillary sinuses.

Frontal Sinus

Ethmoid Sinus

Maxillary Sinus

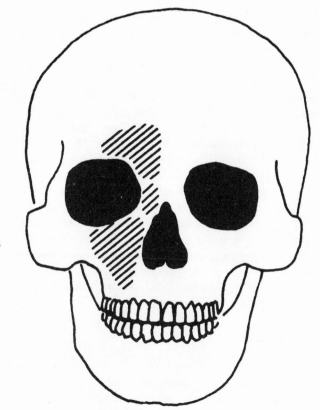

Microbiology

Acute Sinusitis

The bacteria recovered from patients with acute purulent sinusitis are those considered as part of the normal flora of the nose *(Neisseria* species, *S. epidermidis, S. aureus)* and the common respiratory pathogens *(S. pneumoniae,* beta-hemolytic streptococci, and *H. influenzae).*[47] The infection generally is polymicrobial: more than one organism often is recovered. Enteric bacteria are less commonly recovered, but occasionally *E. coli* is recovered. Anaerobic bacteria have been recovered only from a few cases with acute sinusitis.[18]

A variety of viral agents, including the respiratory syncytial virus, rhinovirus, parainfluenzae, ECHO, and Coxsackie viruses have been isolated. Their significance is uncertain; however, bacterial infection is likely to be secondary to one of the viruses mentioned.

Aspergillosis also has been reported as a cause of sinusitis.[48]

Chronic Sinusitis

Anaerobes have been identified in chronic sinus disease whenever techniques for their cultivation were employed.[18] Gram-positive anaerobic cocci, *Bacteroides* species, *Veillonella* species, and *Clostridium* species were recovered in earlier studies.[18]

In studies of adults, anaerobes were recovered in large numbers.[49, 50] Frederick and Braude[49] isolated anaerobes in 52% of patients with paranasal sinusitis, whereas Carenfelt and co-workers[50] recovered anaerobes in 25% to 50% of cases of maxillary sinusitis.

Brook[51] recently reported data concerning anaerobic organisms isolated from inflamed sinuses (table 18.6). Aspiration of chronically inflamed sinuses was aseptically performed in 40 children. Anaerobes were isolated from all 37 culture-positive patients. There were 97 anaerobic and 24 aerobic isolates, with the predominant isolates (in descending order) being *Bacteroides* species (including *B. melaninogenicus, B. oralis,* and *Bacteroides ruminicola* ss. *brevis),* anaerobic Gram-positive cocci, *Fusobacterium* species, alpha-hemolytic streptococci, *S. aureus,* and *Haemophilus* species. The *B. fragilis* group, which has been reported in adults, was not present in the patients. The absence of the *B. fragilis* group in these patients could be attributed to their younger age or the shorter duration of their illness.

Pathogenesis

Since the mucous membranes lining the nasal chambers and the sinuses are alike histologically and are continuous with each other through the natural ostium, upper respiratory infections commonly result in an inflammatory sinusitis. Sinusitis of nondental genesis is considered to be preceded by a viral, mechanical, or allergic stage when the nasal and paranasal mucosa are hyperemic and the permeability of the ostium is decreased. At that stage, the sealed-off sinus that fails to drain freely is prone to secondary infection.

Sinus ostium occlusion is the major predisposing factor causing suppurative infection and most often is the result of viral or upper respiratory infection, a common event in early childhood. Other important contributory factors are the congenital and acquired immune deficiencies.[52, 53]

Mechanical obstruction resulting in sinusitis can be related to various causative factors such as septal dislocation owing to birth trauma,[54] unilateral choanal atresia, foreign bodies placed in the nose, or fractures of the nose following trauma. Up to 30% of cystic fibrosis pa-

Table 18.6. Bacteria Isolated from 37 Children with Chronic Sinusitis

Isolates	No.
Aerobic and Facultative	
Gram-positive cocci (total)	19
Group A beta-hemolytic streptococci	3
S. aureus	7
Gram-negative bacilli (total)	5
E. coli	1
H. influenzae	2
H. parainfluenzae	2
Total	24
Anaerobic	
Anaerobic cocci	34
Gram-positive bacilli	14
Gram-negative bacilli	
Fusobacterium sp.	13
Bacteroides sp.	12
B. melaninogenicus group	14
B. oralis	5
B. ruminicola ss. brevis	5
Total	97

SOURCE: Modified from Brook, I. Bacteriologic features of chronic sinusitis in children. *JAMA* 246:968, 1981. Copyright 1981, American Medical Association. Reprinted by permission.
NOTE: Only the important pathogens are listed in detail. The total number of the groups of organisms is represented.

tients may have polyps complicating the already abnormal sinus secretions that predispose them to sinusitis.[55]

Allergy, especially asthma, is an important predisposing factor in sinusitis.[56] Cyanotic congenital heart disease frequently is complicated by sinusitis.[57] Dental infections also are a source of sinusitis in children.[58]

A recent study showed that the uninfected sinus contains "normal" aerobic and anaerobic bacterial flora similar to those present in the infected sinus.[59] The recovery of these flora in the normal noninflamed sinus may explain the chain of events that lead to formation of empyema and follow the occlusion of the ostium and the pathophysiology of acute and chronic sinusitis.

When sinusitis occurs, oxygen is being absorbed mostly by the sinus mucosa.[60] The possible implication of the oxygen consumption in the diseased sinus is the formation of a bacteria-host relationship in favor of certain bacteria. The mean oxygen tension in serous secretions obtained from acutely inflamed maxillary sinuses was 12.3% (compared to about 17% in the normal sinuses).[61] The bacteria recovered from these aspirates were predominantly *S. pneumoniae*. The oxygen tension in purulent secretion was zero, however, and an accumulation of carbon dioxide was found, particularly when anaerobic bacteria were recovered. It is therefore plausible that the reduced oxygen tension in the sinus during the serous phase better meets the requirements for the growth of those bacteria isolated in acute sinusitis, *S. pneumoniae* and *H. influenzae*,[62] while the complete lack of oxygen in the purulent secretion supports the growth of the anaerobic organisms recovered in chronic sinusitis.

The frequent involvement of anaerobes in chronic sinusitis may be related to the poor drainage and increased intranasal pressure that occur during inflammation.[63] This can reduce the oxygen tension in the inflamed sinus[61] by decreasing the mucosal blood supply[64] and depressing the ciliary action.[65] The lowering of the oxygen content and pH of the sinus cavity supports the growth of anaerobic organisms by providing an optimal-oxidation reduction potential.[62]

Anaerobes frequently are recovered from infectious conditions associated with complications of sinusitis,[18] including periorbital cellulitis, brain abscess, subdural or epidural empyema, cavernous sinus thrombosis, and meningitis. This relationship ascertains their role in sinus infections and warrants appropriate antimicrobial therapy.

Diagnosis

Acute Sinusitis

The child generally presents with edema of the mucous membranes of the nose, mucopurulent nasal discharge, and persistent postnasal drip, fever, and malaise. Tenderness over the involved sinus is present, and so is pain, which can be induced over the affected sinus upon percussion. Cellulitis can be observed in the area overlying the affected sinus. Other occasional findings, especially in acute ethmoiditis, are periorbital cellulitis, edema, and proptosis. Failure to transilluminate the sinus and nasal voice are also evident in many patients. Direct smear of the secretions usually reveals mostly neutrophils and may aid in detection of associated allergy if many eosinophils are present.

Radiologically, clouding, opacity, and thickening of the mucosal interface of the affected sinus usually are present. Fluid level can often be observed.

Chronic Sinusitis

Symptoms of chronic sinusitis vary considerably. Fever may be absent or be of low grade. Frequently symptoms are malaise, easy fatigability, difficulty in mental concentration, anorexia, irregular nasal or postnasal discharge, frequent headaches, and pain or tenderness to palpation over the affected sinus.

Management

Acute Sinusitis

Treatment is aimed at establishing good drainage by use of nasal vasoconstrictors (phenylephrine nose drops or spray) or frequent nasal suction. Systemic decongestants or antihistamines may be helpful, especially in allergic individuals. Humidification may be beneficial. Anatomic deformities should be corrected.

Appropriate antibiotic therapy is of paramount importance. The majority of the organisms recovered from acute sinusitis are susceptible to ampicillin, and it is the drug of choice. In patients allergic to this drug alternative drugs, or drug combinations similar to that described for acute otitis media, can be given. If the patient fails to show significant improvement within 48 hours or shows signs of deterioration in spite of treatment, antral puncture under antibiotic cover is indicated, and sinus irrigation is carried out.

Chronic Sinusitis

Therapy is similar to that for acute sinusitis. Repeated courses of decongestants and antibiotics may be required.

Most of the anaerobic pathogens isolated from inflamed sinuses are sensitive to penicillin. *B. fragilis* and some strains of *B. melaninogenicus* and some of the aerobic organisms (*S. aureus* and *H. influenzae*), however, are resistant to penicillin,[66, 67] and when these organisms are recovered alternative therapy is warranted.[18] The recovery of these penicillin-resistant organisms requires administration of appropriate antimicrobial agents such as clindamycin, chloramphenicol, carbenicillin, or cefoxitin. When the patient does not respond to medical therapy, the physician should consider surgical drainage in conjunction with the use of antimicrobial drugs that are also effective against these aerobic and anaerobic penicillin-resistant organisms.

In contrast to acute sinusitis, which generally is treated vigorously with antibiotics, many physicians believe that surgical drainage and not antibiotics is the mainstay of therapy in chronic sinusitis. The use of antimicrobial therapy alone without surgical drainage of collected pus may not result in clearance of the infection. The chronically inflamed sinus membranes with diminished vascularity may be a poor means of carrying an adequate antibiotic level to the infected tissue, even though the blood level may be therapeutic. Furthermore, the reduction in the pH and oxygen tension within the inflamed sinus may interfere further with the activity of the antimicrobial agents, which can result in bacterial survival despite a high antibiotic concentration.[68]

Complications

Sinus infection when not treated promptly and properly may spread via anastomosing veins or by direct extension to nearby structures. Contiguous spread could reach the orbital area, resulting in periorbital cellulitis, subperiosteal abscess, orbital cellulitis, and abscess. Orbital cellulitis may complicate acute ethmoiditis if a thrombophlebitis of the anterior and posterior ethmoidal veins leads to a spread of infection to the lateral, or orbital, side of the ethmoid labyrinth. Sinusitis may extend also to the central nervous system, causing cavernous sinus thrombosis, retrograde meningitis, and epidural, subdural, and brain abscesses.[69, 70] Orbital symptoms frequently precede intracranial extension of the disease (fig. 18.3).[71]

Brook and associates[71] recently reported eight children who had complications of sinusitis. Subdural empyema occurred in four patients; in one patient it was accompanied by cerebritis and brain abscess and in another by meningitis. Periorbital abscess was present in two children who had ethmoiditis. Alveolar abscess in the upper incisors was present in two children whose infection had spread to the maxillary and ethmoid sinuses. Anaerobic bacteria were isolated from the infected sinuses in all the patients. Three of the four patients with intracranial abscess did not respond initially to appropriate antimicrobial therapy directed against the organisms recovered from their abscesses. They improved only after both the subdural empyema and infected sinus were drained. Surgical drainage and appropriate antimicrobial therapy resulted in complete eradication of the infection in all patients.

Figure 18.3. The route of spread of infection from site of periorbital cellulitis into the cranial cavity through retrograde thrombophlebitis.

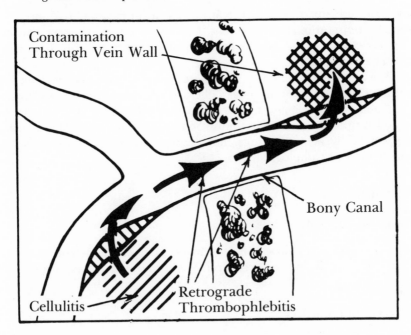

Although the need for judicious selection of antimicrobial agents is of utmost importance, it is essential to note that the treatment of the complications of sinusitis frequently requires surgical intervention. The mortality is reduced when therapy includes surgical drainage, and it is an intregral part of patient management.

Other complications of acute and chronic sinusitis are sinobronchitis, acute maxillary osteomyelitis, and osteomyelitis of the frontal bone.

In persistent sinusitis, bronchitis may occur from the bronchial aspiration of infected material from the draining sinuses. This clinical combination frequently is associated with a chronic cough, and chronic bronchitis may develop.

Acute osteomyelitis of the maxilla may be produced by surgery of an inflamed antrum or by dental abscess or extractions.

Osteomyelitis of the frontal bone generally arises from a spreading thrombophlebitis. A periostitis of the frontal sinus leads to an osteitis and a periostitis of the outer membrane, which gives rise to a tender, puffy swelling of the forehead.

Mastoiditis

Since the advent of antimicrobial agents, acute mastoiditis, once extremely common in childhood, has become quite rare. Chronic mastoiditis, however, still is occasionally encountered in conjunction with chronic otitis media.

Mastoiditis is defined as an inflammation of the mastoid antrum and air cells with bone necrosis. The acute form of the disease manifests itself with fever and tenderness around the mastoid cells, accompanied by pus. Chronic mastoiditis is insidious and generally not accompanied by acute findings, but changes in the mastoid cells are usually evident radiologically.

Microbiology

Acute Mastoiditis

Beta-hemolytic streptococci, *H. influenzae*, and pneumonococci are the most common organisms recovered.[72] Mastoiditis is rarely caused by tuberculosis.

Chronic Mastoiditis

S. aureus, *Proteus* organisms, and *P. aeruginosa* are the isolates that have been recovered most frequently from inflamed mastoids.[73] Occasional reports described the recovery of anaerobes, including *Bacteroides* species, from cases of chronic mastoiditis in children.[74]

In a recent study employing anaerobic methodology, aspirates from 24 children undergoing mastoidectomy for chronic mastoiditis were cultured for aerobes and anaerobes[75] (table 18.7). Bacterial growth occurred in all samples. Anaerobes alone were isolated from four specimens (17%), aerobes alone from one (4%), and mixed aerobic and anaerobic flora were obtained from 19 (79%) of the patients. There were 61 anaerobic isolates (2.5 per specimen). The predominant anaerobic organisms were 22 *Bacteroides* species (including 11 *B. melaninogenicus* and 3 *B. fragilis*), 22 Gram-positive cocci (15 peptococci, 5 peptostreptococci, and 2 microaerophilic streptococci), 6 *Actinomyces* species, 2 *F. nucleatum*, 3 each of *P. acnes* and clostridia, and 2 *Eubacterium limosum*. There were 29 aerobic isolates (1.3 per specimen). The predominant aerobic isolates were *S. aureus* (8), *P. aeruginosa* (7), *E. coli* (5), alpha-hemolytic streptococci (4), and *K. pneumoniae* (2). Beta-lactamase production was noted in 20 isolates recovered from 17 patients (97.1%). These included isolates of *S. aureus* (8), the *B. fragilis* group (3), and *B. oralis* (2), as well as 6 of 10 *B. melaninogenicus* and one of two *Bacteroides* species. This study demonstrated the polymicrobial bacteriology of chronic mastoiditis. Aerobic, facultative, and anaerobic bacteria all play a role in condition.

The lack of proper isolation techniques may account for the relatively low number of anaerobes recovered from chronically inflamed mastoids in certain previous studies.[18, 76] Other studies report the isolation of anaerobic bacteria from inflamed mastoid in almost all patients and thereby reinforce studies done at the turn of the century.[18] Still more evidence for the role of anaerobes in this infection is their recovery from 33% to 55% of patients with chronic otitis media in studies where anaerobic methodology was employed.[36, 39, 77, 78]

Pathogenesis

Infection of the mastoid antrum and cells probably is present with each attack of acute otitis media by virtue of the mucosal continuity between

Table 18.7. Bacteria Isolated from 24 Children with Chronic Mastoiditis

Isolates	No. of Isolates
Aerobic and Facultative	
Gram-positive cocci (total)	15
Group A beta-hemolytic streptococci	2
S. aureus	8
Gram-negative bacilli (total)	14
P. aeruginosa	7
E. coli	5
Total	29
Anaerobic isolates	
Anaerobic cocci	23
Gram-positive bacilli (total)	14
Actinomyces sp.	6
Clostridium sp.	3
Gram-negative bacilli	
F. nucleatum	2
Bacteroides sp.	8
B. melaninogenicus group	11
B. fragilis group	3
Total	61

SOURCE: Modified from Brook, I. Aerobic and anaerobic bacteriology of chronic mastoiditis in children. *Am. J. Dis. Child.* 135:479, 1981. Copyright 1981, American Medical Association. Reprinted by permission.
NOTE: Only the important pathogens are listed in detail. The total number of the groups of organisms is represented.

the tympanum and the mastoid process, but as long as the aditus remains patent an acute mastoiditis does not develop. The factors that lead to an acute otitis media are those that predispose to acute mastoiditis.[79] Therefore, it is not surprising to find a correlation between the aerobic and anaerobic bacteria present in acute or chronic otitis media and cholesteatoma and the organisms recovered from acute or chronic mastoiditis. When mastoiditis is present, it can be considered an abscess for which antibiotic therapy can aid in localization but that often requires surgical drainage.

Anaerobes are the predominant organism in the oropharynx, where they outnumber aerobes at a ratio of 10:1,[80] so their presence is expected in patients with chronic mastoiditis. The predominance of anaerobes in chronic mastoiditis is supported further by their isolation from sites associated with complications of this infection. Complications include brain abscess,[18, 81] subdural and epidural empyema,[82] and meningitis.[83] The frequent involvement of anaerobes in chronic mastoiditis probably is related to the poor drainage and increased pressure that occur during inflammation.[84] This can reduce the oxygen tension in the inflamed sinus[61] by decreasing the mucosal blood[85] and depressing the ciliary action.[62] The lowering of the oxygen content and pH of the sinus cavity supports the growth of anaerobic organisms by providing an optimal oxidation-reduction potential.[80]

Diagnosis

Acute Mastoiditis

This should be suspected when there is pain, tenderness, edema, and erythema of the postauricular area. The pinna is displaced inferiorly and anteriorly, and swelling or sagging of the posterosuperior canal wall also may be present. The eardrum usually shows changes of acute suppurative otitis media, and the child may be irritable and febrile.

Chronic Mastoiditis

The onset is insidious. Clinically, there is a persistent, purulent, foul-smelling, scanty discharge, and it is often the odor that prompts the parent to seek advice. There is conductive hearing loss that is shown audiometrically.

Radiographic films obtained in the acute phase show diffuse inflammatory clouding of the mastoid cells; there is no evidence of bone destruction. With accumulation of the exudate there is resorption of the calcium of the mastoid cells so that they are no longer visible. Subsequently, there is destruction of the cells and areas of radiolucency representing abscesses.

With chronic mastoiditis there is an increase in thickness of the mastoid cells and sclerosis of the bone. This is associated with a reduction in size of the cells. Small abscess cavities may persist in the sclerotic bone.

Management

Acute Mastoiditis

Parenteral antimicrobial therapy should be given to prevent spread to the central nervous system and to aid localization of the disease. Penicillin is the drug of choice for the treatment of group A streptococci or *S. pneumoniae*, but ampicillin is also effective against non-beta-lactamase-producing *H. influenzae*.

If the organisms are susceptible to this treatment the abscess will have decreased in size markedly, or the periosteal thickening will have largely disappeared within 48 hours, and tenderness will be decreased. In this event, treatment should be continued for 7 to 10 days.

In the presence of increasing toxicity and extension of the disease process, surgical intervention and drainage may be necessary. Mastoidectomy seldom is necessary when adequate amounts of antibiotics are employed early in the course of the disease.

If the patient's skin remains red over a fluctuating abscess, or if fever and tenderness persist, the mastoid should be surgically drained. Pus will appear. Osteitis is another indication for surgery to prevent further intratemporal or intracranial complications.

Chronic Mastoiditis

Surgical drainage for chronic mastoiditis still is indicated in many cases. If antimicrobial therapy is to be employed, however, the physician should consider the possible presence of anaerobic bacteria. Some of the anaerobes, such as *B. fragilis* and *B melaninogenicus*,[66] are resistant to penicillin; thus therapy should also include antimicrobial agents effective against *S. aureus* and the Gram-negative bacilli, which were recovered from many of the patients studied. A beta-lactamase-resistant antibiotic, such as methicillin or oxacillin, and an aminoglycoside should be considered.

Clindamycin and third generation cephalosporins have adequate coverage for the beta-lactamase-producing anaerobes and *S. aureus*. An aminoglycoside should be active against Gram-negative enteric organisms. Following surgical drainage and the availability of Gram-stain preparation of the pus and pending the results of the bacteriologic cultures, adjustments in the choice of antimicrobial agents could be made.

Complications

Intracranial complications of acute, and particularly chronic, mastoiditis may occur. These include facial palsy, sinus thrombosis, meningitis, and brain abscess.

Tonsillitis

Tonsillitis is a common disease of childhood. It is extremely infectious in that it spreads easily by droplet. The incubation period is two to four days. The specific cause is usually bacterial, and GABHS are the most frequent infecting organisms. *S. aureus, S. pneumoniae,* and *H. influenzae* also are commonly found, and combinations of these may be recovered on culture.

The role of anaerobic bacteria in this infection is hard to elucidate because anaerobes are normally prevalent on the surface of the tonsils and pharynx, so that cultures taken directly from these areas are difficult to interpret.

The failure to make a microbiological diagnosis in many cases of acute and recurrent acute tonsillitis argues for the possible role of anaerobes in this infection. A possible explanation is that the bacteria sampled by the surface swabbing technique are not an accurate reflection of the flora of the tonsillar tissue.[86]

Discrepancies between the surface and core microflora of tonsils have been reported in the past.[86, 87] It is known that deep tonsillar cultures yielded more GABHS and *S. aureus.* Comparison of surface and core cultures in a recent study of 23 chronically inflamed tonsils[88] showed discrepancies between the surface and core cultures in 30% of the aerobic isolates and in 43% of the anaerobic isolates. Although it is impractical to culture the core of the tonsil in patients, these findings indicate that the routine cultures obtained from the surface of the tonsils do not always represent the nature of the bacterial flora of the core of the tonsil, where potential pathogens such as GABHS or anaerobic bacteria may persist. It has been suggested by several investigators that hitherto unrecognized penicillin-sensitive bacteria may be responsible for many cases of nonstreptococcal tonsillitis. The etiologic role of anaerobic bacteria has received little attention.

Microbiology

Reilly and co-workers[89] have obtained swab cultures from the surface of tonsils from 16 children (aged 2–18 years) with clinical diagnosis of acute tonsillitis. Anaerobic bacteria were isolated from 93.7% of these swabs, of which 66.7% contained more than one anaerobic species. *B. melaninogenicus* was the most prevalent anaerobe, present in 100% of specimens yielding an anaerobic flora, and 60% of the isolates were in large numbers.

Other *Bacteroides* species were recovered from 7 of 16 specimens, and a single *Fusobacterium* species was recovered from five swabs. There were two isolates each of *Veillonella parvula* and *Eubacterium* species. A comparison was made between the flora of acutely inflamed tonsils and "healthy" tonsils: over 90% of both groups yielded anaerobic bacteria, but they were present in significant numbers in 56.2% of swabs taken from acutely inflamed tonsils compared with 24% of swabs from "healthy" children. The isolation rates for aerobic pathogens were 37.5% and 16%, respectively.

Two recent studies[89, 90] were conducted to determine the aerobic and anaerobic flora present in the tonsil core of children with recurrent tonsillitis. Since anaerobes are normal inhabitants of the oropharynx, including the surface of the tonsils, cultures taken directly from this area are difficult to interpret. To avoid this problem cultures were obtained in these studies from the core of excised tonsils.

In the first study by Brook, Yocum, and Friedman,[90] tonsils were obtained from 50 children suffering from recurrent tonsillitis. Patients' mean age was six years. Mixed aerobic and anaerobic flora was obtained from all patients, yielding an average of 7.8 isolates (4.1 anaerobes and 3.7 aerobes) per specimen (table 18.8). There were 207 anaerobes isolated. The predominant isolates were 101 *Bacteroides* species (including 10 *B. fragilis* group and 47 *B. melaninogenicus* group), 39 *Fusobacterium* species, 34 Gram-positive anaerobic cocci (25 peptococci and 9 peptostreptococci), and 16 veillonellae. There were 185 aerobic isolates. The predominant isolates were 41 alpha-hemolytic streptococci, 24 *S. aureus*, 19 beta-hemolytic streptococci (11 group A, 4 group

Table 18.8. Predominant Organisms Isolated in 50 Excised Tonsils from Patients with Recurrent Tonsillitis

Aerobic and Facultative	No. of Isolates	Anaerobic	No. of Isolates
Gram-positive cocci		Gram-positive cocci	34
Group A beta-hemolytic streptococci	11		
Group B beta-hemolytic streptococci	4	Gram-negative bacilli	
Group C beta-hemolytic streptococci	2	*Fusobacterium* sp.	39
Group F beta-hemolytic streptococci	2	*B. melaninogenicus* group	47(15*)
S. aureus	24(24*)	*B. oralis*	12(5*)
		B. fragilis group	10(10*)
Gram-negative bacilli *H. influenzae* type B	12(2*)		

SOURCE: Brook, I.; Yocum, P.; and Friedman, E. M. Aerobic and anaerobic bacteria in tonsils of children with recurrent tonsillitis. *Ann. Otol. Rhinol. Laryngol.* 90:262, 1981.
Reprinted by permission.
*Number of organisms producing beta-lactamase.

B, and 2 each groups C and F), 14 *Haemophilus* species (including 12 *H. influenzae* type B) and 5 *H. parainfluenzae*. Beta-lactamase production was noted in 56 isolates recovered from 37 tonsils. These were all isolates of *S. aureus* and *B. fragilis*, 15 of 47 were *B. melaninogenicus* (32%), 5 of 12 were *B. oralis* (42%), and 2 of 12 were *H. influenzae* type B (17%). These findings indicate the polymicrobial aerobic and anaerobic nature of deep tonsillar flora in children with recurrent tonsillitis.

Reilly and associates[89] have also studied tonsils from 41 children with recurrent tonsillitis who were referred for tonsillectomy. Eighty percent of the tonsils contained more than one anaerobic species. Anaerobes were isolated from 100% of the tonsils. There was moderate to heavy anaerobic growth in 75.6% of specimens.

B. melaninogenicus was the most frequently isolated anaerobic bacterium present in 95% of the tonsils examined. In 46% of these specimens, more than one colonial type of *B. melaninogenicus* was detectable, and the majority belonged to the two subspecies *melaninogenicus* and *intermedius*. Of considerable interest was the observation that many of the isolates were resistant to penicillin.

Other indirect evidence of the role of anaerobes in tonsillar infection is the presence of these organisms as the predominant isolate from cases of peritonsillar abscess.[91]

Other anaerobes that may have a role in tonsillar infection are species of *Actinomyces*. Actinomycetes have been cultured on routine oral examination and are part of the normal oral flora. Mucosal disruption is required for the bacteria to become infective.[92] The most common clinical presentation for the cervicofacial actinomycotic infection is a chronic, slowly progressive indurated mass, usually involving the submaxillary gland and frequently occurring after dental extraction or trauma.[18] Several reports acknowledged the presence of actinomycetes in tonsil tissue.[18]

Pathogenesis

It is known that anaerobic bacteria are abundant among the indigenous flora of the oropharynx.[93] Their pathogenic potential is realized in a variety of localized clinical disorders: alveolar abscesses,[94] peritonsillar abscesses,[91] cervical adenitis,[95] otitis media, and mastoiditis.[96]

Preeminent among the anaerobic isolates is *B. melaninogenicus*[89, 90] whose prevalence in the tonsillar habitat was recognized as early as 1921 by Oliver and Wherry.[97] The isolation rate of this species from the gingival crevice seems to be related to age: figures vary from around 20% for children up to 12 or 13 years to 40% for 5- to 7-year-olds.[98, 99]

This fastidious, nonsporulating, Gram-negative anaerobe that is part of the normal oral and vaginal flora has emerged as the predominating *Bacteroides* species isolated from lung abscesses, empyema, and other anaerobic pleuropulmonary infections.[96] *B. melaninogenicus* is commonly isolated from many other sites of anaerobic infection, such as pelvic infections of women[94] and cutaneous abscesses.[100] Furthermore, this organism appears to play a major role in the pathogenesis of periodontal disease.

Of three designated subspecies of *B. melaninogenicus*, subspecies *asaccharolyticus* is the most frequent clinical isolate. Subspecies *intermedius* is identified somewhat less frequently, and subspecies *melaninogenicus* is the least common.[101] These subspecies were recently promoted to species.

In a recent study Brook and associates[102] demonstrated the pathogenicity of organisms belonging to the *B. melaninogenicus* group that were recovered from tonsillar tissue in animal models. The authors were able to induce subcutaneous and intraperitoneal abscesses by inoculating these organisms alone and were able also to correlate the ability to cause an abscess with the presence of a capsule. Encapsulated and abscess-forming organisms belonging to the *B. melaninogenicus* group were recovered in significantly higher numbers in children with acute tonsillitis, as compared to children with uninflamed tonsils.

Although more studies are needed, these findings support the possible pathogenicity of organisms belonging to the *B. melaninogenicus* group in tonsillar infection in children.

Diagnosis

The patients manifest fever, malaise, and pain on swallowing. On examination the tonsils are enlarged, and in anaerobic tonsillitis have ulceration. A foul-smelling discharge frequently has been observed. Vincent[94] has described the classical findings of anaerobic tonsillitis.

At the early stages of the infection, the tonsil is covered with a thin white or gray film that can be detached to leave a bleeding surface. There may be a superficial ulcer underneath the membrane. By the third or fourth day, the pseudomembrane is thick and caseous in appearance and contributes a foul smell to the breath. With anaerobic tonsillitis enlarged submandibular lymph nodes, periadenitis, edema, and even trismus can be noted.

The differential diagnosis includes diphtheria, GABHS infection, viral pharyngitis, and infectious mononucleosis. The most unique features of anaerobic tonsillitis or tonsillopharyngitis are the fetid or foul odor and the presence of fusiform bacilli, spirochetes, and other organisms that have the unique morphology of anaerobes on direct smear of the membrane. It must be remembered that anaerobic tonsillopharyngitis may coexist with other types of tonsillitis.

Management

Penicillin has been the mainstay for treatment of tonsillar infections because of its effectiveness against GABHS. Penicillin is still the drug of choice in patients with tonsillitis and probably is effective in many cases of nonstreptococcal pharyngitis by virtue of its activity against many organisms, including anaerobes. Recently, however, increasing numbers of patients with tonsillar infections have not shown clinical improvement after treatment with this drug.[103] As a final resource, many of these patients are referred for tonsillectomy. Various theories have been offered to explain this treatment failure. Some investigators suggest that penicillin-resistant alpha-hemolytic streptococci appear in patients receiving prophylactic penicillin therapy[104] or that after repeated oral penicillin administration there is a shift in the oral microflora that selects for an increased incidence of beta-lactamase-producing strains of *H. influenzae, S. aureus,* and *Bacteroides* species.[89, 104, 105] It is quite possible that these beta-lactamase-producing organisms can protect the GABHS from penicillin by inactivating the antibiotic.

Anaerobes and Protection of GABHS

B. melaninogenicus and *B. oralis* are Gram-negative anaerobic rods that are part of the normal flora of the human mouth. Strains of both species have been isolated from a variety of human oral infections.[106] Until recently, *B. melaninogenicus* and *B. oralis* were considered to be susceptible to penicillin; however, penicillin-resistant strains have been reported with increasing frequency.[67]

The appearance of penicillin resistance among these two species has important implications for chemotherapy. Many penicillin-resistant bacteria can produce enzymes that degrade penicillins or cephalosporins. Such organisms, present in a localized soft tissue infection, could degrade penicillin in the area of the infection, thereby protecting not only themselves but also penicillin-sensitive associated pathogens. Thus, penicillin therapy directed against a susceptible pathogen might be rendered ineffective by the presence of a penicillinase-producing organism.

The possibility that penicillin-resistant anaerobic bacteria may protect pathogenic organisms has been recently studied.[89] In this study, 74% of the tonsils obtained from patients with recurrent tonsillitis contained beta-lactamase-producing aerobic and anaerobic bacteria. The beta-lactamase-producing anaerobes belonged to the genus *Bacteroides* and included strains of *B. fragilis, B. melaninogenicus,* and *B. oralis.* Many beta-lactamase-producing strains of *Bacteroides* were found to be associated with other infections in the upper respiratory tract. These include chronic otitis and mastoiditis,[96] periodontal and peritonsillar abscesses, and cervical lymphadenitis.[91, 95, 96] These findings may be due to the selective pressure of repeated administration of penicillin to patients with upper respiratory tract infections, including recurrent tonsillitis.

Beta-lactamase-producing anaerobes may "shield" streptococci from the activity of penicillin, thereby contributing to their persistence. The ability of beta-lactamase-producing organisms to protect penicillin-sensitive microorganisms has been demonstrated in vitro. When mixed with cultures of *B. fragilis* the resistance of GABHS to penicillin increased at least 8500-fold. Simon and Sukair[105] have demonstrated the ability of *S. aureus* to protect GABHS from penicillin. These phenomena are demonstrated in figure 18.4. *S. aureus* was quite resistant to penicillin (it grew close to the penicillin disk), while GABHS were very susceptible to it (i.e., growth on the plate was inhibited to a large extent, as is evident by the zone of the beta hemolysis). When these two organisms were plated mixed together (middle plate), however, GABHS were able to grow in close proximity to the penicillin disk, thus showing resistance to the penicillin.

The importance of this phenomenon in vivo was demonstrated by studies of mixed infections of penicillin-resistant and penicillin-susceptible bacteria in rabbits.[102] Subsequently, Hackman and Wilkins[107, 108]

Figure 18.4. Effect of *S. aureus* on the susceptibility of GABHS to penicillin. A 10-unit (6 μg) penicillin G disk is placed in the center of each blood agar plate. Plate on the left: *S. aureus* is resistant to penicillin. Plate on the right: GABHS is susceptible to penicillin. Middle plate: Mixed with *S. aureus*, GABHS is resistant to penicillin.

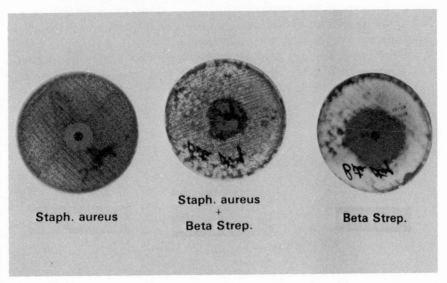

Staph. aureus

Staph. aureus
+
Beta Strep.

Beta Strep.

were able to show that penicillin-resistant strains of *B. fragilis*, *B. melaninogenicus*, and *B. oralis* protected *Fusobacterium necrophorum*, a penicillin-sensitive pathogen, from penicillin therapy in mice.

In recent studies, Brook and co-workers[109] have shown in mice the ability of beta-lactamase-producing strains of *B. fragilis* and *B. melaninogenicus* to protect GABHS from penicillin.

Carriage Elimination of GABHS

Several studies have suggested the possible effectiveness of clindamycin and its parent compound, lincomycin, in the treatment of recurrent streptococcal illness or the streptococcal carrier state.[110, 111] The superiority of these drugs may be due not only to their effectiveness against GABHS but also to the sensitivity of other aerobic and anaerobic organisms that may "protect" the pathogenic streptococci by producing beta-lactamase (such as *S. aureus* and *Bacteroides* species).

Randolph and DeHaan[112] found a a clinical and bacteriological recurrence rate of 13.9% after penicillin treatment as compared to 7.9% after treatment with lincomycin. In a subsequent study Randolph, Redys, and Hibbard[113] reported a 20.8% recurrence rate following penicillin therapy, compared to 6.8% recurrence following clindamycin. Levine and Beman[114] compared clindamycin to erythromycin for treatment of streptococcal infection and found fewer bacteriologic recurrences in the clindamycin group than in the erythromycin group. In another study Breese and colleagues[110] compared lincomycin to penicillin for the eradication of GABHS and found only 16.1% failures in patients treated with lincomycin compared to 41.4% failures in patients treated with penicillin. Massell[111] recently reported a comparative study using clindamycin and penicillin for the prophylaxis of streptococcal infections. Clindamycin was twice as effective as orally administered penicillin for prophylaxis of streptococcal infection.

Brook and Leyva[115] studied 20 children who chronically carried GABHS and had recurrent tonsillitis; they were treated with oral clindamycin for 7 to 10 days. All these patients responded to the therapy and a two-year follow-up showed the elimination of their carrier state for GABHS.

Complications

Peritonsillar abscess, in which anaerobes are the dominant organisms, usually follows acute tonsillitis. Uncommonly, the tonsillar and pharyngeal infection may spread to involve the prevertebral muscles, and this allows a subluxation of the atlantoaxial joint. Other complications of acute tonsillitis may occur because of the size of the tonsils. If the tonsils are very large the child will refuse to swallow solid food. Cor pulmonale can develop following an increase in the size of the inflamed tonsils. Bacteremia and sepsis also can develop following tonsillitis. In a review of the literature from 1925 to 1974 by Finegold[18] more than 200 cases of anaerobic bacteremia and sepsis were preceded with serious tonsillar or nasopharyngeal infection. The organisms most frequently recovered in these cases were *F. nucleatum, Bacteroides* species (including *B. fragilis),* and anaerobic Gram-positive cocci.

In the review of the literature on *Bacteroides* septicemia,[116] nasopharyngeal infection was by far the most common site of the primary lesion in those cases of sepsis present in 54 of 148 reported cases (36%).

The advent of the antimicrobial era had a tremendous impact on this type of infection. While local tonsillar infection still occurs, it is seldom recognized as being due to anaerobes, and the use of antimicrobial therapy has resulted in the prompt response of the infection without later development of the serious complications that were so frequent in the past.

Conclusion

Tonsils can be colonized with various beta-lactamase-producing aerobic and anaerobic organisms. The presence of these organisms in tonsillar tissue of carriers of GABHS may account for failure of treatment of the infection with penicillin. Penicillin therapy could be effective in the therapy of tonsillitis, especially in children who did not develop penicillin-resistant flora after receiving many courses of this drug and should therefore be administered to patients presenting with acute tonsillitis. Data now available suggest that therapy of recurrent tonsillitis, or chronic tonsillitis, should be directed toward the eradication of both the protective organisms and the pathogens.

As more data from in vitro and animal studies accumulate, a logical approach should be found for the eradication of tonsillar and other oral-cavity-associated infections.

Adenotonsillitis

Adenoid tissue arises from the juncture of the roof and posterior wall of the nasopharynx and is composed of vertical ridges of lymphoid tissue separated by deep clefts. It differs from tonsillar tissue in that it contains no crypts, is bounded by no capsule, and is covered by ciliated epithelium. Adenoids are present at birth, continue throughout childhood, and atrophy at puberty, although persistence into adult life is not uncommon. Adenoids probably form part of the body's defense mechanisms against infection.

Adenoids are liable to inflammatory changes and frequently are infected concomitantly with the tonsils. It is, therefore, difficult to differentiate adenoid infection alone from combined infection with the tonsils. Acute adenoiditis may occur alone or in association with rhinitis or tonsillitis. It produces pain behind the nose and postnasal catarrh, lack of resonance of the voice, nasal obstruction, and feeding difficulties in babies, and it is often accompanied by cervical adenitis. Chronic adenoiditis may result from repeated acute attacks or from infection in small adenoid remnants. The main symptom is postnasal drip. This secretion is seen to hang down behind the soft palate as tenacious mucopus.

Adenoid hypertrophy is defined as an enlargement of the adenoids, which may be simple or inflammatory, and the symptoms may be referable to hypertrophy, to infection, or to both. Recurrent adenotonsillitis is defined as a bacterial-viral illness. Microbiologically, these patients carry an abnormal nasopharyngeal and oropharyngeal microflora. Typically, this flora is characterized by the persistent presence of two to five bacterial species that are most frequently associated with clinical infections of the head and neck: group A streptococci, *S. aureus, H. influenzae, S. pneumoniae, Candida albicans,* and the enteric Gram-negative aerobes and anaerobes. The viruses present are adenoviruses and Epstein-Barr virus.[117–119]

The author[120] has compared the bacteria recovered from the core of adenoids obtained from 18 children with chronic adenotonsillitis (group A) and those of 12 children with adenoid hypertrophy and persistent middle ear effusion (group B). The adenoids were sectioned in half after heat searing of the surface, and the core material was cultured for aerobic and anaerobic microorganisms (tables 18.9 and 18.10).

Mixed aerobic and anaerobic flora were obtained from all patients, yielding an average of 7.8 isolates (4.6 anaerobes and 3.2 aerobes) per specimen. There were 97 anaerobes isolated. The predominant isolates in both groups were *Bacteroides* species (including *B. melaninogenicus* and *B. oralis*), *Fusobacterium* species, Gram-positive anaerobic cocci, and *Veillonella* species. There were 138 aerobic isolates. The predominant isolates in both groups were alpha- and gamma-hemolytic streptococci, beta-hemolytic streptococci (groups A, B, C, and F), *S. aureus, S. pneumoniae, Haemophilus* species. *H. influenzae* type B and *S. aureus* were more frequently isolated in group A. *B. fragilis* was recovered only in group A. Beta-lactamase production was noted in 27 isolates obtained from 18 patients. Fifteen (83%) of these patients belonged to group A, while three (25%) were members of group B. These bacteria were all isolates of *S. aureus* (11) and *B. fragilis* (2); 8 of 22 were *B. melaninogenicus*, 4 of 11 were *B. oralis*, and 2 of 8 were *H. influenzae* type B.

Table 18.9. Aerobic and Facultative Organisms Isolated from Excised Adenoids from 18 Children with Chronic Adenotonsillitis (group A) and 12 with Adenoid Hypertrophy (group B)

Isolates	Group A (18 patients)	Group B (12 patients)	Total Number (30 patients)
Gram-positive cocci			
S. pneumoniae	5	4	9
Alpha-hemolytic streptococci	14	9	23
Gamma-hemolytic streptococci	7	5	12
Group A, beta hemolytic streptococci	6	4	10
Group B, beta hemolytic streptococci	2	1	3
Group C, beta hemolytic streptococci		1	1
Group F, beta hemolytic streptococci	1	2	3
S. aureus	9(9*)	2(2*)	11(11*)
Gram-negative cocci			
Neisseria sp.	15	12	27
Gram-positive bacilli			
Lactobacillus sp.	2	3	5
Diphtheroids	7	3	10
Gram-negative bacilli			
H. influenzae type B	7(2*)	1	8(2*)
H. parainfluenzae	3	1	4
E. corrodens	2	1	3
P. aeruginosa	2		2
E. coli	3		3
Yeast			
C. albicans	3	1	4
Total number of aerobes and facultatives	88(11*)	50(2*)	138(13*)

SOURCE: Brook, I. Aerobic and anaerobic bacteriology of adenoids in children: a comparison between patients with chronic adenotonsillitis and adenoid hypertrophy. *Laryngoscope* 9:379, 1980. Reprinted by permission.
*Number of beta-lactamase-producing organisms.

Table 18.10. Anaerobic Organisms Isolated in Excised Adenoids from 18 Children with Adenotonsillitis (group A) and 12 with Adenoid Hypertrophy (group B)

Isolates	Group A (18 patients)	Group B (12 patients)	Total Number (30 patients)
Gram-positive cocci			
Peptococcus sp.	8	5	13
Peptostreptococcus sp.	4	2	6
Gram-negative cocci			
V. parvula	3	2	5
Gram-positive bacilli			
B. adolescentis	1		1
Eubacterium sp.	2	2	4
Actinomyces sp.	2	1	3
Gram-negative bacilli			
Fusobacterium sp.	2	1	3
F. nucleatum	10	6	16
Bacteroides sp.	2	1	3
B. melaninogenicus	1	2	3
B. melaninogenicus ss. *melaninogenicus*	7(4*)	4(1*)	11(5*)
B. melaninogenicus ss. *intermedius*	5(3*)	3	8(3*)
B. oralis	6(3*)	5(1*)	11(4*)
B. ruminicola ss. *brevis*	4	2	6
B. fragilis	2(2*)		2(2*)
B. orchaceus	2		2
Total number of anaerobes	61(12*)	36(2*)	97(14*)
Total number of aerobes, facultatives, and anaerobes	149(23*)	86(4*)	235(27*)

SOURCE: Brook, I. Aerobic and anaerobic bacteriology of adenoids in children: a comparison between patients with chronic adenotonsillitis and adenoid hypertrophy. *Laryngoscope* 9:380, 1980. Reprinted by permission.
*Number of beta-lactamase-producing organisms.

Pathogenesis

As noted by other investigators,[118, 119] the authors have also found *H. influenzae* to be more prevalent in group A; however, the presence of beta-lactamase-producing organisms has been noted in 83% of that group, compared to 25% in group B. Of particular interest is the higher prevalence of *B. fragilis* and the beta-lactamase-producing *B. melaninogenicus* group and *B. oralis* in this group. This could be due to the selective pressure of repeated antimicrobial therapy administered to these patients, which could select these beta-lactamase strains.

The existence of beta-lactamase-producing organisms, many of them anaerobes, within the core of the adenoids may explain the persistence of many pathogenic organisms in that area, where they may be shielded from the activity of the penicillins. The disappearance of these bacteria between episodes of tonsillitis may be only temporary, and their reappearance may be due to their reemergence from the core of adenoids or tonsils. The chronically infected adenoid tissue may also be a factor in the recurrence of middle ear disease by causing Eustachian tube dysfunction and serving as a source for pathogenic organisms.

Clinical Signs and Diagnosis

Mouthbreathing and more or less persistent rhinitis are the most characteristic symptoms. With severe adenoid hypertrophy the mouth is kept open during the day as well as during sleep, and the mucous membranes of the mouth and lips are dry. Chronic nasopharyngitis may be constantly present or recur frequently. The voice is altered, with a nasal, muffled quality. The breath is foul-smelling and frequently offensive, and taste and smell are impaired. A harassing cough may be present, especially at night, resulting from irritation of the larynx by inspired air that has not been warmed and moistened by passage through the nose. Impaired hearing is common. Chronic otitis media may be associated with infected, hypertrophied adenoids and blockage of the Eustachian tube orifices.

Adenoid size can be assessed in the young infant by digital palpation. Fiberoptic bronchoscopy and lateral roentgenogram can assist in evaluating the size of the adenoids.

Management

Adenoidectomy and tonsillectomy frequently are performed to relieve recurrent ear infections and chronic adenoiditis associated with persistent ear effusions in children.[117] Adenoidectomy may be indicated with symptoms such as persistent mouthbreathing, nasal speech, and adenoid facies.

There is no solid data to support adenoidectomy for the treatment of repeated attacks of otitis media, serous otitis media, or recurrent nasopharyngitis. These children usually are treated with multiple courses of antibiotics prior to surgery; however, many continue to harbor pathogenic bacteria in the pharynx.[88, 121, 122]

Various theories were suggested to explain the persistence of these pathogenic organisms in the oropharynx, including appearance of penicillin-resistant alpha-hemolytic streptococci and increased numbers of beta-lactamase-producing organisms such as *S. aureus* and some strains of *H. influenzae*. Removal of the tonsils and adenoids is associated in many instances with a reduction of pathogenic organisms such as GABHS and *S. aureus*.[117]

The isolation of pathogenic beta-lactamase-producing aerobic and anaerobic organisms from chronically inflamed adenoids in children raises the question of whether the therapy of chronic adenotonsillitis is adequate and whether therapy for this infection should be directed also at the eradication of the more prevalent of these potential pathogens.

Although no prospective studies were done of children with adenotonsillitis, when antibiotics such as lincomycin,[123] clindamycin,[113] and oxacillin[105] were administered to patients suffering from chronic recurrent tonsillitis, they were found to be more efficacious than penicillin. This may be due to the effectiveness of those drugs not only against GABHS, but also against other organisms that may "protect" the pathogenic streptococci by producing beta-lactamase.

REFERENCES

1. Mawson, S. R. *Diseases of the ear,* 2nd edition. London: Arnold, 1967, p. 270.

2. Howie, V. M., and Ploussard, J. H. The otitis prone condition. *Am. J. Dis. Child.* 129:675, 1975.

3. Klein, J. O. Middle ear disease in children. *Hosp. Pract.* 11:45, 1976.

4. Coffey, J. D., Jr. Otitis media in the practice of pediatrics: bacteriological and clinical observations. *Pediatrics* 38:25, 1966.

5. Kamme, C.; Lundgren, K.; and March, P.-A. The aetiology of acute otitis media in children. *Scand. J. Infect. Dis.* 3:217, 1971.

6. McLinn, S. E.; Daly, J. F.; and Jones, J. E. Cephalexin monohydrate suspension: treatment of otitis media. *JAMA* 234:171, 1975.

7. Bass, J. W. et al. Ampicillin compared to other antimicrobials in acute otitis media. *JAMA* 202:137, 1967.

8. Schwartz, R. H. et al. The increasing incidence of ampicillin-resistant *Haemophilus influenzae*. A cause of otitis media. *JAMA* 239:320, 1978a.

9. Schwartz, R. H., and Brook, I. Gram-negative rod bacteria as a cause of acute otitis media in children. *Ear Nose Throat J.* 60:9, 1981.

10. Brook, I.; Anthony, B. F.; and Finegold, S. M. Aerobic and anaerobic bacteriology of acute otitis media in children. *J. Pediatr.* 92:13, 1978.

11. Brook, I. Otitis media in children: a prospective study of aerobic and anaerobic bacteriology. *Laryngoscope* 89:992, 1979.

12. Brook, I. A practical technique for tympanocentesis for culturing aerobic and anaerobic bacteria. *Pediatrics* 65:626, 1980.

13. Brook, I., and Schwartz, R. Anaerobic bacteria in acute otitis media. *Acta Otolaryngol.* 91:111, 1981.

14. Brook, I. Microbiological studies of the bacterial flora of the external auditory canal in children. *Acta Otolaryngol.* 91:285, 1981.

15. Dunkle, L. M.; Brotherton, T. J.; and Feigin, R. D. Anaerobic infections in children: a prospective study. *Pediatrics* 57:311, 1976.

16. Everett, E. D.; Eickhoff, T. C.; and Simon, R. H. Cerebrospinal fluid shunt infections with anaerobic diphtheroids. *J. Neurosurg.* 44:580, 1976.

17. Bartlett, J. G., and Finegold, S. M. Anaerobic infections of the lung and pleural space. *Am. Rev. Respir. Dis.* 110:56, 1974.

18. Finegold, S. M. *Anaerobic bacteria in human disease.* New York: Academic Press, 1977.

19. Schwartz, R. H., and Schwartz, O. M. Acute otitis media: diagnosis and drug therapy. *Drugs* 19:107, 1980.

20. Nelson, J. D. et al. Treatment of acute otitis media of infancy with cefactor. *Am. J. Dis. Child.* 132:992, 1978.

21. Syriopoulou, V. et al. Incidence of ampicillin-resistant *Haemophilus influenzae* in otitis media. *J. Pediatr.* 89:838, 1976.

22. Schwartz, R. H. et al. The nasopharyngeal culture in acute otitis media: a reappraisal of its usefulness. *JAMA* 241:2170, 1979.

23. Howard, J. E. et al. Otitis media of infancy and early childhood: a double blind study of four treatment regimens. *Am J. Dis. Child.* 130:965–970, 1976.

24. Teele, D. W., and Klein, J. O. Epidemiology of otitis media during the first two years of life (abstr.). *Pediatr. Res.* 12:385, 1978.

25. Robinson, J. M., and Nicholas, H. O. Catarrhal otitis media with effusion—a disease of a retropharyngeal and lymphatic system. *South. Med. J.* 44:777, 1951.

26. Siirala, U., and Vuori, M. The problem of sterile otitis media. *Prac. Otorhinolaryngol.* 19:159, 1956.

27. Senturia, B. H. et al. Studies concerned with tubo-tympanitis. *Ann. Otol. Rhinol. Laryngol.* 67:440, 1958.

28. Kokko, E. Chronic secretory otitis media in children: a clinical study. *Acta Otolaryngol.* (Suppl.) 327:7, 1974.

29. Healy, G. B., and Teele, D. W. The microbiology of chronic middle ear effusions in children. *Laryngoscope* 87:1472, 1977.

30. Riding, K. H. et al. Microbiology of chronic and recurrent otitis media with effusion. *J. Pediatr.* 93:739, 1978.

31. Liu, Y. et al. Chronic middle ear effusions: immunochemical and bacterial investigation. *Arch. Otolaryngol.* 101:278, 1976.

32. Adlington, P., and Davies, J. E. Virus studies in secretory otitis media. *J. Laryngol. Otol.* 83:161, 1969.

33. Klein, J., and Teele, D. W. Isolation of viruses and mycoplasmas from middle ear effusion: a review. *Ann. Otol. Rhinol. Laryngol.* 85(suppl. 25):140, 1976.

34. Geibink, G. et al. The microbiology of serous and mucoid otitis media. *Pediatrics* 63:915, 1979.

35. Brook, I. et al. The aerobic and anaerobic bacteriology of serous otitis media in children. Submitted for publication.

36. Brook, I., and Finegold, S. M. Bacteriology of chronic otitis media. *JAMA* 241:487, 1979.

37. Bluestone, C. D. et al. Eustachian tube ventilatory function in relation to cleft palate. *Ann. Otol. Rhinol. Laryngol.* 84:333, 1975.

38. Fulghum, R. S.; Daniel, R. J.; and Yarborough, J. G. Anaerobic bacteria in otitis media. *Arch. Otolaryngol.* 103:278, 1977.

39. Jokipii, A. M. M. et al. Anaerobic bacteria in chronic otitis media. *Arch. Otolaryngol.* 103:278, 1977.

40. Brook, I. Chronic otitis media in children: microbiological studies. *Am. J. Dis. Child.* 134:564, 1980.

41. Brook, I. Aerobic and anaerobic bacteriology of cholesteatoma. *Laryngoscope* 91:250, 1981.

42. Liu, Y. S. et al. Microorganisms in chronic otitis media with effusion. *Ann. Otol. Rhinol. Laryngol.* 85:245, 1976.

43. Fernandez, C.; Lindsay, J. R.; and Moskowitz, M. Some observations on the pathogenesis of the middle ear cholesteatoma. *Arch. Otolaryngol.* 69:537, 1952.

44. Juers, A. L. Cholesteatoma genesis. *Arch. Otolaryngol.* 81:5, 1965.

45. Mawson, S. R. *Diseases of the ear*, 3rd edition. Baltimore: Williams & Wilkins, 1975.

46. Brook, I. Bacteriology and treatment of chronic otitis media in children. *Laryngoscope* 89:1129, 1979.

47. Smith, J. M., and Smith, I. M. The medical treatment of sinusitis. *Otolaryngol. Clin. North Am.* 4:39, 1971.

48. Hora, J. F. Primary aspergillosis of the paranasal sinuses and associated areas. *Laryngoscope* 75:768, 1965.

49. Frederick, J., and Braude, A. I. Anaerobic infections of the paranasal sinuses. *N. Engl. J. Med.* 290:135, 1974.

50. Carenfelt, C. et al. Bacteriology of maxillary sinusitis in relation to quality of the retained secretion. *Acta Otolaryngol.* 86:298, 1978.

51. Brook, I. Bacteriologic features of chronic sinusitis in children. *JAMA* 246:967, 1981.

52. Wilson, T. G. Acute rhinitis and sinusitis. In *Diseases of the ear, nose and throat in children*. London: Heinemann, 1962, p. 165.

53. Friedberg, J. Maxillary sinus disease and the pediatric patient. *Otolaryngol. Clin. North Am.* 9(1):163, 1976.

54. Jazbi, B. Subluxation of the nasal septum in newborn; etiology and treatment. *Otolaryngol. Clin. North Am.* 10(1):125, 1977.

55. Kramer, R. Otolaryngologic complications of cystic fibrosis. *Otolaryngol. Clin. North Am.* 10(1):203, 1977.

56. Williams, H. L. The relationship of allergy to chronic sinusitis. *Ann. Allergy* 24:521, 1966.

57. Axelsson, A., and Brorson, J. E. The correlation between bacteriological findings in the nose and maxillary sinus in acute maxillary sinusitis. *Laryngoscope* 83:2003, 1973.

58. Brook, I., and Friedman, E. M. Intracranial complications of sinusitis in children: a sequela of periapical abscess. *Ann. Otol. Rhinol. Laryngol.* 91:41, 1982.

59. Brook, I. Aerobic and anaerobic bacterial flora of normal maxillary sinuses. *Laryngoscope* 91:372, 1981.

60. Aust, R, and Drettner, B. The oxygen exchange through the mucosa of the maxillary sinus. *Rhinology* 12:11, 1974.

61. Carenfelt, C., and Lundberg, C. Purulent and non-purulent maxillary sinus secretions with respect to pO_2, PCO_2 and pH. *Acta Otolaryngol.* 84:138, 1977.

62. Carenfelt, C. Pathogenesis of sinus empyema. *Ann. Otol.* 88:16, 1979.

63. Drettner, B., and Lindholm, C. E. The borderline between acute rhinitis and sinusitis. *Acta Otolaryngol.* 64:508, 1967.

64. Aust, R., and Drettner, B. Oxygen tension in the human maxillary sinus under normal and pathological conditions. *Acta Otolaryngol. (Stockh.)* 78:264, 1974.

65. Reimer, A.; Mereke, U.; and Torlmalm, N. G. Kliniska ciliestudier. *Acta Soc. Med. Suecanae* 84:391, 1975.

66. Sutter, V. L., and Finegold, S. M. Susceptibility of anaerobic bacteria to 23 antimicrobial agents. *Antimicrob. Agents Chemother.* 10:736, 1976.

67. Brook, I.; Calhoun, L.; and Yocum, P. Beta-lactamase-producing isolates of *Bacteroides* species from children. *Antimicrob. Agents Chemother.* 18:164, 1980.

68. Carenfelt, C. et al. Evaluation of the antibiotic effect of treatment of maxillary sinusitis. *Scand. J. Infect. Dis.* 7:259, 1975.

69. Hubert, L. Orbital infection due to nasal sinusitis. *NY State J. Med.* 37:1559, 1937.

70. Blumenfeld, R. J., and Skolnik, E. M. Intracranial complications of sinus disease. *Trans. Am. Acad. Ophthalmol. Otolaryngol.* 70:899, 1966.

71. Brook, I. et al. Complications of sinusitis in children. *Pediatrics* 66:568, 1980.

72. Litton, W. B. Acute and chronic sinusitis. *Otolaryngol. Clin. North Am.* 4:25, 1971.

73. Adams, G. L.; Boies, L. R.; and Paparella, M. M. *Fundamentals of otolaryngology*, 5th edition. Philadelphia: W. B. Saunders, 1978.

74. Bullenger, J. J.; Schull, L. A.; and Smith, W. E. *Bacteroides* meningitis. *Ann. Otol. Rhinol. Laryngol.* 52:895, 1943.

75. Brook, I. Aerobic and anaerobic bacteriology of chronic mastoiditis in children. *Am. J. Dis. Child.* 135:478, 1981.

76. Meyerhoff, W. L., and Gates, G. A. *Pseudomonas* mastoiditis. *Laryngoscope* 87:483, 1977.

77. Fulghum, R. S.; Daniel, H. J.; and Yarborough, J. G. Anaerobic bacterial in otitis media. *Ann. Otol. Rhinol. Laryngol.* 86:196, 1977.

78. Karma, P. et al. Bacteriology of the chronically discharging middle ear. *Acta Otolaryngol.* 86:110, 1978.

79. Ronis, B. J.; Ronis, M. L.; and Liebman, E. P. Acute mastoiditis today. *Eye, Ear, Nose, and Throat Monthly* 47:502, 1968.

80. Rosebury, T. *Microorganisms indigenous to man.* New York: McGraw-Hill, 1966.

81. Swartz, M. N. Anaerobic bacteria in central nervous system infection. *J. Fla. Med. Assoc.* 57:19, 1970.

82. Yoshikawa, T. T.; Chow, A. W.; and Guze, L. B. Role of anaerobic bacteria in subdural empyema: report of four cases and review of 327 cases from the English literature. *Am. J. Med.* 58:99, 1975.

83. Kaufman, D. M.; Miller, M. H.; and Steigbigel, N. H. Subdural empyema: analysis of 17 cases and review of the literature. *Medicine* 54:485, 1975.

84. Drettner, B., and Lindholm, C. E. The borderline between acute rhinitis and sinusitis. *Acta Otolaryngol.* 64:508, 1967.

85. Aust, R., and Drettner, B. Oxygen tension in the human maxillary sinus under normal and pathological conditions. *Acta Otolaryngol. (Stockh.)* 78:264, 1974a.

86. Rosen, G.; Samuel, J.; and Vered, I. Surface tonsillar microflora versus deep tonsillar microflora in recurrent acute tonsillitis. *J. Laryngol. Otol.* 91:911, 1977.

87. Veltri, R. W. et al. Ecological alternatives of oral microflora subsequent to tonsillectomy and adenoidectomy. *J. Laryngol. Otol.* 86:893, 1972.

88. Brook, I.; Yocum, P.; and Shah, K. Surface vs core-tonsillar aerobic and anaerobic flora in recurrent tonsillitis. *JAMA* 244:1696, 1980.

89. Reilly, S. et al. Possible role of the anaerobe in tonsillitis. *J. Clin. Pathol.* 34:542, 1981.

90. Brook, I.; Yocum, P.; and Friedman, E. M. Aerobic and anaerobic bacteria in tonsils of children with recurrent tonsillitis. *Ann. Otol. Rhinol. Laryngol.* 90:261, 1981.

91. Brook, I. Aerobic and anaerobic bacteriology of peritonsillar abscess in children. *Acta Paediatr. Scand.* 70:831, 1981.

92. Bartlett, J. G., and Gorbach, S. Anaerobic infection of head and nose. *Otolaryngol. Clin. North Am.* 9:655, 1976.

93. Socransky, S. S., and Manganiello, S. D. The oral microbiota of man from birth to senility. *J. Pediodontol.* 42:485, 1971.

94. Brook, I.; Grimm, S.; and Keibich, R. B. Bacteriology of acute periapical abscess in children. *J. Endodontics* 7:378, 1981.

95. Brook, I. Aerobic and anaerobic bacteriology of cervical adenitis in children. *Clin. Pediatr.* 19:693, 1980.

96. Brook, I. Anaerobic bacteria in pediatric respiratory disease: progress in diagnosis and treatment. *South Med. J.* 74:719, 1981.

97. Oliver, W. W., and Wherry, W. B. Notes on some bacterial parasites of the human mucous membranes. *J. Infect. Dis.* 28:341, 1921.

98. Kelstrap, J. The incidence of *Bacteroides melaninogenicus* in human gingival sulci, and its prevalence in the oral cavity at different ages. *Periodontics* 4:14, 1966.

99. Bailit, H. L.; Baldwin, D. C.; and Hunt, E. E. The increasing prevalence of gingival *Bacteroides melaninogenicus* with age in children. *Arch. Oral Biol.* 9:435, 1964.

100. Brook, I., and Finegold, S. M. Aerobic and anaerobic bacteriology of cutaneous abscesses in children. *Pediatrics* 67:891, 1981.

101. Holdeman, L. V.; Cato, E. P.; and Moore, W. E. C. Current classification of clinically important anaerobes. In *Anaerobic bacteria: role in disease*, eds. A. Balows et al. Springfield, Ill.: Charles C Thomas, 1974, p. 67.

102. Brook, I. et al. The role of capsule in the pathogenicity of *Bacteroides melaninogenicus* group in subcutaneous and intraperitoneal abscesses in mice. In *Proceedings*, 82nd Annual Conference of the American Society for Microbiology, Atlanta, 1982, p. 818.

103. Ross, P. W. Bacteriological monitoring in penicillin treatment of streptococcal sore throat. *J. Hyg.* 69:355, 1971.

104. Sprunt, E. Penicillin-resistant alpha streptococci in the pharynx of patients given oral penicillin. *Pediatrics* 42:957, 1968.

105. Simon, H. M., and Sukair, W. Staphylococcal antagonism to penicillin group therapy of hemolytic streptococcal pharyngeal infection: effect of oxacillin. *Pediatrics* 31:463, 1968.

106. Takeuchi, H. et al. Oral microorganisms in the gingiva of individuals with periodontal disease. *J. Dent. Res.* 53:132, 1974.

107. Hackman, A. S., and Wilkins, T. D. In vivo protection of *Fusobacterium necrophorum* from penicillin by *Bacteroides fragilis. Antimicrob. Agents Chemother.* 7:698, 1975.

108. Hackman, A., and Wilkins, T. D. Influence of penicillinase production by strains of *Bacteroides melaninogenicus* and *Bacteroides oralis* on penicillin therapy of an experimental mixed anaerobic infection in mice. *Arch. Oral Biol.* 21:385, 1976.

109. Brook, I. et al. In vivo protection of group A beta-hemolytic streptococci by *Bacteroides* sp (abstr. 109). In *Proceedings*, 21st Intersciences Conference on Antimicrobial Agents and Chemotherapy, Chicago, 1981.

110. Breese, B. B.; Disney, F. A.; and Talpey, W. B. Beta-hemolytic streptococcal illness: comparison of lincomycin, ampicillin, and potassium penicillin in treatment. *Am. J. Dis. Child.* 112:21, 1966.

111. Massell, B. F. Prophylaxis of streptococcal infection and rheumatic fever: a comparison of orally administered clindamycin and penicillin. *JAMA* 241:1589, 1979.

112. Randolph, M. F., and DeHaan, R. M. A comparison of lincomycin and penicillin in the treatment of Group A streptococcal infection. *Del. Med. J.* 41:51, 1969.

113. Randolph, M. F.; Redys, J. J.; and Hibbard, E. W. Streptococcal pharyngitis. III. Streptococcal recurrence rates following therapy with penicillin or with clindamycin (7-chlorolincomycin). *Del. Med. J.* 42:87, 1970.

114. Levine, M. K., and Beman, J. D. A comparison of clindamycin and erythromycin in beta-hemolytic streptococcal infections. *J. Med. Assoc. Ga.* 6:108, 1972.

115. Brook, I., and Leyva, F. The treatment of the carrier state of Group A betahemolytic streptococci with clindamycin. *Chemotherapy* 27:360, 1981

116. Gunn, A. A. *Bacteroides* septicemia. *J. R. Coll. Surg. Edinb.* 2:41, 1950.

117. Veltri, R. W. et al. Ecological alterations of oral microflora subsequent to tonsillectomy and adenoidectomy. *J. Laryngol. Otol.* 86:893, 1972.

118. Sprinkle, P. M.; Kirk, B. E.; and Mathias, P. B. *Mycoplasma* species found in naturally occurring adenotonsillitis. *Ann. Otol. Rhinol. Laryngol.* 76:503, 1967.

119. Ruikonen, J.; Sandelin, K.; and Makinen, J. Adenoids and otitis media with effusion. *Ann. Otol.* 88:166, 1979.

120. Brook, I. Aerobic and anaerobic bacteriology of adenoids in children: a comparison between patients with chronic adenotonsillitis and adenoid hypertrophy. *Laryngoscope* 9:377, 1980.

121. Neilson, J. C. Chronic tonsillitis (acute recidivating tonsillitis). Clinical serological and bacteriological examinations. *Acta Otol.* 37:456, 1949.

122. Sprunt, K. et al. Penicillin-resistant alpha streptococci in the pharynx of patients given oral penicillin. *Pediatrics* 42:957, 1968.

123. Breese, B. B. et al. Beta-hemolytic streptococcal infection: comparison of penicillin and lincomycin in the treatment of recurrent infections of the carrier state. *Am. J. Dis. Child.* 117:147, 1969.

CHAPTER 19

Abscesses of the Head and Neck

Tonsillar and Peritonsillar Abscesses

A peritonsillar abscess (or quinsy) occurs much more often in childhood than is generally recognized, but it is seldom diagnosed until tonsillectomy is performed and peritonsillar fibrosis discovered.

Peritonsillar abscess consists of suppuration outside the tonsillar capsule and is situated in the region of the upper pole and involves the soft palate. Infection begins in the intratonsillar fossa, which lies between the upper pole and the body of the tonsil, and eventually extends around the tonsil. A quinsy usually is unilateral; rarely it occurs bilaterally.[1] Bilateral abscess formation is more difficult to diagnose since the classical signs of congestion of the affected side of the palate and edema of the uvula with a shift to the opposite side are absent.

Tonsillar abscess is uncommon and implies an abscess within the tonsil following retention of pus within a follicle to give pain and dysphagia. The tonsil is swollen and inflamed, but the soft palate does not bulge. Treatment is similar to that prescribed for a quinsy.

Microbiology

Group A beta-hemolytic streptococci (GABHS) often are isolated from tonsillar and peritonsillar infections, followed in frequency by *Staphylococcus aureus*, *Streptococcus pneumoniae*, and, rarely, Gram-negative organisms.[2] Anaerobes have been identified in peritonsillar abscess whenever appropriate techniques for their cultivation have been employed.[3] The results of previous studies of the bacteriology of peritonsillar abscess may be misleading owing to lack of appropriate sampling techniques to prevent contamination of specimens by oral flora, the failure to culture adequately for strict anaerobes, and the collection of specimens by swabs rather than by aspiration with a syringe. Finegold[3] provided a thorough review of the literature, summarizing many studies of the bacteriology of peritonsillar abscess. Hansen[4] studied 153 aspirates from peritonsillar abscesses. He recovered 151 strains of anaerobic Gram-negative bacteria, including anaerobic Gram-negative cocci, *Bacteroides funduliformis*, fusiform bacilli, and *Bacteroides fragilis*. Hallander, Flodstrom, and Holmberg[5] isolated anaerobic bacteria from 26 of 30 patients studied. Isolates recovered included *Bacteroides* species, fusobacteria, peptostreptococci, peptococci, microaerophilic cocci, veillonellae, and bifidobacteria. Sprinkle, Veltri, and Kantor[6] recovered anaerobes from four of six individuals with peritonsillar abscess. Anaerobes only were isolated in one instance, and the others yielded mixed aerobic and anaerobic flora. Lodenkämper and Stienen[7] recovered *Bacteroides* organisms from six patients with retrotonsillar abscess, and Baba, Mamiya, and Suzuki[8] recovered anaerobic Gram-positive cocci from four patients.

Several single-case reports described the recovery of anaerobes in peritonsillar abscess. Prevot[9] recovered *Ramibacterium pseudoramosum*. Alston[10] obtained *Bacteroides necrophorus*. Beerens and Tahon-Castel[11] recovered *B. funduliformis* and *Fusiformis fusiformis*. Gruner isolated *Actinomyces* species,[12] and Rubinstein, Onderdonk, and Rahal[23] and Oleske, Starr, and Nahmias[24] isolated fusobacteria.

Aseptic aspiration of peritonsillar abscess (quinsy) performed in 16 children was reported in a recent study.[15] Anaerobes were isolated from all patients. There were 91 anaerobic and 32 aerobic isolates (table 19.1). The predominant isolates were, in descending order of frequency: *Bacteroides melaninogenicus*, anaerobic Gram-positive cocci, *Fusobacterium* species, gamma-hemolytic streptococci, alpha-hemolytic streptococci, group A beta-hemolytic streptococci, *Haemophilus* species, clostridia, and *S. aureus*. Beta-lactamase production was noted in 13 isolates recovered from 11 patients (68%). These included all three isolates of *S. aureus*, eight (35%) of the 23 isolates of *B. melaninogenicus*, and two (40%) of the five isolates of *Bacteroides oralis*.

Pathogenesis

The isolation of anaerobic bacteria mixed with aerobic and facultative organisms from peritonsillar abscess is not surprising since anaerobes are the predominant organisms in the oropharynx, where they outnumber aerobes at a ratio of 10:1.[16] Anaerobic bacteria have also been found to be present in the core of chronically inflamed tonsils.[17] Whether these organisms had any role in the chronic inflammation is not certain, but their presence in the pus obtained from peritonsillar abscess supports their pathogenic role.

Table 19.1. Bacteria Isolated in 16 Children with Peritonsillar Abscesses

Aerobic and Facultative Isolates	No. of Isolates	Anaerobic Isolates	No. of Isolates
Gram-positive cocci (total)	27	Anaerobic cocci	22
Group A beta-hemolytic streptococci	4	Gram-positive bacilli (total)	12
S. aureus	3	Clostridium sp.	3
Gram-negative bacilli (total)	5	Gram-negative bacilli (total)	57
H. influenzae	4	Fusobacterium sp.	15
		Bacteroides sp.	14
		B. melaninogenicus group	23
		B. oralis	5
Total number of aerobes	32	Total number of anaerobes	91

SOURCE: Modified from Brook, I. Aerobic and anaerobic bacteriology of peritonsillar abscess in children. *Acta Paediatr. Scand.* 70:832, 1981. Reprinted by permission.
NOTE: Only the important pathogens are listed in detail. The total number of the groups of organisms is represented.

Diagnosis

Examination may be difficult because the patient can only open his jaws to a slight extent, but with good illumination the affected side of the plate is seen to be congested and bulging. The uvula is edematous and pushed toward the opposite side; the affected tonsil usually is hidden by the swelling but may have some mucopus on its surface. The ipsilateral cervical glands are enlarged and tender.

With the development of a peritonsillar abscess there is acute pain in one side of the throat and a considerable constitutional disturbance. The child may be apprehensive and pale, and the temperature and pulse rate rise, often preceded by a rigor. Pain increases in severity, radiates to the ear and causes trismus. It gives rise to dysphagia, which is aggravated by the swelling, and the voice is muffled. The breath has a foul odor. Saliva may dribble from the mouth because of pain on swallowing. If not relieved either by antibiotics or by surgery the abscess may burst or leak slowly in about a week.

Management

Systemic penicillin antimicrobial therapy should be given in large doses whenever the diagnosis is made. Frank pus forms on about the fifth day, so that if the patient is not seen until then, or if the antibiotic therapy fails to relieve the condition, the abscess must be opened.

If treatment is started within the first 24 to 48 hours following the onset of pain there is every chance of the condition resolving by fibrosis without abscess formation. If the child is not seen until pus has formed then the abscess must be opened. The tonsils should be removed six to eight weeks following a quinsy because of the high frequency of recurrence. A recent report, however, has indicated that this is not always necessary in children.[18] These authors found a recurrence rate of only 7% in children, compared to 16% in adults.

Penicillin G is the drug of choice for the treatment of this infection, but the presence of the beta-lactamase-producing organisms may prevent the resolution of the infection by "protecting" the other organisms.[17] This phenomenon has been observed in patients who received penicillin but show no resolution of infection. Since anaerobic bacteria frequently are associated with quinsy in pediatric patients, physicians should consider their presence when antimicrobial therapy is used. Some anaerobes are resistant to penicillin, and therapy therefore should also include appropriate coverage of such organisms. Although surgical drainage is still the therapy of choice, the presence of penicillin-resistant anaerobic bacteria such as *B. fragilis*[19] and some strains of *B. melaninogenicus*[20] may warrant the administration of appropriate antimicrobial agents such as clindamycin, chloramphenicol, cefoxitin, carbenicillin, ticarcillin, or metronidazole.

Complications

Surgical drainage and antimicrobial therapy of peritonsillar abscesses are essential for the prompt recovery and prevention of complications such as bacteremia, aspiration pneumonia, and lung abscess after spontaneous rupture.

Acute Suppurative Parotitis

The parotid gland is the salivary gland most commonly affected by inflammation. Acute suppurative parotitis may arise from a septic focus in the mouth, such as chronic tonsillitis or dental sepsis, and may be found in patients taking tranquilizer drugs or antihistamines, both of which tend to suppress saliva excretion.

It occurs mostly in elderly persons who are debilitated by systemic illness or previous surgical procedures, although persons of all ages may be affected.[21, 22] Other predisposing factors include dehydration, malnutrition, neoplasms of the oral cavity, tracheostomy, immunosuppression, sialectasis, and medications that diminish salivary flow such as antihistamines and diuretics.[21, 23–25]

Microbiology

S. aureus is by far the most common pathogen associated with acute parotitis; however, streptococci (including *S. pneumoniae*) and Gram-negative bacilli (including *Escherichia coli*) have also been reported.[21, 23, 25] Although anaerobic organisms are commonly isolated from patients with infections around the face, they have seldom been isolated from patients with acute suppurative parotitis or parotid abscess.[3]

Only a few reports describe anaerobic isolates from parotid infections.[26-30] A recent report described the recovery of *B. melaninogenicus* and *Peptostreptococcus micros* from the blood culture of a young adult with acute suppurative parotitis.[31]

There are two reports of recovery of anaerobes from infections of other salivary glands. Bock[32] described a patient with sublingual gland inflammation and a bad taste in the mouth. Numerous spirochetes and a few fusiform bacilli were seen on smears. Baba, Mamiya, and Suzuki[8] obtained a *Peptococcus* in pure culture from a purulent submaxillary gland infection.

Brook and Finegold recently treated two patients with acute suppurative parotitis.[33] In one case, the cultures yielded mixed culture of *B. melaninogenicus* ss. *intermedius* and alpha-hemolytic streptococci. In the other child, no aerobes were recovered and the specimen yielded growth of *Fusobacterium nucleatum* and *Peptostreptococcus intermedius*. Of interest is that both of these patients were institutionalized mentally retarded children, and one had Down's syndrome.

It should be noted that children with Down's syndrome have a striking incidence of severe periodontal disease and have a greater prevalence of *B. melaninogenicus* in the gingival sulcus in comparison with normal children.[34]

Pathogenesis

Although acute parotitis from anaerobic bacteria has not been reported previously, its occurrence should not be surprising. Both clinicopathologic correlations in humans and experimental studies in dogs have shown that bacteria can ascend Stensen's duct from the oral cavity and thus infect the parotid glands.[35] Improved techniques for isolation and identification of anaerobic bacteria have shown that the flora of the mouth is predominantly anaerobic, and normal adults harbor about 10^{11} microorganisms per gram of material in gingival crevices.[36] Saliva contains many genera of anaerobic bacteria, including *Peptostreptococcus, Veillonella, Actinomyces, Propionibacterium, Leptotrichia, Bacteroides,* and *Fusobacterium.*[36] Diminution in salivary flow could allow the ascent of any of the indigenous bacterial flora, thereby triggering acute parotitis.

B. melaninogenicus is the most common *Bacteroides* species found in oral flora and, like *Peptostreptococcus* species, are frequently isolated from odontogenic orofacial infections.[36] The paucity of reports of involvement of such organisms in bacterial infections of the parotid gland probably indicates that anaerobic cultures have not been done, or that inadequate anaerobic transport or culture techniques accounted for failure to recover such organisms.

Diagnosis

Acute suppurative parotitis is characterized by the sudden onset of an indurated, warm, erythematous swelling of the cheek extending to the angle of the jaw. Acute bacterial parotitis usually is unilateral, the gland becomes swollen and tender, and patients frequently have toxemia with marked fever and leukocytosis. The mouth of the parotid duct is red and pouting, and pus may be seen exuding, or may be produced by gentle pressure on the duct. Pus rarely points externally because of the dense fibrous capsule of the gland.

Acute suppurative parotitis should be differentiated from viral parotitis (mumps), which usually is endemic and produces no pus.

Percutaneous aspirates of the inflamed gland is the method of choice for obtaining cultures. Specimens for anaerobic culture should not be taken from Stensen's duct because oropharyngeal contamination is certain.

Management

Most cases respond to antimicrobial therapy; however, some inflamed glands may reach a stage of abscess formation that requires surgical drainage. Broad antimicrobial therapy is indicated to cover all possible aerobic and anaerobic pathogens, including adequate coverage for *S. aureus*, hemolytic streptococci, and anaerobic bacteria.

Penicillin is active against most strains of *B. melaninogenicus*, peptostreptococci, and anaerobic bacteria other than the *B. fragilis* group and would provide additional coverage for *S. aureus*; however, growing resistance to penicillin was recently reported in some strains of *B. melaninogenicus*.[37] Clindamycin or a cephalosporin would be an appropriate alternative drug for patients allergic to penicillin.

Cervical Lymphadenitis

Cervical lymphadenitis is common in children. It is characterized by enlarged, tender lymph nodes in the neck. Usually involved are the anterior cervical, the submandibular nodes, or the posterior cervical nodes. Although many patients without evidence of local inflammation have an infectious cause of the adenopathy, noninfectious causes also should be considered.

Microbiology

Previous studies of the bacterial causes of this infection reported the recovery of aerobic organisms, mainly *S. aureus*[38] and GABHS[39] and, rarely, *S. pneumoniae* and Gram-negative aerobic rods.[39] Other rare causes of infection are atypical mycobacteria,[40] from which *Mycobacterium scrofulaceum*[40, 41] is the most frequently isolated. Cervical lymphadenitis also has been associated with actinomycosis of the jaw,[42] histoplasmosis,[39] cat-scratch fever,[43] infectious mononucleosis, and mumps.

Anaerobic bacteria were isolated rarely.[38, 39] Appropriate methodology for the cultivation and isolation of anaerobic organisms was not used in these studies, however.

Anaerobic bacteria such as *Bacteroides* species[39, 44] and *Peptostreptococcus*[38, 45] have, however, also been isolated from children presenting with this condition. Brook[46] recently studied 53 children who presented with cervical lymphadenitis (table 19.2). Bacterial growth was noted in 45 patients (85%). A total of 66 bacterial isolates (35 aerobes and 31 anaerobes) were recovered. Aerobic organisms alone were recovered from 27 aspirates (60%) of the 45 culture-positive aspirates, anaerobic bacteria alone from 8 (18%), and mixed aerobic and anaerobic bacteria from 9 specimens (20%).

Recovery of these organisms is not surprising, since anaerobic bacteria outnumber aerobic organisms in the oropharynx by 10:1[3] and frequently are recovered from infection adjacent to the oral cavity.[45]

Two previous reports described the recovery of anaerobes from cervical adenitis in children.[39, 45] Barton and Feigin[39] isolated four *Peptostreptococcus* species from 74 children. The microbiological techniques used in that study probably were not optimal for the recovery of anaerobes. Bradford and Plotkin[45] have reported the recovery of anaerobes from two children, one with alpha-hemolytic streptococci, *Bacteroides* species, and *Peptostreptococcus* species and the other with *Bacteroides* species.

Only 15% of the cultures in the Brook study[46] were negative. The large number of sterile lymph node cultures in past studies (24% to 35%) may be due to failure of isolation of fastidious organisms.

Table 19.2. Bacterial Isolates Recovered from 53 Aspirates Obtained from Pediatric Patients with Cervical Lymphadenitis

Aerobic and Facultative Isolates	Number	Anaerobic Isolates	Number
Gram-positive cocci		Gram-positive cocci	
Alpha-hemolytic streptococci	4	*Peptococcus* sp.	6
		Peptostreptococcus sp.	3
Group A beta-hemolytic streptococci	8	Gram-negative cocci	
Group C streptococci	2	*V. parvula*	2
S. aureus	14	Gram-positive bacilli	
S. epidermidis	3	*P. acnes*	5
Gram-negative bacilli		*Bifidobacterium* sp.	2
K. pneumoniae	1	*Lactobacillus* sp.	1
E. coli	2	Gram-negative bacilli	
M. scrofulaceum	1	*F. nucleatum*	4
		Bacteroides sp.	2
		B. melaninogenicus	3
		B. ruminicola ss. *brevis*	1
		B. corrodens	1
		B. asaccharolyticus	1
Total	35	Total	31

SOURCE: Brook, I. Aerobic and anaerobic bacteriology of cervical adenitis in children. *Clin. Pediatr.* 19:694, 1980. Reprinted by permission.

Pathogenesis

Invasion occurs commonly at the site of pharyngitis or tonsillitis. Other entry sites for pyogenic adenitis are periapical dental abscess (usually producing a submandibular adenitis), impetigo of the face, infected acne, or otitis externa (usually producing preauricular adenitis). The problem is most prevalent among preschool children.

The predominant anaerobes recovered were anaerobic Gram-positive cocci and *Bacteroides* species. These organisms are inhabitants of the oral pharyngeal cavity and have been recovered also from various upper and lower respiratory infections.[3] The isolation of these anaerobic and aerobic organisms, all of which are part of the normal mouth flora, from lymph nodes aspirates suggests the oropharynx as the major port of entry into the lymphatic system for these organisms.

No significant correlation was found between the bacteria isolated from cervical lymphadenitis aspirate and the age, sex, history, prior antibiotic therapy, or clinical presentation.[46] The only exception was the presence of a higher prevalence of dental caries and dental abscesses in children from whom anaerobic bacteria were recovered (10 of 17 with anaerobes) than in those with aerobes (3 of 36) ($P<0.05$). This association between anaerobes and dental abscess was observed before.[38]

Diagnosis

The patients generally present with a swollen neck and high fever. The mass is often the size of a walnut or even an egg; it is taut, firm, and exquisitely tender. If left untreated, it may develop an overlying erythema. Each tooth should be examined for a periapical abscess and percussed for tenderness.

The white count usually is about 20,000/cu mm with a shift to the left. A tuberculin skin test should be given and a throat culture obtained.

The differential diagnosis should include evaluation for all other causes of cervical lymphadenitis mentioned, including bacterial (beta-hemolytic streptococci, anaerobes), viral (infectious mononucleosis, mumps) cat-scratch fever, atypical mycobacteria, tumors (sarcoma, leukemia, lymphoma, or Hodgkin's disease), or cysts (thyroglossal or bronchial cleft).

Management

Local heat may be of value for symptomatic relief in mild cases. Penicillin is the drug of choice unless *S. aureus* or resistant anaerobes are suspected. The patient should be referred to a dentist if a periapical abscess is suspected. Analgesics (even codeine) are necessary during the first few days of treatment.

Early treatment with antibiotics prevents most cases of pyogenic adenitis from progressing to suppuration. If there is no improvement within 48 hours and the tuberculin skin test is negative, it can be safely assumed that the infecting organism is penicillin-resistant. Aspiration of the node with an 18-gauge needle and 0.5 ml of normal saline in the syringe to obtain material for Gram's stain and culture may be helpful at this stage. Once fluctuation occurs, however, antibiotic therapy alone is insufficient. When fluctuation or pointing is present, the abscess should be incised and drained.

Since almost all the anaerobes recovered were susceptible to penicillin, it is likely that this drug would be effective in treatment of the infection; however, penicillin resistance recently has been reported in some strains of *B. melaninogenicus*.[20] Moreover, *S. aureus*, the predominant aerobic isolate, usually is resistant to that drug. When aspiration cultures are not available and/or the patient does not respond to therapy, the physician should consider the use of other antimicrobial agents, such as oxacillins, clindamycin, or a cephalosporin.

Acute Suppurative Thyroiditis

Acute suppurative thyroiditis is far less common, particularly in children, than the clinical types of subacute thyroiditis and Hashimoto's thyroiditis. Kirkland and colleagues[47] reported in 1973 that only five cases of this disease in children have been documented in the literature in the English language since 1950.

Microbiology

The aerobic organisms implicated in acute thyroiditis in children include *S. aureus, S. pneumoniae, Klebsiella* species, *H. influenzae,* and *Streptococcus viridans*.[48–50] Anaerobic bacteria such as *Bacteroides* organisms and anaerobic Gram-positive cocci also may cause this infection.[50–52] Abe and colleagues[51] reported two children with recurrent episodes of acute suppurative thyroiditis. Anaerobic bacteria such as *Bacteroides, Peptostreptococcus,* and *Peptococcus* were identified as causative agents. *Eikenella corrodens* (previously named HB-1) is a Gram-negative, facultatively anaerobic or capnophilic rod that occurs as normal flora in the mouth and has been reported also in two cases of thyroiditis in children.[53, 54]

Pathogenesis

Acute suppurative thyroiditis is rare in children, which may reflect resistance of the thyroid gland to local infection.[51, 55] Because the thyroid is encapsulated and without direct communication with neighboring structures, it may also be resistant to infection by direct extension from contiguous organs.[55]

The rarity of acute suppurative thyroiditis may be due to the remarkable degree of local resistance of the thyroid gland to bacterial infection. Live streptococci and staphylococci injected directly into the thyroid gland of dogs are reported to result rarely in suppuration.[56] The relatively high concentration of the iodine within the thyroid gland may provide an unfavorable environment for bacterial growth. Bacteria may reach the thyroid via the bloodstream, the lymphatic system, direct trauma to the gland, direct invasion from neighboring structures, or a thyroglossal cyst or fistula.[55]

The anaerobic bacteria recovered from inflamed thyroid are part of oral flora, and may, therefore, reach the gland in the same fashion as the aerobic pathogens. The recovery of these organisms as the only isolate of inflamed gland suggests that anaerobic bacteria may play an important role in the pathogenesis of acute suppurative thyroiditis, and they indicate the need for clinical awareness of these anaerobic bacteria as potential causes of this disease.

Diagnosis

Suppurative thyroiditis can occur as part of a cellulitis in the neck or because of infection of a cyst in a multinodular goiter. Usually the patient presents with fever, pain in the neck, dysphagia, and a mass involving the thyroid area. The area is erythematous and tender to palpation. Often only one portion of the thyroid is involved, and contiguous infection is evident. The leukocyte count is elevated. The serum thyroxine is normal. On scintiscan there may be some depression of radioiodine uptake in a portion of the thyroid, but radioactive iodine uptake usually is normal. Thyroid function tests show mild increases in T-3 and T-4 caused by hormone release from the inflamed gland.[48, 57, 58]

Lateral soft tissue radiographs of the neck will show evidence of tissue edema, and the tracheal air column may be deviated or compressed. The presence of anaerobic infection may be associated with the presence of soft tissue gas.[52, 57, 59, 60]

Thyroid scanning may not visualize the organ with diffuse inflammation, although "patchy" uptake or a "cold" area may be present with localized or less severe involvement.

Differentiation from other, more common, thyroid conditions can be difficult, especially in the early stage of the disease.[57] Subacute thyroiditis may have similar local signs, but systemic manifestations are not as severe. Leukocytosis may occur but is infrequent and mild in degree. Subacute thyroiditis generally subsides with time, whereas untreated suppurative thyroiditis generally will result in signs of increasing toxicity.[58]

Diagnosis can be facilitated by needle aspiration of the neck mass and Gram stain of the specimen.[48]

Management

An appropriate antibiotic may be selected on the basis of the results of Gram stain of the aspirated pus. Alterations in therapy can be made when final culture and sensitivities are reported. Because of the wide range of different bacteria that can be involved in this infection, a broad coverage of antimicrobial agents is indicated, at least until culture results are available. Most of the anaerobes recovered from this infection are susceptible to penicillin; however, some resistant strains may occur among some of the *Bacteroides* species.

Operative therapy is indicated when antibiotics fail to control sepsis promptly, as evidenced by leukocytosis, continued fever, and progressive signs of local inflammation. In addition, a fluctuant area palpated in the thyroid on physical examination should be incised and drained.[48, 56] Debridement of necrotic tissue should be performed and the wound allowed to heal by secondary intention.

The prognosis following appropriate medical and surgical therapy is excellent. Hypothyroidism rarely occurs and the thyroid function tests return to normal with eradication of infection.[48]

Cervicofacial *Actinomyces* Infection

Actinomycosis is an uncommon chronic bacterial infection characterized by abscesses and sinus tract formation that involve the cervicofacial, thoracic, or abdominal regions.[61] Cervicofacial actinomycosis, the most common clinical form of infection, seldom is encountered in pediatric patients.[62]

Microbiology

Actinomyces israelii is the most prevalent etiologic agent, with occasional instances of human disease attributed to other species such as *Actinomyces viscosum*.[63]

Members of the genus *Actinomyces* are characterized as Gram-positive, branching, filamentous, anaerobic-to-microaerophilic microorganisms. These species contain cell wall constitutents (e.g., muramic acid) that are found in bacterial cell walls and are susceptible to a variety of antibiotics. They are, therefore, considered bacteria rather than fungi.[64]

Special anaerobic techniques are required for culture of the causative microorganisms. Actinomycetes are indigenous to the oral and intestinal microflora, and recovery of the microorganisms from these sites per se does not establish the diagnosis; actinomycotic lesions frequently involve other bacteria that render the primary isolation of *Actinomyces* organisms more difficult.

Pathogenesis

Actinomycosis frequently produces a different type of lesion than is found with other anaerobes causing infection in the same area. Actinomycosis tends to spread along connective tissue planes with little tendency toward ulceration or lymphatic involvement. As part of the inflammatory reaction, there is characteristically produced a very hard fibrosis, and draining sinuses or fistulas are found relatively frequently. Chronic suppuration also is very common. Discrete colonies of the organism are formed in tissues with some frequency. These "sulfur granules" are discharged along with purulent material by way of sinuses.

Diagnosis

Cervicofacial actinomycosis is the most common form of actinomycosis.[65] The lesion generally begins as a painful, indurated swelling a few weeks after dental extraction or trauma to the mouth. The mass is frequently located at the angle of the jaw (lumpy jaw); and suppurates with multiple draining skin sinuses. Sulfur granules may be seen in the exudate. There is little tendency toward ulceration or lymphatic involvement. Osteomyelitis and periostitis of the mandible occasionally may result from direct extension of infection. Direct extension into the orbit or paranasal sinuses also has been described. The overlying skin may become fixed to the inflammatory mass, often with a violaceous discoloration. Poor oral hygiene, dental caries, and minor endoral trauma are the major predisposing conditions. *Actinomyces* species also may cause periodontal disease, lacrimal canaliculitis, and actinomycotic lesions of the tongue.

Exudate and biopsy material should be anaerobically cultured and stained with hematoxylin and eosin. The presence of sulfur granules is highly suggestive of actinomycosis; it is not diagnostic. Similar forms can be seen with other organisms such as aspergilli, Nocardia, and *Coccidioides*.[66]

Management

Penicillin is the drug of choice for treatment of patients with actinomycosis. Erythromycin, clindamycin, minocycline, cephalothin, ampicillin, lincomycin, tetracycline, and chloramphenicol are active also.[67] Actinomycetes generally are resistant to metronidazole. Antimicrobial therapy should be given for two to three weeks beyond subsidence of all clinical signs of the disease. In severe cases, it usually is necessary to continue treatment for several months. Actinomycosis may not always require drainage in order to obtain cure. If large areas are involved, however, surgical excision may be a helpful adjunct to antibiotic therapy. Surgery alone is of little value in achieving complete eradication of the infection.

REFERENCES

1. Brook, I., and Shah, K. Bilateral peritonsillar abscess: an unusual presentation. *South. Med. J.* 74:514, 1981.

2. Adams, G. L.; Boies, L. R.; and Paparella, M. M. *Boies's fundamentals of otolaryngology.* Philadelphia: W. B. Saunders, 1978.

3. Finegold, S. M. *Anaerobic bacteria in human disease.* New York: Academic Press, 1977.

4. Hansen, A. *Nogle undersøgelser over gramnegative aerobe ikke-spore-dannende bacterier isolerede fra peritonsillere abscesser hos mennesker.* Copenhagen: Ejnar Munksgaard, 1950.

5. Hallander, H. O.; Flodstrom, A.; and Holmberg, K. Influence of the collection and transport of specimens on the recovery of bacteria from peritonsillar abscesses. *J. Clin. Microbiol.* 2:504, 1975.

6. Sprinkel, P. M.; Veltri, R. W.; and Kantor, L. M. Abscesses of the head and neck. *Laryngoscope* 84:1143, 1974.

7. Lodenkämper, H., and Stienen, G. Importance and therapy of anaerobic infections. *Antibiotic Medicine* 1:653, 1955.

8. Baba, S.; Mamiya, K.; and Suzuki A. Anaerobic bacteria isolated from otolaryngologic infections. *Jpn. J. Clin. Pathol.* 19 (suppl.):35, 1971.

9. Prévot, A. R. *Biologies des maladies dués aux anaerobies.* Paris: Éditions Medicales Flammarion, 1955.

10. Alston, J. M. Necrobacillosis in Great Britain. *Br. Med. J.* 2:1524, 1955.

11. Beerens, H., and Tahon-Castel, M. *Infections humaines à bactéries anaerobies nontoxigènes.* Brussels: Presses Acad Eur, 1965.

12. Gruner, O. P. N. Actinomyces in tonsillar tissue: a histological study of tonsillectomy material. *Acta Pathol. Microbiol. Scand.* 76:239, 1969.

13. Rubenstein, E.; Onderdonk, A. B.; and Rahal, J., Jr. Peritonsillar infection and bacteremia caused by *Fusobacterium gonidiaformans. J. Pediatr.* 85:673, 1974.

14. Oleske, J. M.; Starr, S. E.; and Nahmias, A. J. Complications of peritonsillar abscess due to *Fusobacterium necrophorum. Pediatrics* 57:570, 1976.

15. Brook, I. Aerobic and anaerobic bacteriology of peritonsillar abscess in children. *Acta Paediatr. Scand.* 70:831, 1981.

16. Rosebury, T. *Microorganisms indigenous to man.* New York: McGraw-Hill, 1966.

17. Brook, I.; Yocum, P.; and Friedman, E. M.; Aerobic and anaerobic bacteria in tonsils of children with recurrent tonsillitis. *Ann. Otol. Rhinol. Laryngol.* 90:261, 1981.

18. Holt, G. R., and Tinsley, P. P., Jr. Peritonsillar abscess in children. *Laryngoscope* 91:1226, 1981.

19. Sutter, V. L., and Finegold, S. M. Susceptibility of anaerobic bacteria to 23 antimicrobial agents. *Antimicrob. Agents Chemother.* 10:736, 1976.

20. Murray, P. R., and Rosenblatt, J. E. Penicillin resistant and penicillinase production in clinical isolates of *Bacteroides melaninogenicus. Antimicrob. Agents Chemother.* 11:605, 1977.

21. Krippaehne, W. W.; Hunt, T. K.; and Dunphy, J. E. Acute suppurative parotitis: a study of 161 cases. *Ann. Surg.* 156:251, 1962.

22. Ragheb, M. Parotid infection caused by dryness of mouth: report of 3 cases after use of tranquilizers. *Geriatrics* 18:627, 1963.

23. Ham, J. M. Acute bacterial parotitis. *Aust. NZ J. Surg.* 32:220, 1963.

24. Kaban, L. B.; Mulliken, J. B.; and Murray, J. E. Sialadenitis in childhood. *Am. J. Surg.* 135:570, 1978.

25. Petersdorf, R. G.; Forsyth, B. R.; and Bernanke, D. Staphylococcal parotitis. *N. Engl. J. Med.* 259:1250, 1958.

26. Shevky, M.; Kohn, C.; and Marshall, M. S. *Bacterium melaninogenicum. J. Lab. Clin. Med.* 19:689, 1934.

27. Heck, W. E., and McNaught, R. C. Periauricular *Bacteroides* infection, probably arising in the parotid. *JAMA* 149:662, 1952.

28. Heinrich, S., and Pulverer, G. Uber den Nachweis des Bacteroides melaninogenicus in Krankheitsprozessen bein Mensch und Teir. *Ztschr. f. Hyg.* 146:331, 1960.

29. Beigelman, P. M., and Rantz, L. A. Clinical significance of *Bacteroides. Arch. Intern. Med.* 84:605, 1949.

30. Coleman, R. M., and Georg, L. K. Comparative pathogenicity of *Actinomyces naeslundii* and *Actinomyces israelii. Appl. Microbiol.* 18:427, 1969.

31. Anthes, W. H.; Blaser, M. J.; and Reller, L. B. Acute suppurative parotitis associated with anaerobic bacteremia. *Am. J. Clin. Pathol.* 75:250, 1981.

32. Bock, E. Ueber isolierte Entzundung der Glandula sublingualis durch Plaut-Vincentsche Infektion. *Munch. Med. Wochenschr.* 85:786, 1938.

33. Brook, I., and Finegold, S. M. Acute suppurative parotitis caused by anaerobic bacteria: report of two cases. *Pediatrics* 62:1019, 1978.

34. Meskin, L. H.; Farsht, E. M.; and Anderson, D. L. Prevalence of *Bacteroides melaninogenicus* in the gingival crevice area of institutionalized trisomy 21 and cerebral palsy patients and normal children. *J. Periodontol.* 39:326, 1968.

35. Berndt, A. L.; Buck, R.; and Buxton, R. L. The pathogenesis of acute suppurative parotitis. *Am. J. Med. Sci.* 182:639, 1931.

36. Chow, A. W.; Roser, S. M.; and Frady, F. A. Orofacial odontogenic infections. *Ann. Intern. Med.* 88:392, 1978.

37. Brook, I.; Calhoun, L.; and Yocum, P. Beta-lactamase-producing isolates of *Bacteroides* species from children. *Antimicrob. Agents Chemother.* 18:164, 1980.

38. Dajini, A. S.; Garcia, R. E.; and Wolinsky, E. Etiology of cervical lymphadenitis in children. *N. Engl. J. Med.* 268:1329, 1963.

39. Barton, L. L., and Feigin, R. D. Childhood cervical lymphadenitis: a reappraisal. *J. Pediatr.* 84:846, 1974.

40. Black, B. G., and Chapmann, J. S. Cervical adenitis in children due to human and unclassified mycobacteria. *Pediatrics* 33:887, 1964.

41. Altman, R. P., and Margileth, A. M. Atypical mycobacterial disease in children. *J. Pediatr. Surg.* 10:419, 1975.

42. Eastridge, C. E. et al. Actinomycosis: a 24-year experience. *South. Med. J.* 65:839, 1972.

43. Margileth, A. M. Cat scratch disease: nonbacterial regional lymphadenitis. The study of 145 patients and a review of the literature. *Pediatrics* 42:803, 1968.

44. Beewokes, H.; Vismans, J.; and Smeets, A. H. *Bacteroides* infections. *Ned. Tijdschr. Geneeskd.* 95:1143, 1951.

45. Bradford, B. J., and Plotkin, S. A. Cervical adenitis caused by anaerobic bacteria. *J. Pediatr.* 89:1060, 1976.

46. Brook, I. Aerobic and anaerobic bacteriology of cervical adenitis in children. *Clin. Pediatr.* 19:963, 1980.

47. Kirkland, R. T. et al. Solitary thyroid nodules in 30 children and report of a child with a thyroid abscess. *Pediatrics* 51:85, 1973.

48. Hazard, J. B. Thyroiditis: a review. *Am. J. Clin. Pathol.* 25:289, 1955.

49. Olambiwonnu, N. D.; Penny, R.; and Frasier, S. D. Thyroid abscess in childhood. *Pediatrics* 52:465, 1973.

50. Taguchi, T. et al. Four cases of acute pyogenic thyroiditis. *Rinsho Shoni Iyaka* 21:213, 1973.

51. Abe, K. et al. Recurrent acute suppurative thyroiditis. *Am. J. Dis. Child.* 132:990, 1978.

52. Bussman, Y. C. et al. Suppurative thyroiditis with gas formation due to mixed anaerobic infection. *J. Pediatr.* 90:321, 1977.

53. Kaplan, J. M.; McCracken, G. H., Jr.; and Nelson, J. D. Infections in children caused by the HB group of bacteria. *J. Pediatr.* 82:398, 1973.

54. Applebaum, P. C., and Cohen, I. T. Thyroid abscess associated with *Eikenella corrodens* in a 7-year-old child. *Clin. Pediatr.* 21:241, 1982.

55. Abe, K. et al. Acute suppurative thyroiditis in children. *J. Pediatr.* 94:912, 1979.

56. Womack, N. A. Thyroiditis. *Surgery* 16:770, 1944.

57. Adler, M. E.; Jordan, G.; and Walter, R. M., Jr. Acute suppurative thyroiditis. *West. J. Med.* 128:165, 1978.

58. Olin, R.; LeBien, W. E.; and Leigh, J. E. Acute suppurative thyroiditis. *Minn. Med.* 56:586, 1973.

59. Gaafar, H., and El-Garem, F. Acute thyroiditis with gas formation. *J. Laryngol.* 89:323, 1975.

60. Alteimeier, W. A. Acute pyogenic thyroiditis. *Arch. Surg.* 61:76, 1950.

61. Georg, L. K. et al. A new pathogenic anaerobic *Actinomyces* species. *J. Infect. Dis.* 115:88, 1965.

62. Drake, D. P., and Holt, R. J. Childhood actinomycosis—report of three recent cases. *Arch. Dis. Child.* 51:979, 1976.

63. Larsen, J. et al. Cervicofacial *Actinomyces viscosum* infection. *J. Pediatr.* 93:797, 1978.

64. Harvey, J. C.; Cantrell, J. R.; and Fisher, A. M. Actinomycosis: its recognition and treatment. *Ann. Intern. Med.* 46:868, 1957.

65. Leafstedt, S. W., and Gleeson, R. M. Cervicofacial actinomycosis. *Am. J. Surg.* 130:496, 1975.

66. Graybill, J. R., and Silverman, B. D. Sulfur granules. Second thoughts. *Arch. Intern. Med.* 123:430, 1969.

67. Lerner, P. I. Susceptibility of pathogenic actinomycetes to antimicrobial compounds. *Antimicrob. Agents Chemother.* 5:302, 1974.

Anaerobic Pulmonary Infections

Aspiration Pneumonia and Lung Abscess

Aspiration pneumonia is common in pediatric patients who tend to aspirate because of debilitation, tracheoesophageal malformations, central nervous system disorders, and altered consciousness. The management of aspiration pneumonia in children has been complicated by the scarcity of information concerning the bacteria involved in those infections. This relates to failure to obtain reliable specimens for culture.

The bacteriology of aspiration pneumonia in adults has been extensively studied recently, with the use of transtracheal aspiration (TTA) to bypass normal oral flora.[1, 2] Anaerobic organisms were isolated from most cases of aspiration pneumonia in adults, but mixed infection with aerobic and anaerobic organisms was common with aspiration in the hospital setting.

This section is devoted to the different types of childhood anaerobic pulmonary infections that usually develop following aspiration. The use of the term *aspiration pneumonia* has led to some confusion. There are four major clinical pictures associated with aspiration: aspiration of particulate matter, chemical pneumonitis (from gastric contents, chemicals, etc.), infectious pneumonitis, and drowning.

Microbiology

For more than 50 years, anaerobic microorganisms have been known to play a role in lung abscess.[3, 4] The organisms recovered in these studies included anaerobic or microaerophilic streptococci, *Bacteroides melaninogenicus*, *Fusobacterium* species, *Clostridium ramosum*, and *Bacte-*

Table 20.1. Analysis of the Clinical and Radiologic Features of 74 Pediatric Patients with Aspiration Pneumonia

Findings	Total	No. of Patients		
		Pneumonitis (52)	Necrotizing Pneumonia (12)	Lung Abscess (10)
Clinical features				
Mean age, years	8.25	7.33	9.81	9.33
underlying conditions				
altered consciousness	42	31	8	3
dysphagia	25	15	8	2
seizure disorder	32	20	4	8
periodontal disease	48	33	9	6
observed aspiration	44	28	9	7
peak peripheral WBC count	17,460	14,200	18,800	22,860
mean peak temperature	103.1	102.8	103.9	103.8
putrid sputum	28	15	7	6
duration of symptoms prior to presentation (days) 1 day	30	29	1	—
1–3 days	25	13	6	6
≥4 days	9	—	5	4
Roentgenographic findings				
Location of lesions				
Right upper lobe				
anterior segment	4	2	1	1
posterior segment	18	9	4	5
Right middle lobe	8	7	1	
Right lower lobe superior segment	9	5	2	2
basilar segments	25	23	2	
Left upper lobe apical posterior segment	12	10	1	1
Left lower lobe superior segment	9	3	4	2
basilar segments	24	21	3	
Length of therapy (days)	18.4	11.4	34	30.2
Response to therapy				
Duration of fever (days)	4.0	2.8	8.2	5.2
Time for roentgenologic clearance (days)	20	13	41	31

SOURCE: Brook, I., and Finegold, S. M. Bacteriology of aspiration pneumonia in children. *Pediatrics* 65:1115–1120, 1980. Copyright 1980, American Academy of Pediatrics. Reprinted by permission.

roides fragilis. Most later reports dealing with the bacteriology of lung infections have based their findings on aerobic culture of expectorated sputum. Recent studies involving adult patients and using the TTA method show anaerobes in 70% to 90% of cases of pneumonitis, necrotizing pneumonia, and lung abscess.[1, 5] Anaerobes, either alone or in combination with aerobes,[6] have been recovered from approximately 30% of lung abscesses. The anaerobes most frequently isolated are *B. melaninogenicus, Fusobacterium nucleatum,* anaerobic Gram-positive cocci, microaerophilic streptococci, and *B. fragilis* (which can be found in 10% to 20% of the patients). The major aerobic pathogens that are usually isolated mixed with anaerobic bacteria are *Staphylococcus aureus, Klebsiella pneumoniae,* and *Pseudomonas aeruginosa.*[5]

Using TTA, Brook and Finegold[8] recently evaluated 74 institutionalized children suffering from aspiration pneumonia.[7] There were 52 patients with pneumonitis, 12 with necrotizing pneumonia, and 10 with lung abscess (table 20.1). Anaerobes were present in 90%. There was no difference in the quantity of isolates recovered among these three groups, and the tracheal aspirate cultures yielded an average of 4.9 organisms per patient (2.7 anaerobes and 2.2 aerobes). The predominant anaerobic isolates were Gram-positive cocci, *B. melaninogenicus,* and *Fusobacterium* species. Ten patients yielded members of *B. fragilis* group. The predominant aerobic bacteria were alpha-hemolytic streptococci, *P. aeruginosa, Streptococcus pneumoniae, Escherichia coli, K. pneumoniae,* and *S. aureus.*

No correlation between the patient's age and the isolation of most anaerobic bacteria was detected, with the exception of fusobacteria and Gram-negative enteric rods, which were more frequently isolated in children younger than 4 years, and *B. fragilis* group, which was absent in children younger than two years (tables 20.2–20.4).

The organisms involved in aspiration pneumonia in children are similar to those found in adults. *B. fragilis,* which was isolated in 14% of patients, is rarely isolated from the oropharynx,[8, 9] but was isolated from 10% to 20% of adults with aspiration pneumonia. Since most of the patients studied had poor oral hygiene, this organism might have colonized their upper respiratory tract.[8]

Pathogenesis

A breakdown of the normal host protective mechanisms predisposes to anaerobic infection and is the common denominator of pulmonary infection. Specific predisposing conditions include reduced levels of consciousness, dysphagia, alcoholism, seizure disorders, general anesthesia, cerebrovascular accidents, esophageal disease, nasogastric tube feeding, and drug addiction. All of the patients studied were institutionalized children who had convulsive disorders, chronic neurologic

Table 20.2. Aerobic Bacterial Isolates from 94 Patients with Aspiration Pneumonia

	Patient Age (Years) No. Patients					Total Pediatric Patients	Total Patients
Aerobic Isolates:	0–1	2–5	6–11	12–18	>18		
	10	24	12	28	20	74	94
Gram-positive cocci							
S. pneumoniae	5	5	4	6	3	20	23
Alpha-hemolytic streptococci	3	11	5	11	10	30	40
Group A beta-hemolytic streptococci		5	3	1	1	9	10
Non-group A beta-hemolytic streptococci				2		2	2
S. aureus		7	1	3	1	11	12
S. epidermidis	3	4	3	3	3	13	16
Gram-negative bacilli							
Proteus sp.		1	1	1	2	3	5
P. aeruginosa	5	11	5	5	5	26	31
K. pneumoniae	2	8	3	3	5	16	21
E. coli	3	9	2	3	2	17	19
S. marcescens		1		5	5	6	11
Citrobacter sp.					1		1
Enterobacter sp.		1		1		4	5
H. influenzae		2	2			3	3
H. parainfluenzae	1	1	1	2	1	4	5
E. corrodens	1			1		2	2
Candida sp.				1		1	1
Total no. of patients with no aerobes				3	1	3	4
Total no. of aerobic isolates	23	66	30	48	40	167	207
Aerobes per specimen	2.3	2.8	2.5	1.6	2.0	2.2	2.2
Total no. of bacteria	48	129	59	129	109	365	474
Bacteria per specimen	4.8	5.4	4.9	4.6	5.4	4.9	5.0

Source: Brook, I., and Finegold, S. M. Bacteriology of aspiration pneumonia in children. *Pediatrics* 65:1115–1120. 1980. Copyright 1980, American Academy of Pediatrics. Reprinted by permission.

Table 20.3. Anaerobic Bacterial Isolates from 94 Patients with Aspiration Pneumonia

Anaerobic Isolates	Patient Age (Years) No. Patients					Total Pediatric Patients	Total Patients
	0–1	2–5	6–11	12–18	>18		
	10	24	12	28	20	74	94
Anaerobic cocci							
Peptococcus sp.	3	11	8	15	10	37	47
Peptostreptococcus sp.	2	9	1	13	8	25	33
Veillonella sp.	3	4	2	3	2	12	14
Microaerophilic streptococci		1		1		2	2
Gram-positive bacilli							
Bifidobacterium sp.	1		1	1	1	3	4
P. acnes	1			3	3	4	7
Eubacterium sp.				1	1	1	2
Lactobacillus sp.	1	4		3	1	8	9
Leptotrichia sp.				1		1	1
Actinomyces sp.	2				1	2	3
Clostridium sp.				1		1	1
Gram-negative bacilli							
F. nucleatum	4	8		11	8	23	31
F. mortiferum		1			1	1	2
B. melaninogenicus	4	10	8	17	12	39	51
B. corrodens		3		5	4	8	12
B. ruminicola ss. brevis	1	2	1	1	2	5	7
B. oralis	2	4	1	2	5	9	14
Bacteroides sp.	1	2	1	4	1	8	9
B. fragilis ⎫		1	1		1	2	3
B. vulgatus ⎬ B. fragilis group		2	4		2	6	8
B. distasonis ⎭		1	1		5	2	7
Total no. of anaerobic isolates	25	63	29	82	68	199	267
No. of patients with no anaerobes	2		1	2		5	5
No. anaerobes per specimen	2.5	2.6	2.4	3.0	3.4	2.7	2.8

Source: Brook, I., and Finegold, S. M. Bacteriology of aspiration pneumonia in children. *Pediatrics* 65:1115–1120, 1980. Copyright 1980, American Academy of Pediatrics. Reprinted by permission.

Table 20.4. Bacteriologic Results in 10 Cases of Lung Abscess

Aerobic and Facultative Isolates	No. of Patients	Anaerobic Isolates	No. of Patients
Gram-positive cocci		Cocci	
S. pneumoniae	2	Peptococcus sp.	5
Group A β-hemolytic streptococci	4	Peptostreptococcus sp.	8
		Veillonella sp.	3
Alpha-hemolytic streptococci	5	Microaerophilic streptococci	1
Group D streptococci	1		
S. aureus	1	Gram-positive bacilli	
		Bifidobacterium sp.	2
Gram-negative bacilli		Actinomyces sp.	1
E. coli	4		
K. pneumoniae	4	Gram-negative bacilli	
P. aeruginosa	2	F. nucleatum	2
S. marcescens	1	B. melaninogenicus	6
E. corrodens	1	B. oralis	1
		B. corrodens	1
		B. fragilis	1
		B. distasonis	1
		B. vulgatus	1
		B. ruminicola ss. brevis	2
		Bacteroides sp.	2
Total	25	Total	37

SOURCE: Brook, I., and Finegold, S. M. Bacteriology and therapy of lung abscess in children. *J. Pediatr.* 94:10, 1979. Reprinted by permission.

conditions, and regurgitation. All of these predisposing conditions have been observed in adult patients in the past.[1] Poor oral hygiene, gingivitis, and periodontitis were common in these patients; diphenylhydantoin contributed to poor oral hygiene in some (table 20.1).

Pneumonitis

Most anaerobic pulmonary infections occur in patients with a clinical condition that predisposes to aspiration.[1] Since human saliva and oropharyngeal secretions contain many anaerobic bacteria,[10, 11] their aspiration may contaminate the lower respiratory tract. The anaerobic infection that usually occurs after aspiration of oropharyngeal secretion into a dependent segment of the lung commences as pneumonitis with relatively mild symptoms. If untreated, liquification and abscess formation occur within 7 to 14 days.

Necrotizing Pneumonia and Lung Abscess

Characterized by necrosis, this suppurative infection creates numerous small cavities or abscesses (less than 2 cm in diameter) in the lung. Initially, it usually is limited to a single pulmonary segment or lobe, but it may progress rapidly to other lobes. Necrotizing pneumonia may progress to lung abscess, defined as a cavity larger than 2 cm in diameter.

The initial lesion following aspiration is pneumonitis without distinctive features except for the predisposition to aspiration, a relatively insidious onset in many patients, and involvement of dependent segments of the lung. After a week to 10 days, tissue necrosis leading to abscess formation or empyema occurs in many patients. Excavation may lead to solitary lung abscess or multiple small areas of necrosis of the lung, with or without air-fluid levels (necrotizing pneumonia). Following cavitation, putrid discharge may be noted in 50% or more of patients. The severity of the illness varies considerably. Patients with acute necrotizing pneumonia are often quite ill, however. The course is relatively prolonged. Patients with only parenchymal disease require an average of three to eight weeks for complete cure. A much longer time—perhaps four to five months—is required for cases with empyema.

Diagnosis

The Use of Transtracheal Aspiration

Therapeutic decisions involving the use of antibiotics are best made with the identification of specific organisms causing the infection. The selection of antimicrobial agents for the treatment of pneumonia in children is largely based on age, history, physical and radiographic findings, and by recovering an organism from the blood or pleural space. Nasopharyngeal or sputum aspirates cannot provide reliable specimens for the identification of pathogens causing this disease since the samples so obtained are contaminated by bacteria present in the oropharynx.[1] Attempts have been made to avoid such contamination by sampling the lower respiratory tract by direct lung puncture,[12, 13] bronchoscopy,[14] repeated washing of the expectorated sputum,[16] or by quantitative culture of the sputum[16]; however, contamination of the specimen by oropharyngeal organisms can occur with all of these techniques, except the direct lung puncture.

Transtracheal aspiration (TTA) (fig. 20.1) has been used for the diagnosis of pneumonia in adults since 1959.[17] It is a relatively safe and reliable means of diagnosing pneumonias caused by aerobic or anaerobic organisms in adult[1, 18] and pediatric[19, 20] patients.

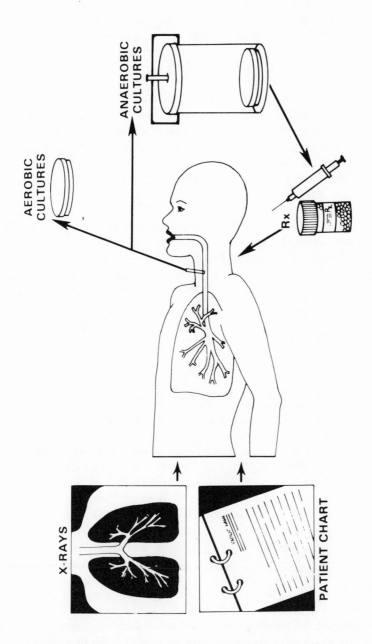

Figure 20.1. Use of transtracheal aspiration in the diagnosis of pneumonia.

TTA has been a relatively safe technique in children, providing valuable information for selection of appropriate antimicrobial therapy.[20] This procedure should, however, be performed by an experienced person and only when the benefit derived from the information is likely to outweigh the potential risks.

Caution is advised also in selection of patients for the procedure. TTA is contraindicated in uncooperative patients and in those who have bleeding diatheses, severe coughing, and serious dyspnea and hypoxemia requiring positive pressure ventilatory aid.[21] The last group of patients is at higher risk for developing mediastinal emphysema. Special consideration should also be given to performing TTA on infants in respiratory distress, since introduction of the catheter can further compromise the small airway and increase the cyanosis in such patients.

The Gram stain of TTA specimens provided immediate tentative information about the causative organisms in more than 90% of patients treated by Brook and Finegold.[22] It is recommended that all TTA specimens be Gram stained. This technique provides a presumptive diagnosis and a guide to initial therapy, indicates the validity of the specimen, and permits an evaluation of culture technique. If large, squamous epithelial cells are present, accidental passage of the catheter into the oropharynx or aspiration during the procedure should be suspected.

Indications of Anaerobic Lung Infection

Important clues to the diagnosis of anaerobic lung infection are observed aspiration or predisposition to aspiration; disease in a dependent segment; cavitation or abscess formation, with or without empyema; foul-smelling sputum or empyema fluid; and distinctive microscopic morphology of organisms from empyema fluid, transtracheal aspirate, or other source free of normal flora. Discharges with foul odors are definitive evidence of involvement of anaerobes in the infective process. The absence of such odor does not exclude this possibility, however, since the odor appears only after cavitation or abscess formation has taken place, and certain organisms, particularly microaerophils and some anaerobic cocci, may not produce an odor.

Conditions that predispose to aspiration are present in many children with aspiration pneumonia (table 20.4), and include periodontitis, altered or compromised consciousness, seizure disorder, and dysphagia. An incident of aspiration can be observed in two-thirds of the patients.

In the group of 74 children studied,[7, 22] the location of the parenchymal involvement was the basilar segments of the lower lobes in 49 patients, the posterior segment of the upper lobe in 30 patients, and the superior segments of the lower lobes in 18 patients (table 20.1). The posterior segments of the upper lobes were the most commonly involved in these patients, undoubtedly owing to the recumbent position (in which most of the patients lie) of the dependent segments.

The duration of the pulmonary symptoms prior to the diagnosis was less than one day in 30 patients, one to three days in 25 patients, and 4 to 13 days in 9 patients. Foul-smelling sputum was noted in 28 patients. There was no association, however, between the presence of foul-smelling sputum and the isolation of any organism or combination of organism. The mean peak temperature was 103.1°F, and the mean peak peripheral white blood cell (WBC) count was 17,460/cu mm (range 6200 to 38,000). Blood cultures were obtained from 15 patients, and all were negative.

The patients generally presented with a fairly sudden onset of rapidly rising fever, chills, rapid respiration, cough, vomiting and diarrhea, and abdominal distention. The onset of disease is sometimes much more insidious than acute pneumonia. Weeks to months of malaise, low-grade fever, and cough, with significant weight loss and anemia, may precede consolidation. Examination may reveal dyspnea with frequent expiratory grunts, dilated nostrils during respiration, flushed cheeks, cyanosis (occasionally), dullness, diminished breath sounds, rales, and prolonged expiration phase. Chest x-rays that localize a pneumonic process to a posterior upper lobe or superior lower lobe segment should suggest the possibility of a lung abscess. The demonstration of a cavitation with air-fluid level establishes the diagnosis.

Management

Antimicrobial therapy is of utmost importance in treatment. Prolonged therapy is important to prevent relapse; the actual duration of treatment can vary and must be individualized, but periods of more than two months may be required.

Therapy for anaerobic pleuropulmonary infection generally is prolonged to prevent relapse. In the uncomplicated case, therapy should continue until the patient has clinically improved, has been afebrile for five to seven days, and has shown improvement on chest roentgenogram. It is important to remember that radiographic changes can lag up to 10 days behind clinical improvement.

In addition to effective antimicrobial therapy, anaerobic pleuropulmonary infections may require drainage. Since lung abscess and necrotizing pneumonitis can drain spontaneously through postural drainage, surgical evacuation is not necessary if diagnosis is made early and appropriate therapy is instituted.[22, 23] Bronchoscopy may be helpful in relieving obstruction by carcinoma or foreign body, but prolonged antimicrobial therapy is usually necessary.

Antimicrobial therapy may be guided by Gram stain of appropriate material, but should not be withheld pending culture results in severely ill patients. Parenteral penicillin G is still the drug of choice in almost all anaerobic pleuropulmonary infections, since most of the anaerobes isolated, with the exception of *B. fragilis* group and some strains of *B. melaninogenicus*,[24] are highly sensitive to penicillin.

Whether the presence of *B. fragilis*,[1, 7] which is resistant to penicillin, should alter the therapeutic approach is undetermined. This question was addressed in the study[22, 23] of 74 patients who received either penicillin G, carbenicillin, or clindamycin. It is important to note that although patient selection was not randomized, the study in children confirms findings in adults,[1, 25] showing penicillin G to be efficacious in the treatment of anaerobic pleuropulmonary infections, even when the *B. fragilis* group is isolated. It should be noted that a recent study showed clindamycin (which is more effective against beta-lactamase-producing anaerobes) to be more effective than penicillin in the treatment of lung abscesses in adults.[26]

There is, however, some difference in the rate of recovery depending on the type of pulmonary involvement. Brook[23] observed that patients with necrotizing pneumonia and lung abscess needed longer courses of therapy (mean 28 days) than those with pneumonitis (mean 15 days). Penicillin G is effective in the treatment of pleuropulmonary infections even when the *B. fragilis* group isolated is mixed with other aerobic and anaerobic bacteria in adults[1, 6, 25] and pediatric patients.[23] It is possible that eradication of other bacteria enhances the clearance of the *B. fragilis* group by the body defense mechanisms.

Clindamycin is an effective alternative to penicillin in the treatment of anaerobic pleuropulmonary infections.[27] It is also effective against various aerobic organisms, including *S. aureus*. Carbenicillin is an effective agent against many anaerobic organisms, including *B. fragilis*, and has been successfully used in the treatment of aspiration pneumonia in children.[28] It is also active against many aerobic Gram-negative rods and may be synergistic with aminoglycosides against many of them. This factor should be considered when such organisms, especially *Pseudomonas*, are recovered.

Although no statistically significant difference was noted between the three modes of therapy among the pediatric patients studied,[23] consideration should be given to the choice of therapy directed against these penicillin-resistant anaerobic organisms in seriously ill patients. This requires use of agents such as clindamycin, carbenicillin, cefoxitin, chloramphenicol, or metronidazole. The choice of antibiotics and the addition of an aminoglycoside should be based on results of the Gram stain, the culture growth, and clinical judgment.

Although the reading of direct Gram stain of the transtracheal aspirate may be misleading, it allows the clinician to suspect the presence of aerobic Gram-negative enteric organisms and to initiate appropriate therapy without delay. When culture result is available, confirmation of the preliminary Gram stain can be done, and therapy can be modified when indicated.

Gentamicin is an appropriate agent for the treatment of most Gram-negative infections and should be added to the agents directed against the anaerobes when Gram-negative enteric rods are present. Emergence of resistance to gentamicin has been a concern in recent years, however.[29] Other aminoglycosides such as amikacin[30] or tobramycin[31] are also available for the treatment of such infections. Carbenicillin or ticarcillin also are active and possess synergistic qualities with aminoglycosides against many of these organisms, especially *P. aeruginosa.*[32]

Infections with Cystic Fibrosis

The bacteria most often isolated from children suffering from cystic fibrosis are *P. aeruginosa* and *S. aureus.* Studies to identify anaerobic bacteria in the lower respiratory tract of patients with cystic fibrosis have not been reported. Since anaerobic organisms recently were recovered from children with aspiration pneumonia by TTA, an attempt to isolate these organisms from children with cystic fibrosis was warranted. Expectorated sputum or pharyngeal swab are generally contaminated by the mouth flora, and therefore are unreliable representatives of the flora of the lower respiratory tract. Anaerobes that are part of the normal mouth flora cannot be identified by these techniques.[1] It is, therefore, imperative to employ techniques that bypass the normal mouth flora when anaerobic bacteria are to be identified.

Use of TTA for the diagnosis of pulmonary infection in children is not as common as its use in adults.[18] Several investigators[7, 19] have used it in the past, however. In 1973 Baran and Cordier[19] used TTA for the identification of infecting organisms in children with cystic fibrosis and met no major complications. This study reported a good correlation between the organisms isolated in the sputum and TTA in patients with cystic fibrosis, although anaerobic culture techniques were not employed in this study.

Brook and Finegold[7] have performed TTA in 74 pediatric and 20 adult patients with aspiration pneumonia and encountered a complication (subcutaneous emphysema) in only one child. Performing this procedure in those patients permitted isolation of the infecting organisms in 92 of the 94 patients. Reliance on sputum cultures alone could be misleading, since they do not always indicate the bacteria present below the cricothyroid membrane.[20]

TTA was used recently in a small study of the diagnosis of pulmonary infection, also in children with cystic fibrosis.[33] Six transtracheal aspirations and expectorated sputum specimens were collected from four children suffering from cystic fibrosis who had pulmonary infection. Specimens obtained from both sites were cultured for aerobic bacteria, and TTA aspirates were also cultured for anaerobes. Differences in bacteria isolated in TTA and sputum aspirates were present in all instances. Six isolates were recovered from both sites (three *P. aeruginosa,* two *S. aureus* and one *Aspergillus flavus*). Five aerobic isolates were recovered only from the expectorated sputum and from TTA aspirates (two *K. pneumoniae* and one each of *P. aeruginosa, E. coli* and *Proteus mirabilis*). Nine organisms were isolated only from the TTA (two each of *Veillonella parvula* and alpha-hemolytic streptococci, and one each of *B. fragilis, B. melaninogenicus, Lactobacillus* species, *Haemophilus influenzae* and gamma-hemolytic streptococci). The recovery of anaerobic organisms from four of the six TTA specimens suggests a possible role for these organisms in the etiology of pulmonary infection in cystic fibrosis.

Although the number of the patients with cystic fibrosis studied so far is small, a few conclusions can be drawn relating to the efficacy of TTA in the diagnosis and management of pulmonary infection in these patients. It is evident that a discrepancy existed between the bacteria recovered from the expectorated sputum and those recovered by TTA in the six transtracheal aspirations performed. Since the pathogen recovered from transtracheal aspirate more accurately represents the organisms present below the cricothyroid membrane, the therapy administered to the patients was directed only against these isolates.

Transtracheal aspirations prevented the use of unnecessary and potentially toxic antimicrobial agents in many patients who had a number of potential pathogens in their expectorated sputum but not in the transtracheal aspirates. In other instances, the results of the TTA prompted specific therapy directed against organisms that otherwise would not have been treated optimally, since they either had been not isolated in the sputum, or if recovered, would have been considered to be contaminants.

In four instances, TTA also confirmed the presence of various anaerobic bacteria in the tracheal secretions. Since anaerobic organisms are part of the normal oropharyngeal flora and would, therefore, contaminate any expectorated sputum specimen, the TTA specimen was adequate for their cultivation. The role of these bacteria in the pathogenesis of the pulmonary infection in patients with cystic fibrosis is not yet clear. Since anaerobic bacteria are known pathogens in aspiration pneumonitis in adults,[1] and children,[7] more studies are warranted to investigate their role in the infectious process in children with cystic fibrosis.

Colonization and Infection Following Tracheostomy and Intubation

Bacterial colonization of the tracheobronchial tree almost always follows tracheal intubation after tracheostomy.[34] It is sometimes difficult to evaluate the clinical significance of the isolation of pathogenic bacteria from tracheal cultures of patients with tracheostomy, to differentiate between colonization or clinical infection,[35] and to assess various factors influencing the acquisition of those bacteria.[36]

Microbiology

The role of anaerobes in pediatric patients intubated for prolonged periods was recently studied.[37] Serial tracheal cultures for aerobic and anaerobic bacteria were obtained from 27 patients who required tracheostomy and prolonged intubation for periods ranging from 3 to 12 months. Tracheal cultures yielded pathogenic aerobic and anaerobic bacteria. Of the 1508 isolates (969 aerobes and 539 anaerobes) recovered from 444 tracheal aspirates, the most common were *K. pneumoniae*, *S. aureus*, anaerobic Gram-positive cocci, *F. nucleatum*, and *B. fragilis*. This accounts for 2.2 aerobes and 1.2 anaerobes isolated per specimen. Cultures from all 27 patients grew aerobic bacteria. Twenty-one (78%) patients yielded both aerobic and anaerobic bacteria from the tracheal aspirates, and from six patients (22%), only aerobes were isolated.

All of the 27 patients developed colonization with aerobic or anaerobic bacteria (or both). Three patients developed chronic colonization after intubation but never developed infection. Twenty-four (89%) of the patients appeared to have developed chronic tracheobronchitis with recurrent episodes of pneumonia (table 20.5).

Eleven of the patients had one or two episodes of pneumonia in one year, seven patients had three to five episodes, and six patients had more than five episodes of pneumonia. There were 68 episodes of pneumonia noted in those 24 patients (2.8 episodes per patient). In about half of the episodes, a change in the bacterial flora occurred during the episode of pneumonia, with the appearance of new pathogens; while in the other half, no change in the bacterial isolates was noted. Although all of the patients responded favorably to the therapy, the bacterial pathogens usually persisted or were replaced by others.

All the patients became colonized by more than two organisms. Peptostreptococci and *B. melaninogenicus* were more frequently isolated during episodes of pneumonia than during periods when the patients were only colonized ($P < 0.05$). The data suggest that anaerobic bacteria are also a part of the bacterial flora causing colonization, tracheobron-

Table 20.5. Bacteria Isolated from the Tracheal Secretions
in the 68 Episodes of Pneumonia

Aerobic and facultative isolates	
Gram-positive cocci	
S. pneumoniae	5
alpha-hemolytic streptococci	...
Group A beta-hemolytic streptococci	4
S. aureus	13
Gram-negative bacilli	
H. influenzae	3
H. parainfluenzae	3
P. mirabilis	2
P. rettgeri	1
P. aeruginosa	1
S. marcescens	5
E. coli	7
K. pneumoniae	15
E. cloacae	3
C. diversus	2
Total aerobic isolates	64
Anaerobic isolates	
Gram-positive cocci	
Peptococcus sp.	4
Peptostreptococcus sp.	16
Gram-negative bacilli	
F. nucleatum	9
B. melaninogenicus	1
B. fragilis	4
B. vulgatus	3
Total anaerobic isolates	37

chitis, and pneumonia in children who require tracheostomy and prolonged intubation.

Pathogenesis

Since anaerobic bacteria are part of the normal oral flora, their presence in the tracheal aspirates of those patients is not surprising. Similar
anaerobic bacteria were previously isolated from adults[1] and pediatric[7]
patients with aspiration pneumonia. The acquisition of the aerobic and
anaerobic organisms that are part of the normal oral flora occurs in
patients who undergo tracheostomy and intubation because of their inability to clear their secretions and their dependency on mechanical
suctioning.

B. fragilis, which usually is not a part of the normal oral flora, was isolated from many of these patients; however, the occurrence of this pathogen in pleuropulmonary infections was noted by other investigators,[5] especially in patients with poor oral hygiene. Peptostreptococci and *B. melaninogenicus* were more frequently isolated from patients with pneumonia than from patients with colonization, suggesting the possible role of these organisms in those infections.

With the increase in prevalence of Gram-negative enteric bacilli in the oropharyngeal flora of seriously ill hospitalized patients, these organisms became the most common cause of hospital-acquired pneumonia.[38-40] Since tracheobronchitis and pneumonia generally follow the inhalation or aspiration of organisms present in the upper respiratory tract, the alteration of the pharyngeal flora of seriously ill patients may be an important first step in the pathogenesis of hospital-acquired pneumonia caused by Gram-negative bacilli.[38]

Organisms that appeared in the tracheal secretions prior to the acquisition of pneumonia were also present in episodes of pneumonia in half of the patients. These findings confirm data obtained by previous investigators,[34] although newly acquired pathogens appeared in many other cases of pneumonia.

Diagnosis

Colonization is defined as the isolation of a potential pathogen from tracheal cultures for at least four weeks, in the absence of purulent tracheobronchial secretions or clinical evidence of infection. Tracheobronchitis should be considered to be present when purulent secretions appear, but when physical examination and chest films show no evidence of pneumonia. The diagnosis of pneumonia can be made only when unequivocal clinical and radiographic evidence of pulmonary parenchymal involvement is present and when a patient has leukocytosis and develops fever.

Management

The patient should be examined daily, with particular attention to the quantity and character of tracheal secretions. Chest films should be made when indicated. The patient should be treated by postural drainage and frequent suctioning and cleaning of tracheostomy tubes, which should be changed once a week. Treatment should include antibiotic administration when pneumonia is suspected. The choice and changes in the therapy with antimicrobial agents are based on the patient's clinical condition and the results of the tracheal cultures.

Routine cultures of the tracheal secretions for surveillance of aerobic and anaerobic bacteria would enable the clinician to predict changes in the tracheal flora and facilitate the selection of appropriate antimicrobial therapy whenever the patient is infected. Repeated tracheal cultures for aerobic and anaerobic bacteria during the course of the pneumonia would allow for adjustment of the therapy if and when the bacteria present change or become resistant to the antibiotics used. Prophylaxis against acquisition of pneumonia is not recommended, since this would only facilitate the selection and acquisition of resistance by the bacteria, which would make it more difficult to treat the patients if and when they did become infected.

Antimicrobial therapy may be guided by Gram stain of appropriate material, but should not be withheld pending culture results in severely ill patients. Parenteral penicillin G is still the drug of choice in almost all anaerobic pleuropulmonary infections, since most of the anaerobes isolated, with the exception of B. *fragilis* group and some strains of B. *melaninogenicus*,[24, 41] are highly sensitive to penicillin.

Discussion of the choice of antibiotics for anaerobes is included in the section on aspiration pneumonia. Since Gram-negative bacilli were recovered mixed with other organisms in almost half of the cases studied, the institution of combined therapy of an aminoglycoside and one of the other drugs is recommended as an initial therapy of lower respiratory infection.

Gentamicin is an appropriate agent for the treatment of most Gram-negative infections. Emergence of resistance to gentamicin has been a concern in recent years, however.[29] Other aminoglycosides such as amikacin[30] or tobramycin[31] are also available for the treatment of such infections. Carbenicillin or ticarcillin are also active and possess synergistic qualities with aminoglycosides against many of these organisms, especially P. *aeruginosa*.[32]

Colonization in Intubated Newborns

Bacterial colonization of the tracheobronchial tree almost always follows tracheal intubation.[34] It is difficult not only to differentiate between colonization and clinical infection,[35] but also to try to assess the various factors that may influence the acquisition of these bacteria.[36]

The newborn infant who presents with respiratory distress syndrome (RDS) may require intubation for extended periods of time. Studies of the bacterial colonization in newborns who require intubation have rarely been done,[42] and studies of the role of anaerobic bacteria in this setting are rare.

Microbiology

The bacteriology of tracheal aspirates from intubated newborns was studied.[43] Specimens were obtained twice weekly from 127 newborns as long as they were intubated. Each newborn had between one and eight specimens taken (average 1.7). One specimen was taken from each of 127 babies, and 38 had two, 25 had three, 12 had four, and 10 had more than four specimens taken, for a total of 212 specimens. No bacterial or fungal growth was obtained from 65 specimens, whereas the remaining specimens (147) yielded 209 bacterial and fungal isolates accounting for 1.4 isolates per specimen. The total isolates recovered were 168 aerobes, 36 anaerobes, and 5 *Candida albicans*. Of this total, 70 specimens yielded one isolate, 48 two isolates, 6 three isolates, 5 four isolates, and one aspirate yielded five isolates. Seventy-eight (61%) newborns received antimicrobial therapy. A higher incidence of positive cultures and the presence of more than one organism per culture were found in those infants not receiving antibiotics. More isolates per specimen were noted with increasing time of incubation. The rate of isolation of *S. aureus*, *P. aeruginosa*, and *K. pneumoniae* remained constant with increased length of intubation, the rate of recovery of *Staphylococcus epidermidis*, streptococcus viridans, and *Propionibacterium acnes* increased, and the rate of isolation of *E. coli* and anaerobic organisms decreased.

Anaerobic bacteria were found to play a role in three of the five cases of pneumonia.[44] These three infants presented with premature rupture of membranes and neonatal pneumonia caused by organisms belonging to members of the *B. fragilis* group. In all three instances, the organisms were recovered from tracheal aspirates and in two from blood cultures as well.

Pathogenesis

Data obtained in several studies[42, 45] demonstrate the occurrence of microbial colonization immediately after intubation in 70% of newborns. Whether these organisms are acquired before or during delivery, or during the intubation process, is undetermined. The bacteria recovered from the first specimens obtained from newborns, which were obtained immediately after intubation and usually within 24 hours after delivery, may reflect microbial contamination acquired upon passage through the birth canal. Organisms recovered at that time were primarily Gram-positive cocci and *Bacteroides* species. These bacteria tend to decrease in numbers and are replaced by organisms such as streptococcus viridans, *S. epidermidis*, and *P. acnes*.

The use of systemic antibiotics in newborns can alter the bacterial flora of their respiratory tract, which may result in an overgrowth of Gram-negative bacteria.[46–48] Bacterial colonization and superinfection are also common in adults treated with antimicrobial agents for pneumonia.[49] It is noteworthy that organisms such as *S. aureus, P. aeruginosa,* and a variety of anaerobes tend to increase in numbers in chronically intubated adults[36] and older children.[37] These organisms did not predominate in the newborn population studied, however. This observation could be due to a variety of factors, such as the relatively shorter intubation period in the neonate (which usually does not exceed one week), the relatively low levels of colonization with resistant bacteria,[42, 45] the relatively short courses of antimicrobial agents, and the occurrence of early infant death.

S. *epidermidis,* streptococcus viridans, and *P. acnes* were the predominant isolates also in patients receiving antimicrobial therapy; however, the administration of antimicrobial agents appeared to reduce not only the number of bacteria isolated per specimen, but also the number of positive cultures as well.

Since anaerobic bacteria are part of the normal flora of the cervix,[50] their presence in tracheal aspirates of neonates is not surprising. Similar anaerobic bacteria were isolated from conjunctiva[51] and gastric aspirates of newborns[50] and represent acquisition during passage through the birth canal.

The microbial colonization of the trachea in intubated neonates with different aerobic and anaerobic bacteria could be due to their acquisition from the mother's cervical flora. This flora tends to decrease in proportion with time and is replaced by normal skin flora. It is also evident that intubated neonates treated with antibiotics show reduced numbers of bacteria colonizing their trachea. It is evident that some of the acquired anaerobes can cause pneumonia in the newborn (see chapter 10).

Diagnosis

The technique of tracheal aspiration culture plus the Wright's staining procedure is effective in defining infective and noninfective conditions in newborns with respiratory distress.[51] Moreover, it seemed to be effective in early recognition of perinatal pneumonia caused by both aerobic and anaerobic bacteria. Although the technique of obtaining tracheal cultures by aspiration of material from an endotracheal tube that is used for ventilation is not ideal, it seemed to be a simple and safe procedure with almost no side effects or risks. It is clear that anaerobes, along with facultative and aerobic bacteria, may play a role in perinatal pneumonia. This must be considered in devising therapeutic regimens.

The presence of polymorphonuclear leukocytes on Wright's stain of the aspirated material correlated with the presence of pathogenic organisms and an inflammatory process. In cases where pathologic examination was done, inflammatory changes were noted in the lungs;

thus, the use of appropriate staining procedures provides another tool for determining the pathogenicity of the recovered bacteria. Additional evidence for the significance of the organisms in tracheal aspirates from babies with perinatal pneumonia was an accompanying bacteremia with at least one of the same organisms in two of the five patients.[44] Clinical signs of pneumonia should also alert the clinician to the presence of this infection.

Management

Whenever neonatal pneumonia is present, appropriate antimicrobial therapy should be administered. A penicillin derivative and one of the aminoglycosides are generally effective for treatment of infection or pneumonia in newborns. This combination will provide adequate coverage for the majority of organisms causing neonatal pneumonia such as Gram-negative enteric rods and group B streptococci. While most anaerobic organisms are susceptible to penicillin G, members of the *B. fragilis* group, and some strains of *B. melaninogenicus*[52] are known to be resistant to that agent.

Because of the generally short duration of neonatal tracheal intubation, tracheal colonization generally does not present as a management problem. Prompt termination of the intubation will usually be followed by rapid resolution of the condition. The same caution in management as indicated in the management of older children (see previous section on long-term intubation) is required. This requires daily examination of the patient, with particular attention to the quantity and character of the tracheal secretion, frequent suctioning and cleaning of tubes, and change of tubes when indicated.

REFERENCES

1. Bartlett, J. G., and Finegold, S. M. Anaerobic infections of the lung and pleural space. *Am. Rev. Respir. Dis.* 110:56, 1974.

2. Gorbach, S. L., and Bartlett, J. G. Anaerobic infections (second of three parts). *N. Engl. J. Med.* 290:1237, 1974.

3. Varney, P. L. The bacterial flora of treated and untreated abscesses of the lung. *Arch. Surg.* 19:1602, 1920.

4. Lambert, A. V. S., and Miller, J. A. Abscess of the lung. *Arch. Surg.* 8:446, 1924.

5. Finegold, S. M. *Anaerobic bacteria in human disease.* New York: Academic Press, 1977, p. 223.

6. Bartlett, J. G. et al. Bacteriology and treatment of primary lung abscess. *Am. Rev. Respir. Dis.* 109:510, 1974.

7. Brook, I., and Finegold, S. M. Bacteriology of aspiration pneumonia in children. *Pediatrics* 65:1115, 1980.

8. Rosebury, T. *Microorganisms indigenous to man*. New York: McGraw-Hill, 1962.

9. Socransky, S. S., and Mangeniello, S. O. The oral microbiota of man from birth to senility. *J. Periodontol.* 42:485, 1971.

10. Gibbons, R. J. et al. Studies of the predominant cultivable microbiota of dental plaque. *Arch. Oral Biol.* 9:365, 1964.

11. Gibbons, R. J. Aspects of the pathogenicity and ecology of the indigenous oral flora of man. In *Anaerobic bacteria: role in disease*, eds. A. Ballow et al. Springfield, Ill.: Charles C Thomas, 1974.

12. Klein, J. O. Diagnostic lung puncture in the pneumonias of infants and children. *Pediatrics* 44:486, 1969.

13. Mimica, I. et al. Lung puncture in the etiological diagnosis of pneumonia. A study of 543 infants and children. *Am. J. Dis. Child.* 122:278, 1971.

14. Laurenzi, G. A.; Potter, R. T.; and Kass, E. H. Bacteriologic flora of the lower respiratory tract. *N. Engl. J. Med.* 265:278, 1961.

15. Lapinski, E. M.; Flakas, E. D.; and Taylor, B. C. An evaluation of some methods for culturing sputum from patients with bronchitis and emphysema. *Am. Rev. Resp. Dis.* 89:760, 1964.

16. Louria, D. B. Uses of quantitative analyses of bacterial populations in sputum. *JAMA* 182:1082, 1962.

17. Pecora, D. V. A method of securing uncontaminated tracheal secretions for bacterial examination. *J. Thorac. Cardiovasc. Surg.* 37:653, 1959.

18. Bartlett, J. G.; Rosenblatt, J. E.; and Finegold, S. M. Percutaneous transtracheal aspiration in the diagnosis of anaerobic pulmonary infections. *Ann. Intern. Med.* 79:535, 1973.

19. Baran, D., and Cordier, N. Usefulness of transtracheal puncture in the bacteriological diagnosis of lung infections in children. *Helv. Paediatr. Acta* 28:391, 1974.

20. Brook, I. Percutaneous transtracheal aspiration in the diagnosis and treatment of aspiration pneumonia in children. *J. Pediatr.* 96:1000, 1980.

21. Hoeprich, P. D. Etiologic diagnosis of lower respiratory tract infections. *Calif. Med.* 112:1, 1970.

22. Brook, I., and Finegold, S. M. Bacteriology and therapy of lung abscess in children. *J. Pediatr.* 94:10, 1979.

23. Brook, I. Aspiration pneumonia in institutionalized children, a retrospective comparison of treatment with penicillin G, clindamycin, and carbenicillin. *Clin. Pediatr.* 20:117, 1981.

24. Sutter, V. L., and Finegold, S. M. Susceptibility of anaerobic bacteria to 23 antimicrobial agents. *Antimicrob. Agents Chemother.* 10:736, 1976.

25. Bartlett, J. G., and Gorbach, S. L. Treatment of aspiration pneumonia and primary lung abscess: penicillin G vs clindamycin. *JAMA* 234:935, 1975.

26. Levison, M. E. et al. Penicillin v.s. clindamycin treatment of anaerobic lung abscess (abstr. 365). *Proceedings of the 21th Interscience Conference on Antimicrobial Agents and Chemotherapy*, 1981.

27. Brook, I. Clindamycin in treatment of aspiration pneumonia in children. *Antimicrob. Agents Chemother.* 15:342, 1979.

28. Brook, I. Carbenicillin in treatment of aspiration pneumonia in children. *Curr. Ther. Res.* 23:136, 1973.

29. Bryan, L. E.; Shahrbade, M. W.; and Van den Elzen, H. M. Gentamicin resistance in *Pseudomonas aeruginosa*. R-factor mediated resistance. *Antimicrob. Agents Chemother.* 6:19, 1974.

30. Bartlett, J. G. Amikacin treatment of pulmonary infections involving gentamicin resistant Gram-negative bacilli. *Am. J. Med.* 62:245, 1977.

31. Moellering, R. C., Jr.; Wennerstin, C.; and Kunz, J. L. Emergence of gentamicin-resistant bacteria: experience with tobramicin therapy of infections due to gentamicin-resistant organisms. *J. Infect. Dis.* 134:540, 1976.

32. Prior, R. B., and Fass, R. J. Comparison of ticarcillin and carbenicillin activity against random and selected population of *Pseudomonas aeruginosa*. *Antimicrob. Agents Chemother.* 13:189, 1979.

33. Brook, I., and Fink, R. Transtracheal aspiration in pulmonary infection in children with cystic fibrosis. *Eur. J. Resp. Dis.*, in press.

34. Aass, A. S. Complications to tracheostomy and long term intubation: a follow-up study. *Acta Anaesthesiol. Scand.* 19:127, 1975.

35. Gotsman, M. S., and Whilby, J. L. Respiratory infection following tracheostomy. *Thorax* 19:89, 1964.

36. Bryant, L. R. et al. Bacterial colonization profile with tracheal intubation and mechanical ventilation. *Arch. Surg.* 104:647, 1972.

37. Brook, I. Bacterial colonization tracheobronchitis and pneumonia, following tracheostomy and long-term intubation in pediatric patients. *Chest* 74:420, 1979.

38. Johanson, E. G., Jr. et al. Nosocomial respiratory infections with Gram-negative bacilli. The significance of colonization of the respiratory tract. *Ann. Intern. Med.* 77:701, 1972.

39. Johanson, W. G.; Pierce, A. K.; and Sanford, J. P. Changing pharyngeal bacterial flora of hospitalized patients. Emergence of Gram-negative bacilli. *N. Engl. J. Med.* 281:1137, 1969.

40. Statford, B. et al. Alteration of superficial bacterial flora in severely ill patients. *Lancet* 1:68, 1968.

41. Brook, I.; Calhoun, L.; and Yocum, P. Beta lactamase-producing isolates of *Bacteroides* species from children. *Antimicrob. Agents Chemother.* 18:164, 1980.

42. Harris, H.; Wirtschafter, D.; and Cassady, G. Endotracheal intubation and its relationship to bacterial colonization and systemic infection of newborn infants. *Pediatrics* 56:816, 1976.

43. Brook, I., and Martin, W. J. Bacterial colonization in intubated newborns. *Respiration* 40:323, 1980.

44. Brook, I.; Martin, W. J.; and Finegold, S. M. Neonatal pneumonia caused by members of *Bacteroides fragilis* group. *Clin. Pediatr.* 19:541, 1980.

45. Sprunt, K.; Leidy, G.; and Redman, W. Abnormal colonization and infection in neonates. *Pediatr. Res.* 8:429, 1974.

46. Eitzman, D. V., and Smith, R. T. The significance of blood cultures in the newborn period. *Am. J. Dis. Child.* 94:601, 1957.

47. Dalton, H. P. et al. Pulmonary infection due to disruption of the pharyngeal bacterial flora by antibiotics in hamsters. *Am. J. Pathol.* 76:469, 1974.

48. Farmer, K. The influence of hospital environment and antibiotics on the bacterial flora of the upper respiratory tract of the newborn. *NZ Med. J.* 67:541, 1968.

49. Tillotson, J. R., and Finland, M. Secondary pulmonary infections following antibiotic therapy for primary bacterial pneumonia. *Antimicrob. Agents Chemother.* 8:326, 1968.

50. Brook, I. et al. Aerobic and anaerobic flora of maternal cervix and newborns with conjunctiva and gastric fluid: a prospective study. *Pediatrics* 63:451, 1979.

51. Brook, I.; Martin, W. J.; and Finegold, S. M. Effect of silver nitrate application on the conjunctival flora of the newborn and the occurrence of clostridial conjunctivitis. *J. Pediatr. Ophthalmol. Strabis.* 15:179, 1978.

52. Brook, I.; Martin, W. J.; and Finegold, S. M. Bacteriology of tracheal aspirates in intubated newborn. *Chest* 78:875, 1980.

CHAPTER 21

Intraabdominal Infections

Peritonitis

Secondary peritonitis and intraabdominal abscesses generally are due to the entry of enteric microorganisms into the peritoneal cavity through a defect in the wall of the intestines or other viscus as a result of obstruction, infarction, or direct trauma. In children, peritonitis is associated primarily with appendicitis but may occur with intussusception, volvulus, incarcerated hernia, or rupture of a Meckel's diverticulum. Although less common in pediatrics, peritonitis may occur also as a complication of intestinal mucosal disease, including peptic ulcers, ulcerative colitis, and pseudomembranous enterocolitis.

Intraabdominal infections in the neonatal period are generally a complication of necrotizing enterocolitis but may be associated with meconium ileus or spontaneous rupture of the stomach or intestines. The peritonitis following appendicitis usually is a synergistic infection in which more than one organism is involved. Characteristically, the more types of bacteria that can be isolated, the graver the morbidity. The specific microorganisms involved in peritonitis are generally those of the normal flora of the gastrointestinal tract where anaerobic bacteria outnumber aerobes in the ratio 1:1000.[1]

Microbiology

Anaerobic bacteria are the predominant organisms in the gastrointestinal tract,[1] and this accounts for their predominance in infections associated with perforation of the bowel. Perforated appendicitis, inflammatory bowel disease with perforation, and gastrointestinal surgery often are associated with infections caused by anaerobic bacteria.

Studies in adults demonstrate the presence of mixed aerobic and anaerobic flora in the peritoneal cavity of patients with ruptured appendix or intestinal viscus[2] and show that these organisms may occasionally be recovered from the postoperative wound.[3]

A few studies of the bacterial flora of the peritoneal cavity and postoperative wounds following perforated appendix in children have been conducted.[4, 5] Anaerobic organisms were isolated from almost all of the peritoneal cavity cultures and from two-thirds of the complicating wounds in children who underwent surgery for perforation of the appendix or other viscus.[4] *Clostridium* species were recovered from 43%, and *Bacteroides fragilis* was present in 93% of the peritoneal fluids of these patients, along with aerobic Gram-negative bacteria and enterococci. Similar isolates were recovered also from liver, pelvic and subphrenic abscesses, surgical wounds, and blood cultures of these patients.[5]

A recent study reported the bacteria recovered from peritoneal specimens obtained from 100 children who presented with a ruptured appendix (table 21.1). Additional samples were studied from 11 of these patients who developed drainage from the postoperative surgical wound. Bacterial growth occurred in 100 peritoneal fluid specimens.

Table 21.1. Organisms Isolated from Peritoneal Fluid from 100 Patients with Perforated Appendix and 11 with Postoperative Wound Infection

Aerobic and Facultative Isolates	No. of Isolates (No. from Wound Infection)	Anaerobic Isolates	No. of Isolates (No. from Wound Infection)
Gram-positive cocci (total)	53(6)	Gram-positive cocci (total)	62(9)
Group D streptococci	12(1)	Gram-positive bacilli (total)	52(7)
Gram-positive bacilli	4(1)	*Clostridium* sp.	16(2)
Gram-negative bacilli (total)	87(10)	Gram-negative bacilli	
P. aeruginosa	9(3)	*Fusobacterium* sp.	27(3)
E. coli	57(6)	*Bacteroides* sp.	42(4)
K. pneumoniae	7	*B. melaninogenicus* group	26(2)
Total number of aerobes and facultatives	144(17)	*B. fragilis* group	92(8)
		Total number of anaerobes	301(33)

SOURCE: Modified from Brook, I. Bacterial studies of peritoneal cavity and postoperative wound infection following perforated appendix in children. *Ann. Surg.* 192:208, 1980. Reprinted by permission.
NOTE: Only the important pathogens are listed in detail. The total number of the groups of organisms is represented.

Anaerobic bacteria alone were present in 14 specimens, aerobes alone in 12, and mixed aerobic and anaerobic flora in 74. There were 144 aerobic isolates (1.4 per specimen). The predominant isolates were *Escherichia coli*, alpha-hemolytic streptococci, gamma-hemolytic streptococci, group D streptococci, and *Pseudomonas aeruginosa*. There were 301 anaerobic isolates (three per specimen). The predominant isolates were *Bacteroides* species (*B. fragilis* group and *Bacteroides melaninogenicus* group), Gram-positive anaerobic cocci, *Fusobacterium* species, and *Clostridium* species. *B. fragilis* and *E. coli* in combination occurred in 39 instances, *B. fragilis* and *Peptococcus* species occurred in 23. Beta-lactamase production was detectable in 98 isolates recovered from 74 patients. These included all isolates of *B. fragilis* group and 6 of the 37 *Bacteroides* species.

Forty-nine organisms (16 aerobic and 33 anaerobic) were recovered from the draining surgical wounds and were predominantly *B. fragilis*, *E. coli*, *Peptostreptococcus* species, *P. aeruginosa*, and *Peptococcus* species. Most of these isolates were recovered also from the peritoneal cavity of the patients.

These findings demonstrate the polymicrobial aerobic and anaerobic nature of peritoneal cavity and postoperative wound flora in children with perforated appendix, and demonstrate the presence of beta-lactamase-producing organisms in three-fourths of the patients.

Pathogenesis

Peritonitis is an excellent example of a synergistic infection between aerobic and anaerobic microorganisms. The two types of bacteria have opposite oxygen requirements, and the alteration each causes in its environment allows for the rapid proliferation of their partners.[7-9] The results of appropriate culture techniques have consistently documented that the great majority of intraabdominal infections are based on this symbiotic relationship.[10-12] As more types of bacteria are isolated from patients with peritonitis, the postsurgical morbidity increases.[13, 14]

Although more than 400 bacterial species reside in the colon, and more than 200 are thought to colonize healthy oral cavities, the average number of bacterial species in infections associated with colonic perforation is five.[15] The dominant anaerobic bacteria in this type of disease include *B. fragilis*, *B. melaninogenicus*, *Fusobacterium nucleatum*, *Clostridium perfringens*, *Peptostreptococcus anaerobius*, and *Peptococcus asaccharolyticus*—six species that probably account for the great majority of anaerobic isolates in clinical laboratories.[16] Thus, from the multiple anaerobic bacteria present in the normal flora, only a few are common in septic processes; it is likely that virulence is an important factor in their selection.

Of all the anaerobes, *B. fragilis* is the most frequently encountered in intraabdominal sepsis or bacteremia. Organisms classified as *B. fragilis* were subdivided formerly into six subspecies: *fragilis, distasonis, vulgatus, thetaiotaomicron, ovatus,* and an unspecified group, subspecies "other." These subspecies share many phenotypic characteristics, including resistance to penicillins, and their separation was based on minor variations in biochemical reactions. The distribution of the *B. fragilis* subspecies is markedly different in normal flora and infected sites. In the colon, the usual source of *B. fragilis* in septic processes, the numerically dominant subspecies are *distasonis, vulgatus,* and *thetaiotaomicron;* subspecies *fragilis* accounts for only about 0.5% of the colonic microflora.[15] In clinical specimens, however, subspecies *fragilis* is most often encountered. Its predominance in exudate and blood strongly suggests that this subspecies has unique virulence properties.

One of the important virulence factors of *B. fragilis* is its capsule. When unencapsulated *B. fragilis* were injected intraabdominally into mice, an aerobic organism was required to form an abscess. The aerobe was unnecessary as an adjunct for abscess development, however, when encapsulated *B. fragilis* was used as the anaerobe for infection of animals.[17] Subsequently, it was shown that heat-killed *B. fragilis* produced abscesses indistinguishable from those resulting from infection with viable organisms. Finally, when purified capsular material from *B. fragilis* was implanted, abscesses again resulted.

The pathogenic importance of anaerobes, and especially *B. fragilis,* was further demonstrated in models of treatment of the anaerobic-aerobic infection. In the studies by Weinstein and Onderdonk and their associates,[18, 19] peritonitis was induced in rats by introducing gelatin capsules containing cecal contents into their abdominal cavities. The animals that survived the initial septicemic stage caused by coliforms developed intraabdominal abscesses caused by anaerobes. An evaluation of the effect of therapy with clindamycin, gentamicin, or a combination of both was done. It was shown that the untreated control and the clindamycin-treated group had identical mortality rates of about 35%; however, administration of gentamicin alone or in combination with clindamycin led to greater than 92% survival. These data suggest that the early mortality in the peritonitis and septicemic phase is attributable to gentamicin-sensitive coliform bacteria. The effect of treatment on abscess formation was entirely different. All untreated animals that survived developed abscesses, as did those treated with gentamicin alone. The use of clindamycin alone or in combination with gentamicin was associated with a greatly reduced incidence and size of the abscesses, which occurred only in 5% of the animals. These findings indicate that anaerobes may be responsible for complications following abdominal perforation, such as intraabdominal abscess formation, and show that optimal treatment of intestinal perforation requires a drug to control both aerobic and anaerobic bacteria.

Diagnosis

Clinical Manifestations

The clinical manifestations of secondary peritonitis are a reflection of the underlying disease process. Fever, diffuse abdominal pain, nausea, and vomiting are characteristic. Physical examination reveals signs of peritoneal inflammation, including rebound tenderness, abdominal wall rigidity, and decrease in bowel sounds. These early findings may be followed by signs and symptoms of shock owing to loss of protein-rich fluids into the peritoneal cavity and bowel lumen.

The manifestations of shock from a ruptured viscus merge with those of peritonitis and may be followed by toxemia, restlessness and irritability, by a higher temperature, by an increase in the pulse rate, and by chills and convulsions. In early infancy, the temperature may be normal or subnormal.

Laboratory studies reveal an elevated blood leukocyte count in excess of 12,000 with a predominance of polymorphonuclear forms. Roentgenograms of the abdomen may reveal free air in the peritoneal cavity, evidence of ileus or obstruction, and obliteration of the psoas shadow.

Measurement of levels of lactic acid in the ascitic fluid is a potentially useful tool for establishing a diagnosis of peritonitis and for differentiating it from other conditions that it can simulate. Concentrations of lactic acid of greater than 33 mg/100 ml were found in all patients with infectious ascites, regardless of the organism responsible.[20]

Diagnostic ultrasound[21] or gallium scan may be useful in detecting appendiceal or other intraabdominal abscesses. Postoperative wound infections in children can occur after appendectomy.

Management

The mainstay of therapy is stabilization of the patient by correcting fluid and electrolyte deficiencies with parenteral fluids, alleviation of intestinal obstruction with nasal suction, and controlling the peritoneal infection with antibiotics.

The treatment of abdominal infection should always include surgical correction and drainage. The surgical intervention should be performed as soon as possible, preferably when the patient is stabilized. The medical therapy should supplement the surgical approach by attempting to eradicate both aerobic and anaerobic microorganisms. Aminoglycosides are effective in eliminating enteric Gram-negative rods, although growing numbers of strains are resistant to some of these drugs. Antibiotics effective against *B. fragilis* group include chlor-

amphenicol, carbenicillin, ticarcillin, clindamycin, cefoxitin, and metronidazole.[22] Since some strains of *B. fragilis* may acquire resistance to
one of these antibiotics,[15] susceptibility testing of the organism should
be performed in serious infections.

As noted in the section on pathogenesis, peritonitis is an example
of a synergistic infection in which aerobic and anaerobic microorganisms each promote the growth of the other.[23] Infections in the abdominal cavity usually are caused by gastrointestinal tract contamination.
The principle anaerobic pathogens are *B. fragilis*, clostridia, and anaerobic Gram-positive cocci. Coliforms and facultative streptococci were
frequent cohabitors. The recovery of multiple bacteria from infected
sites poses important practical questions, such as which organisms require specific therapy and whether treatment should incorporate drugs
to deal with both the aerobic and the anaerobic bacteria present. There
is general agreement that aminoglycosides are appropriate treatment
for coliforms. The necessity for treating both components of mixed infections has now been adequately documented in experimental and
clinical studies. A recent study[12] compared two groups of patients with
trauma to the abdomen and perforation. One group was treated with
cephalosporin and gentamicin, and the other was treated with clindamycin and gentamicin. More complications occurred in the cephalo-
sporin-treated group, suggesting that complications such as intraabdominal abscesses are avoided in patients treated for anaerobic
bacteria including *B. fragilis*.

Bartlett and co-workers[24] have examined the efficacy of 29 different antimicrobial regimens in the treatment of experimental intraabdominal sepsis. They concluded that optimal results were obtained
with several regimens that showed good in vitro activity against both
coliforms and *B. fragilis*.

Complications

The complications following perforation of viscus include septic shock,
respiratory failure, retroperitoneal or intraabdominal abscesses, small
bowel obstruction from adhesions, fistula formation, and infection of
the postsurgical wounds.[15] Anaerobic bacteria are major pathogens in
the infections and were recovered from all of these infectious sites.

In a recent study, Brook[6] recovered anaerobes from 91% of the
exudates of the draining wound, which in children corresponds to
findings in adult patients.[3] *Bacteroides* species and peptostreptococci
were recovered as the only isolates from an adrenal abscess in a neonate.[25] It is of interest that the presence of free gas detected inside the
abscess served as a clue to the presence of anaerobic infection.

Pyogenic Liver Abscess

Pyogenic liver abscesses, which can have devastating consequences, are relatively rare in infants and children. Prior to the advent of antibiotics, liver abscesses mainly followed unmanageable infections in otherwise normal children. Since the 1940s, most of the reported cases are in children with leukemia or chronic granulomatous disease, or in children who are immunosuppressed. Recently, the incidence of hepatic abscess appears to be increasing, probably because of the increasing awareness of the disease and availability of better diagnostic techniques.[26]

Microbiology

Review of the literature disclosed a total of 73 cases of hepatic abscess in childhood.[27-29] The microorganisms commonly isolated from the liver abscess include *Staphylococcus aureus, E. coli, Streptococcus faecalis, Klebsiella* organisms, *Enterobacter* species, *Pseudomonas* organisms, and salmonellae.

Recently, anaerobic microorganisms have been recognized as causes of liver abscess in adults,[30] but in children, only two cases of hepatic abscess caused by anaerobic bacteria have been reported.[31, 32] The true incidence of liver abscess from anaerobic organisms may be higher if anaerobic cultures are performed with proper techniques.

Data from adults have demonstrated that anaerobes may be involved in at least 50% of cases of pyogenic liver abscess. With proper transport of specimens and suitable anaerobic methodology, anaerobes are the exclusive isolates in two-thirds of the cases yielding anaerobic bacteria. The anaerobes most prevalent in liver abscess are anaerobic and microaerophilic streptococci, *Fusobacterium nucleatum, B. fragilis,* and *B. melaninogenicus.*[15] In many patients the infection is polymicrobial, and anaerobes are present mixed with aerobes.

Pathogenesis

The liver may be invaded by pyogenic microorganisms in several ways. Embolic abscesses, usually multiple, may originate from foci anywhere in the body via the hepatic artery. Direct extension of infection, or extension by way of the lymphatics, may develop from such situations as an infected intraabdominal site of appendicitis, diverticulitis, perforated bowel, or pelvic infection. In the newborn period, septic phlebitis of the umbilical vein secondary to bacterial omphalitis may spread to the portal vein, causing liver abscess. Catheterization of the umbilical vein may result in septic thrombophlebitis leading to hepatic abscess as a result of direct extension of infection.[27, 33] Extrahepatic biliary obstruction and cholangitis may cause hepatic abscess. Occasionally, liver abscess may follow a penetrating or blunt hepatic trauma. The disease is particularly common in children with immunodeficiency states such as acute leukemia, aplastic anemia, chronic granulomatous disease (CGD), or in patients receiving immunosuppressive drugs. In children, most cases of pyogenic liver abscess are either secondary to generalized septicemia or associated with underlying immune disorders. Since anaerobes are the predominant organisms present in the normal flora of the gastrointestinal tract, outnumbering aerobes at a ratio 1000:1,[15] their predominance in the pyogenic hepatic abscess is not surprising.

Diagnosis

Patients with solitary or multiple liver abscesses generally present with fever accompanied by chills and sweats. Aching pain and tenderness localized over the liver or epigastrium are also common. Laboratory studies reveal leukocytosis, anemia, elevated alkaline phosphatase, and positive blood culture.

Since the clinical and routine laboratory findings in hepatic abscess are nonspecific (fever, abdominal pain, hepatomegaly, leukocytosis), the diagnosis of this infection can be missed, especially in patients with multiple small abscesses.

Diagnosis of solitary hepatic abscesses has been greatly enhanced by the development of effective radionuclide liver scanning procedures. These techniques allow detection of hepatic lesions as small as 2 cm in diameter.[34] Celiac angiography has been employed occasionally but offers no advantage over radionuclide liver scan.

Roentgenographic studies may show elevation, change in contour, and reduced mobility of the diaphragm. Abscess of the left lobe of the liver may produce pressure deformities in the barium- or gas-filled stomach, or it may displace the duodenal cap. Pleural effusion or thickening also may be noted, and occasionally a gas-fluid level may be noted within the liver.

Amebic abscess should be excluded in every child suspected of liver abscess. Amebic abscess has an insidious onset, and the patients are less acutely ill. The diagnosis may be suggested by finding amebas in the stools or by finding a high titer of antibodies by hemagglutination or complement fixation tests for amebiasis.

Management

The therapy of hepatic abscess is based on two major elements: surgical drainage of the localized lesion and long-term antibiotic therapy.

Once the abscess has been localized, adequate surgical drainage must be performed. Simple percutaneous needle aspiration alone is not sufficient. Evacuation of the abscess cavity serves two major purposes: to obtain good bacteriologic specimens for maximal antibiotic efficiency, and to remove and thus prevent local spread of purulent material. In addition to surgical drainage, appropriate broad-spectrum antibiotics must be started parenterally and continued for at least four to six weeks. A careful attempt should be made to identify the causative microorganisms, including anaerobes. If anaerobic organisms are isolated, chloramphenicol, metronidazole, or clindamycin are the drugs of choice.[15] Aminoglycosides should be added if Gram-negative enteric bacteria are present, and if *S. aureus* is present antistaphylococcal agents should be administered.

Complications

An unrecognized and untreated pyogenic liver abscess is invariably fatal. Even with therapy, mortality from pyogenic liver abscess in adults has been reported to vary from 30% to 90%.[35, 36] The mortality in infants less than 1 month of age is 75%. In older children, mortality is 25%. The overall mortality in all patients without CGD is 42%, and in patients with CGD it is 27%. The adult literature suggests there is a markedly higher mortality with multiple as opposed to single abscesses, but this has not been confirmed in children.[37]

REFERENCES

1. Gorbach, S. L. Intestinal microflora. *Gastroenterology* 60:1110, 1971.

2. Stone, H. H.; Kolb, L. D.; and Geheber, C. E. Incidence and significance of interperitoneal anaerobic bacteria. *Ann. Surg.* 181:705, 1975.

3. Sanderson, P. J.; Wren, M. W. P.; and Baldwin, A. W. F. Anaerobic organisms in postoperative wounds. *J. Clin. Pathol.* 32:143, 1979.

4. Marchildon, M. B., and Dudgeon, D. L. Perforating appendicitis: a current experience in Children's Hospital. *Ann. Surg.* 185:84, 1977.

5. Stone, J. H. Bacterial flora of appendicitis in children. *J. Pediatr. Surg.* 11:37, 1976.

6. Brook, I. Bacterial studies of peritoneal cavity and postoperative wound infection following perforated appendix in children. *Ann. Surg.* 192:208, 1980.

7. Meleney, F. L. Hemolytic streptococcus gangrene. *Arch. Surg.* 9:317, 1924.

8. Rea, W. J., and Wyrick, W. J., Jr. Necrotizing fasciitis. *Ann. Surg.* 172:957, 1970.

9. Stone, H. H., and Martin, J. D., Jr. Synergistic necrotizing cellulitis. *Ann. Surg.* 175:702, 1972.

10. Gorbach, S. L., and Bartlett, J. G. Anaerobic infections. *N. Engl. J. Med.* 290:1177, 1974.

11. Thadepalli, H. et al. Prospective study of infections in penetrating abdominal trauma. *Am. J. Surg.* 25:1405, 1972.

12. Thadepalli, H. et al. Abdominal trauma, anaerobes and antibiotics. *Surg. Gynecol. Obstet.* 137:270, 1973.

13. Meleney, F. L. et al. Peritonitis. II. Synergism of bacteria commonly found in peritoneal exudates. *Arch. Surg.* 25:709, 1932.

14. Altemeier, W. A. The bacterial flora of acute perforated appendicitis with peritonitis. *Ann. Surg.* 107:517, 1938.

15. Finegold, S. M. Anaerobic bacteria in human disease. New York: Academic Press, 1977.

16. Finegold, S. M.; Shepard, W. E.; and Spaulding, E. H. Practical anaerobic bacteriology. In *CUMITECH*, no. 5. Washington, D.C.: American Society for Microbiology, April, 1977, p. 1.

17. Onderdonk, A. B. et al. The capsular polysaccharide of *B. fragilis* as a virulence factor: comparison of the pathogenic potential of encapsulated and unencapsulated strains. *J. Infect. Dis.* 136:82, 1977.

18. Weinstein, W. M. et al. Experimental intraabdominal abscesses in rats. I. Development of an experimental mode. *Infect. Immun.* 10:1250, 1974.

19. Onderdonk, A. B. et al. Experimental intraabdominal abscesses in rats. II. Quantitative bacteriology of infected animals. *Infec. Immun.* 10:1256, 1974.

20. Brook, I. et al. Measurement of lactic acid in peritoneal fluid: a diagnostic aid in infectious peritonitis with emphasis on spontaneous peritonitis of the cirrhotic. *Dig. Dis. Sci.* 26:1089, 1981.

21. Friday, R. O.; Barriga, P.; and Crummy, A. B. Detection and localization of intraabdominal abscesses by diagnostic ultrasound. *Arch. Surg.* 110:335, 1975.

22. Sutter, V. L., and Finegold, S. M. Susceptibility of anaerobic bacteria to 23 antimicrobial agents. *Antimicrob. Agent Chemother.* 10:736, 1976.

23. Rea, W. J., and Wyrick, W. J: Necrotizing fasciitis. *Ann. Surg.* 172:957, 1970.

24. Bartlett, J. G. et al. Therapeutic efficacy of 29 antimicrobial regimens in experimental intraabdominal sepsis. *Rev. Infect. Dis.* 3:535, 1981.

25. Bekdash, B. A., and Slim, M. S. Adrenal abscess in a neonate due to gas-forming organism: a diagnostic dilemma. *Zeit Zeitschrift Fuer Kinderich Granzgeb* 32:184, 1981.

26. Young, A. E. The clinical presentation of pyogenic liver abscess. *Br. J. Surg.* 63:216, 1976.

27. Chusid, M. J. Pyogenic hepatic abscess in infancy and childhood. *Pediatrics* 62:554, 1978.

28. Arya, L. S. et al. Pyogenic liver abscesses in children. *Clin. Pediatr.* 21:89, 1982.

29. Moss, T. J., and Pysher, T. J. Hepatic abscess in neonates. *Am. J. Dis. Child.* 135:726, 1981.

30. Sabbaj, J.; Sutter, V. L.; and Finegold, S. M. Anaerobic pyogenic liver abscess. *Ann. Intern. Med.* 77:629, 1972.

31. Shulman, S. T., and Beem, M. O. A unique presentation of sickle cell disease: pyogenic hepatic abscess. *Pediatrics* 47:1019, 1971.

32. Asnes, R. S. Shaking chills and fever. *Clin. Pediatr.* 10:334, 1971.

33. Brans, Y. W.; Ceballos, R.; and Cassady, G. Umbilical catheters and hepatic abscesses. *Pediatrics* 53:264, 1974.

34. O'Mara, R. E., and McAfee, J. G. Scintillation scanning in the diagnosis of hepatic abscess in children. *J. Pediatr.* 77:211, 1970.

35. Preimesberger, K. F., and Goldberg, M. E. Acute liver abscess in chronic granulomatous disease of childhood. *Radiology* 110:147, 1974.

36. Samuels, L. D. Liver scans in chronic granulomatous disease of childhood. *Pediatrics* 48:41, 1971.

37. Pitt, H. A., and Zuidema, G. D. Factors influencing mortality in the treatment of pyogenic hepatic abscess. *Surg. Gynecol. Obstet.* 140:228, 1975.

CHAPTER 22

Urinary Tract Infections

Acute urinary tract infection may be limited to the lower urinary tract, but persistent or recurrent cases often progress to involve the renal pelvis and parenchyma, producing pyelonephritis. Urinary tract infections are most common between two months and two years of age and are much more frequent in girls than in boys.

Microbiology

Most bacterial urinary tract infections (UTI) have been ascribed to large groups of Gram-negative aerobic or facultative anaerobic bacilli, including *Escherichia, Klebsiella, Aerobacter, Proteus,* and *Pseudomonas* species.[1] Other organisms usually not considered pathogenic, such as *Staphylococcus epidermidis,* may also be responsible. The clinical significance of other specific groups of organisms including the obligate anaerobe, many strains of which are present in the cecal, vaginal, and cervical flora, has received even less attention in urinary tract disease,[2] and anaerobes have been reported only rarely to cause UTI in children.[3]

Several reports describe the recovery of anaerobes in UTI in adults,[4] but many lack sufficient clinical bacteriologic detail to judge the reliability of the data; however, there are a good number of well-documented reports of infections of all types in adults. The types of infections of the urinary tract in which anaerobes have been involved include para- or periurethral cellulitis or abscess, acute and chronic urethritis, cystitis, acute and chronic prostatitis, prostatic abscess, periprostatic phlegmon, ureteritis, periureteritis, pyelitis, pyelonephritis, renal abscess, metastatic renal infection, pyonephrosis, perinephric abscess, retroperitoneal abscess, and other infections.[4]

The anaerobes recovered from these infections as reported in many studies[4] were *Bacteroides* species (including *Bacteroides fragilis* and

Bacteroides melaninogenicus), *Clostridium* species (including *Clostridium welchii* and *Clostridium perfringens*), anaerobic Gram-positive cocci, and *Actinomyces* species. In many cases they were recovered mixed with coliforms or streptococci.

Brook[3] recovered anaerobic bacteria from five young girls with UTI. Three had pyelonephritis, and two had cystitis. Two of the patients had a history of prior recurrent UTI. Urine samples were collected using suprapubic aspiration. The anaerobic organisms recovered were three isolates of *B. fragilis* and one each of *B. melaninogenicus*, *Peptococcus asaccharolyticus*, and *Bifidobacterium adolescentis*. Mixed infection was present in three children. In two patients *B. fragilis* was present with *Escherichia coli*, and in the other patient two anaerobes were present. All patients were treated with antimicrobial agents for 10 to 14 days and responded well to therapy. Two of the children had a recurrence of UTI with aerobic organisms recovered from their urine within six to eight months.

Pathogenesis

The source of bacteria causing UTI usually is the patient's fecal flora. Since anaerobes are another part of the fecal flora, it is not surprising to find them in some cases of UTI. Congenital anomalies of the urinary tract, especially those that obstruct the flow of urine, predispose to urinary tract infection. Foreign bodies, urethral catheters, and nephrolithiasis also predispose to infection. Most urinary tract infections, however, are not related to a structural or functional abnormality. The consistently higher incidence in girls beyond infancy may result from the short female urethra; the usual route of infection is an ascending one from external genitalia rather than a hematogenous one.

The periurethral region of healthy girls probably forms a barrier against UTI, and the bacterial flora at that region has been found to influence the acquisition of infections.[5] Anaerobes recently were found to constitute 95% of the total colony-forming units of organisms per square centimeter of the periurethral area of healthy girls.[6] The presence of anaerobes in the periurethral region may explain the mode of infectivity of these organisms.

Anaerobes may also gain access to the urinary tract, other than the urethra, by the ascending route, by direct extension from adjacent organs, such as the uterus or bowel, or by way of the bloodstream. Bran, Levinson, and Kaye[7] showed that urethral trauma may introduce organisms from the urethra to the bladder. Alling and colleagues[8] demonstrated that patients with indwelling urethral catheters have a high incidence of anaerobes recovered from urine. Sapico, Wideman, and Finegold[9] have shown that, on occasion, patients with indwelling

Foley catheters will show anaerobes along with aerobes and facultative organisms.

The growth conditions for anaerobes may be at times favorable in the urinary tracts of patients. Requirements are the availability of nutrients[10] and oxygen tension low enough to permit the growth of certain anaerobic bacteria. A low oxygen tension may be found when facultative anaerobes or aerobes are present, which consume the available oxygen for their growth and so create ideal conditions. Once introduced into the bladder or other parts of the urinary tract, certain anaerobes are capable of growing well in the urine itself.[10]

The low medullary blood flow, plasma skimming, and countercurrent flow all promote decreased oxygen supply to the medullary tissues, thus assisting the growth of anaerobes in cases of pyelonephritis. Medullary tissues derive their metabolic energy from anaerobic glycolysis to a greater extent than does cortical tissue. Anaerobic glycolysis of the inner medulla is relatively unaffected by the hypertonic environment of the medulla.[11] The state of dehydration further disposes a patient to anaerobic UTI, because the oxygen tension of the urine is sharply decreased in the dehydrated patient.[12]

Diagnosis

Symptoms may be absent, particularly in the chronic form of the disease. Onset may be gradual or abrupt. Fever may be as high as 40.3°C (104.5°F), accompanied by chills. Urinary frequency, urgency, incontinence, dysuria, prostration, anorexia, and pallor may occur. Vomiting may be projectile. There may be irritability and sometimes convulsions.

Signs include dull or sharp pain and tenderness in the kidney area or abdomen. Hypertension and evidence of chronic renal failure may be present in long-standing and severe cases. Jaundice may occur, particularly in early infancy. Anemia is found in cases of long-standing infection. Leukocytosis is usually in the range of 15,000 to 35,000/cu mm.

The diagnosis of acute pyelonephritis should be based on at least two consecutive positive urine cultures showing growth, and on a history of fever, chills, flank pain, nausea and vomiting, frequency, urgency, dysuria, and elevated sedimentation rate (above 30 mm/hr). Diagnosis of lower UTI (cystitis) should be based on at least two consecutive positive urine cultures and signs of urgency and dysuria.

The early detection of pyelonephritis and its differentiation from cystitis is of great clinical importance. Numerous studies have attempted to differentiate between lower and upper UTI in adults and children.[13-17] In addition to the evaluation of symptoms and signs such as fever and flank pain, several other methods have been proposed for determining the level of urinary tract infection,[13-17] but no single method is both simple and reliable. Ureteric catheterization is an invasive and unjustifiable procedure for children who have acute urinary tract infection.[14] The bladder washout technique[13] is less elaborate but requires trained personnel. In addition, the reliability of this test for diagnosing the level of involvement has been questioned.[18] Identification of antibody-coated bacteria[14] is simple but has been found to have little value for young children.[19]

Differences recently have been reported in urinary lactic dehydrogenase isoenzyme levels in the two types of infection.[20] Preliminary evidence suggests that the concentration of lactic acid in urine may be a good means of distinguishing lower UTI (cystitis) from upper UTI (pyelonephritis) and may be helpful in detecting urinary tract obstruction.[21]

Since the level of infection cannot be determined accurately with any of these tests, the best way to detect involvement of renal parenchyma seems to be the evaluation of clinical findings supplemented by a battery of laboratory tests.

Children with proved urinary infection should be examined by voiding cystourethrography and intravenous pyelography to identify anomalies of the urinary tract or vesicoureteral reflux. These studies should be delayed when possible until infection has been cleared for a few weeks. Although data on UTI in children is limited, it seems that these patients' radiologic studies show abnormalities that are indistinguishable from UTI caused by other bacteria. Examination of the urine generally reveals pyuria.

Slight or moderate hematuria occasionally occurs. There may be slight proteinuria. Pathogenic organisms and casts of all types may be present in the urine, but the urine may be normal for long periods of time.

Since anaerobes are found as normal flora in the urethra, it is seldom satisfactory or reliable to obtain voided specimens for diagnosis of UTI caused by anaerobic bacteria. In the study reported by Finegold and co-workers,[20] anaerobes were recovered from 14 of 100 random urine specimens. Relatively high counts of anaerobes were recovered in certain cases. In follow-up studies, these authors failed to recover any obligate anaerobes from 19 specimens of "urethral" urine and "midstream" urine yielded anaerobes in mixed culture in 13 instances. The anaerobes recovered from the voided specimens clearly represented normal urethral flora. In this study, anaerobes were recovered in counts of 10^3 to 10^4/ml or greater on a number of occasions.[10] Thus, even quantitative anaerobic culture is not helpful in distinguishing between infection and the presence of anaerobes as normal flora.

The report of Segura and colleagues[22] confirmed the validity of suprapubic bladder puncture for documentation of anaerobic UTI. In their study suprapubic bladder aspirations were performed in two groups of patients: one group whose aerobic cultures did not reveal organisms that were present in significant numbers on Gram stain and a second group that required suprapubic bladder aspiration for other reasons, such as an inability to void. Of 5781 patients studied, at least 1.3% of patients with significant bacteriuria had anaerobic organisms involved. Of the 10 suprapubic bladder taps that were positive for anaerobes, there was one instance in which an anaerobe was recovered in pure culture; this was an isolate of *B. fragilis* in a patient with known renal tuberculosis. Five of the subjects had two anaerobes recovered.

It is possible that with the improvements and simplification of the techniques of recovery of anaerobic organisms and proper methods of their collection and transportation to the laboratory, the yield of anaerobes in UTI in children may increase.

The data presented herein suggest the role of anaerobic organisms in UTI in children. It is therefore recommended that in symptomatic cases in which routine aerobic cultures fail to yield bacterial growth, and Gram stain shows bacteria to be present in the urine sediment, appropriate cultures for anaerobic bacteria be obtained.

Management

Increased fluid intake can assist in clearing the infection in the acute stage. Although there is no substantial evidence that routine surgical correction alters the course of recurrent UTI to any significant degree, repair of clearly obstructive lesions is indicated.

Eradication of infection with appropriate antibiotic therapy is of utmost importance. A prolonged course of urinary tract antisepsis (two to six months or longer) may be indicated, especially for repeated infections. Repeated urinalysis and culture should be obtained 48 hours after starting treatment and at intervals of one to two months for at least a year.

Acute uncomplicated infection, which is commonly caused by enteric organisms such as *E. coli*, generally is treated by oral sulfonamides, trimethoprim-sulfamethoxazole, or ampicillin. Acutely ill patients may be treated with intravenously administered drug—one of the antibiotics mentioned above or an aminoglycoside such as gentamicin. The recovery of aerobic or facultative anaerobic organisms from the urine of a patient with UTI does not exclude the possibility of the concomitant presence of an anaerobe.

The recovery of anaerobes in UTI may have important implications on the choice of antimicrobial agents. Most anaerobic organisms are sensitive to penicillin and cephalosporins. Most anaerobes, however, are resistant to sulfonamides, and all are highly resistant to aminoglycosides. Furthermore, *B. fragilis* and some strains of *B. melaninogenicus* are also resistant to penicillin and cephalosporins.[23]

The recovery of anaerobes requires the choice of an agent that is effective against these organisms. Penicillin or cephalosporins can be used against most anaerobic organisms; however, the recovery of penicillin-resistant organisms requires administration of appropriate antimicrobial agents such as clindamycin, chloramphenicol, carbenicillin, ticarcillin, or cefoxitin.[4]

Complications

In patients with uncomplicated cystitis or pyelonephritis, treatment ordinarily results in complete resolution of symptoms. Cystitis may occasionally result in upper tract infection or bacteremia, especially during instrumentation. Cases of anaerobic bacteremia following urologic procedures have been reported.[9] Repeated symptomatic UTI in children with obstructive uropathy, neurogenic bladder, structural renal disease, or diabetes more often progresses to chronic renal disease. Untreated UTI can progress to renal abscess, pyonephrosis, perinephric or retroperitoneal abscess. Anaerobes have been recovered in each of these disease states.

REFERENCES

1. Kass, E. H. Pyelonephritis and bacteremia: a major problem in preventive medicine. *Ann. Intern. Med.* 56:46, 1962.

2. Kumazawa, J. et al. Significance of anaerobic bacteria isolated from the urinary tract. I. Clinical studies. *J. Urol.* 112:257, 1974.

3. Brook, I. Urinary tract infection caused by anaerobic bacteria in children. *Urology* 16:596, 1980.

4. Finegold, S. M. *Anaerobic bacteria in human disease.* New York: Academic Press, 1977, p. 314.

5. Fair, W. R. et al. Bacteriologic and hormonal observations of the urethra and vaginal vestibule in normal, premenopausal women. *J. Urol.* 104:426, 1970.

6. Bollgren, I.; Kallenius, G.; and Nord, C. E. Periurethral anaerobic microflora of healthy girls. *J. Clin. Microbiol.* 10:419, 1979.

7. Bran, J. L.; Levinson, M. E.; and Kaye, D. Entrance of bacteria into the female urinary bladder. *N. Engl. J. Med.* 286:626, 1972.

8. Alling, B. et al. Aerobic and anaerobic microbial flora in the urinary tract of geriatric patients during long-term care. *J. Infect. Dis.* 127:34, 1973.

9. Sapico, F. L.; Wideman, P. A.; and Finegold, S. M. Aerobic and anaerobic bladder urine flora of patients with indwelling urethral catheters. *Urology* 7:382, 1976.

10. Finegold, S. M. et al. Significance of anaerobic and capnophilic bacteria isolated from the urinary tract. In *Progress in pyelonephritis,* 1st edition, ed. E. M. Kass. Philadelphia: F. A. Davis, 1965, p. 159.

11. Editorial. Oxygen tension of the urine and renal function. *N. Engl. J. Med.* 269:159, 1963.

12. Leonhardt, K. O., and Landes, R. R. Oxygen tension of the urine and renal structures. Preliminary report of clinical findings. *N. Engl. J. Med.* 269:115, 1963.

13. Fairley, K. P. et al. Site of infection in acute urinary-tract infection in general practice. *Lancet* 2:615, 1971.

14. Hewstone, A. S., and Whitaker, J. The correlation of ureteric urine bacteriology and homologous antibody titer in children with urinary infection. *J. Pediatr.* 70:540, 1969.

15. Steele, R. E.; Leadbetter, G. W.; and Crawford, J. D. Prognosis of childhood urinary-tract infection. *N. Engl. J. Med.* 169:883, 1963.

16. Thomas, V.; Shelokov, A.; and Forland, M. Antibody-coated bacteria in the urine and the site of urinary-tract infection. *N. Engl. J. Med.* 290:588, 1974.

17. Winberg, J. et al. Studies of urinary tract infection in infancy and childhood. I. Antibody response in different types of infections caused by coliform bacteria. *Br. Med. J.* 2:524, 1963.

18. Jodal, U.; Lindberg, U.; and Lincoln, K. Level diagnosis of symptomatic urinary tract infections in childhood. *Acta Paediatr. Scand.* 64:201, 1975.

19. Hellerstein, S. et al. Localization of the site of urinary tract infections by means of antibody-coated bacteria in the urinary sediments. *J. Pediatr.* 92:188, 1978.

20. Devaskar, U., and Montgomery, W. Urinary lactic dehydrogenase isoenzymes IV and V in the differential diagnosis of cystitis and pyelonephritis. *J. Pediatr.* 93:789, 1978.

21. Brook, I.; Belman, A. B.; and Controni, G. Lactic acid in urine of children with lower and upper urinary tract infection and renal obstruction. *Am. J. Clin. Pathol.* 75:110, 1981.

22. Segura, J. W. et al. Anaerobic bacteria in the urinary tract, *Mayo Clin. Proc.* 47:20, 1972.

23. Sutter, V. L., and Finegold, S. M. Susceptibility of anaerobic bacteria to 23 antimicrobial agents. *Antimicrob. Agents Chemother.* 10:736, 1976.

CHAPTER 23

Female Genital Tract Infections

With earlier arrival of physiologic and sexual maturity a larger number of adolescent patients are contracting sexually transmitted diseases and their complications.[1] The highest incidence of pelvic inflammatory disease, which is the most serious complication of sexually transmitted diseases, occurs between the ages of 15 and 20.[2] Pediatricians, and especially those dealing with adolescents, must be aware of the clinical presentation and management of female genital tract infections.

Pathogenesis

With only a few exceptions, such as group A beta-hemolytic streptococci (GABHS) and certain sexually transmitted organisms, the bacterial pathogens involved in gynecologic infections reflect the normal microflora of the vagina and cervix. This flora is complex and includes obligate anaerobes of the Peptococcaceae and Bacteroidaceae families, aerobic Gram-negative bacilli of the Enterbacteriaceae family, and aerobic as well as microaerophilic streptococci.

Many studies have documented that the vagina and cervix of healthy women harbor a sparse indigenous microflora. Obligate anaerobes were recovered in 70% of cervical cultures from healthy women.[3] *Bacteroides* species, the most common anaerobes, was recovered from 57% of specimens. Several species of *Bacteroides* were encountered, including *Bacteroides fragilis, Bacteroides capillosus, Bacteroides clostridiformis, Bacteroides oralis,* and *Bacteroides melaninogenicus*. Although the latter two species are believed to be confined to the oral cavity, they could also be recovered from the cervical flora.

In addition, peptostreptococci, clostridia, facultative lactobacilli, and streptococci are a part of the normal vaginal flora. These host factors may greatly influence the composition of the microbiota of established pelvic infections. The concentration of obligate anaerobes, particularly *Bacteroides* species, increases substantially in certain situations, for example, during the first half of the menstrual cycle, in the post-partum period, after pelvic surgery, with pelvic malignancy, and during immunosuppression.

Anaerobes can be cultured in 50% to 90% of females with a variety of genital infections and are the exclusive isolates in 20% to 50%.[4] Obligate anaerobes are particularly common in closed space infections, such as tubo-ovarian and vulvovaginal abscesses. The most common anaerobes found in these infections are *Bacteroides* species (especially *B. bivius*) and anaerobic cocci. Although *B. fragilis* is cultured less frequently, it is more important in closed-space infections.

Aerobes generally are not the only pathogens found, but are usually mixed with aerobes. The most common aerobic pathogens are members of the Enterobacteriaceae family, especially *Escherichia coli*, and aerobic or microaerophilic streptococci.

Specific Infections

Vulvovaginal Pyogenic Infections

Vulvovaginal pyogenic infections include abscesses of Bartholin's and Skene's glands, infected labial inclusion cysts, labial abscesses, furunculosis, and hidradenitis. Most infections are due to both aerobic and anaerobic organisms arising from the normal vaginal and cervical flora. *Neisseria gonorrhoeae* is responsible for approximately 10% of these infections. The majority of nonvenereal abscesses are caused by anaerobic bacteria.

Parker and Jones[5] recovered anaerobes in two-thirds of 75 patients with such infections. Similarly, Swenson and associates[6] recovered anaerobes from 10 of 15 patients with Bartholin's gland abscess. Anaerobic streptococci and *Bacteroides* species were cultured from these abscesses. The clinical course of such infections is indistinguishable from that associated with other pathogens.[7]

In diabetic patients, the inflammation can extend to deeper structures of the perineum, the lower extremities, or back and cause extensive necrosis.[8] Other pathogens in addition to *Peptostreptococcus* species and *B. fragilis* are *Staphylococcus aureus* and facultative streptococci, particularly group A *Streptococcus pyogenes*.

Therapy consists primarily of surgical drainage; antibiotics are of secondary importance. In the absence of cultural and antibiotic susceptibility data, initial selection of drugs should include those effective against both aerobic and anaerobic bacteria of vaginal-cervical origin. Broad-spectrum antibiotics such as ampicillin or the cephalosporins are often useful. If *B. fragilis* is suspected, however, then clindamycin, chloramphenicol, cefoxitin, or metronidazole should be administered.[9]

Endometritis and Pyometra

Although endometritis and pyometra are seen more commonly in older women who suffer from cervical canal obstruction or carcinoma or following delivery, they can be seen occasionally in adolescent females. Endometritis occurs when bacteria invade the uterine cavity, and pyometra develops when pus is collected within the uterus. Regardless of the etiology, anaerobes are predominant in endometritis and pyometra.

Carter and colleagues,[10] who studied 133 patients with endometritis and pyometra, isolated obligate anaerobes from 75% of the patients. The most frequent anaerobic isolates were anaerobic streptococci and *Bacteroides* species. Swenson and co-workers[6] studied 14 women with this diagnosis and recovered anaerobes from 13, often associated with facultative bacteria, but in pure culture in six.

Muram, Drouin, and Thompson[11] recovered anaerobes from only 5 of 15 patients with pyometra they have studied, and from 7 they have recovered mixed aerobic and anaerobic flora.

Pyometra should be considered an abscess and treated promptly and vigorously with drainage of the uterine cavity followed by curettage to debride the necrotic tissue.[12] The most serious fatal complication of these conditions is spread of the organisms from the uterus into the blood.[1, 7]

Antibiotics effective against aerobic and anaerobic bacteria should be given. This is especially important for patients with signs of systemic infection, such as fever, peritonitis, tachycardia, or leukocytosis. Appropriate specimens for cultures should be obtained prior to initiation of therapy. Combined therapy with an aminoglycoside and an agent against anaerobes (clindamycin, metronidazole, chloramphenicol, cefoxitin) will be adequate in most patients. Evacuation of the uterus remains the mainstay of management, however.

Acute Salpingitis and Pelvic Inflammatory Disease

Acute salpingitis and pelvic inflammatory disease (PID) occur after extension of the infection from the lower parts of the female genital tract to higher structures.

Organisms infecting the cervix can spread to involve the uterus and fallopian tubes by two routes: by causing a transient endometritis that extends to involve the endosalpinx, or they may reach the tubes via lymphatic spread.

Acute salpingitis and PID may be gonococcal or nongonococcal, according to presence or absence of associated endocervical gonorrhea. Acute pelvic salpingitis and PID is predominantly a disease of adolescent sexually active nonparous women.

The recovery of *N. gonorrhoeae* from the upper genital tract is variable. Many species of aerobes and anaerobes that are related to the normal vaginal flora can be isolated. Rarely, chlamydiae and mycoplasmae also have been implicated. It is generally suspected that *N. gonorrhoeae* paves the way to anaerobic PID and that the anaerobic bacteria travel through the endometrium and salpinges to the tubo-ovarian junction.[13] Presumably, it explains the rarity of pelvic infections during the full-term pregnancy. The isolation of gonococci from the endocervix does not necessarily account for upper genital tract disease. Moreover, the eradication of gonococci may not be adequate treatment for acute salpingitis. The morbidity and sequelae of both gonococcal and nongonococcal salpingitis may be attributed to repeated ascending infection by the aerobic and anaerobic microorganisms as secondary invaders.

Recent investigations[4, 13, 14] have documented the polymicrobial etiology of acute salpingitis. Culdocentesis and laparoscopy have revealed mixed aerobic and anaerobic bacterial flora in addition to gonococci in patients with acute salpingitis. The most frequent pathogens appear to be gonococci and anaerobic bacteria (most commonly *Peptostreptococcus*, *Peptococcus*, and *Bacteroides* species).

A characteristic pattern has evolved from these studies. In approximately one-third of patients, only gonococci could be recovered from the intraabdominal site; another third had gonococci plus anaerobic and aerobic bacteria; and the final third had both aerobic and anaerobic bacteria, but not gonococci, recovered from their abdominal cavity.

Chlamydia trachomatis has received attention recently as an etiologic agent in acute salpingitis. Studies from Sweden show a 30% incidence of *Chlamydia* isolation from the fallopian tubes of patients with acute salpingitis.[15] Scandinavian serologic studies suggest that *C. trachomatis* is associated with 40% to 60% of acute salpingitis cases.[16]

Although mycoplasmae have been recovered frequently from the lower genital tract of women with salpingitis, no difference exists between the rates of isolation from the cervix of such patients and that of control patients.[17]

The clinical picture of gonococcal PID is similar to that of the nongonococcal PID; the latter is predominantly anaerobic. Acute pelvic inflammatory disease causes fever, chills, malaise, anorexia, nausea, and severe bilateral lower abdominal pain. Adynamic ileus is present if associated pelvic peritonitis has occurred. Pelvic examination reveals a purulent discharge oozing from an inflamed cervical os, and exquisite cervical motion tenderness. The adnexal regions are tender and thickened, and an adnexal or cul-de-sac mass may be palpable if infection is recurrent or chronic.

PID must be differentiated from other acute lower abdominal processes such as acute appendicitis, pelvic endometrosis, ovarian tumors, rupture of an ovarian cyst, or a ruptured ectopic pregnancy. Diagnosis of acute salpingitis and PID should also include visual confirmation of tubal inflammation by such procedures as colposcopy and laparoscopy.

Although an accurate bacteriologic diagnosis is of great importance, the relative inaccessibility of pelvic structures and the likelihood of external contamination of cultures obtained through the vagina limits the value of such cultures, especially for anaerobes. Procedures such as colposcopy, laparoscopy, or culdocentesis to obtain culture specimens can increase diagnostic accuracy. Material obtained for culture should be Gram stained and cultured aerobically and anaerobically.

Salpingitis and PID are managed primarily with antimicrobial therapy. Because endocervical gonorrhea frequently is present, initial treatment should be at least adequate for gonococcal salpingitis. This can be achieved by penicillin plus probenecid, ampicillin, or tetracycline. In areas where resistance of gonococci to penicillin has been observed, spectinomycin can be used. Surgical intervention may be required if the patient fails to respond to medical therapy.

Severely ill patients should be admitted to the hospital, particularly if an adnexal mass or peritonitis is present. The antimicrobial regimen of choice is, in addition to penicillin, the combination of an aminoglycoside with either clindamycin or cefoxitin, given intravenously. The use of these antimicrobial agents is required because of the high frequency of involvement by *Bacteroides* species and the poor prognosis without optimal therapy. This combination is effective against anaerobic bacteria, aerobic Gram-negative bacilli, enterococci, and staphylococci, as well as gonococci.[18]

Patients with an intrauterine device (IUD) have a higher incidence of acute salpingitis, and the clinical presentation of infection in this group may be different. Unilateral adnexal infection occurs more frequently, and the infections may be more severe. In addition, serious *Actinomyces* infections generally are associated with this form of contraception. It is important to make a precise microbiologic diagnosis of pelvic actinomycosis, since penicillin or tetracycline is the agent of choice, and prolonged therapy is necessary.[19]

Long-term sequelae commonly are observed following nongonococcal salpingitis and include recurrent exacerbations, tubo-ovarian abscess, sterility, chronic pain, and dysfunctional bleeding.

Tubo-ovarian and Pelvic Abscess

Tubo-ovarian abscess (TOA) generally is a consequence of pelvic inflammatory disease of acute or chronic nature. Other conditions associated with pelvic abscess formation include endometritis, pyelonephritis, uterine fibroids, and malignancy in the pelvic area.

Most pelvic abscesses are caused by anaerobic bacteria, with *Bacteroides* species predominating, followed by peptostreptococci and peptococci and, rarely, clostridia. They often are found in association with aerobic bacteria.

Swenson and colleagues[6] recovered anaerobes from 8 of 10 pelvic abscesses, and they were the exclusive pathogens in five patients. Similarly, Thadepalli[20] recovered anaerobes from all 13 patients with pelvic abscess, and these organisms were the only isolates in nine patients. The specimens for culture were obtained in both studies either at operation or by culdocentesis, thereby avoiding contamination by the normal vaginal flora.

The bacteriology of TOA is somewhat different from that of other pelvic abscesses. Whereas pelvic abscesses are caused by mixed aerobic and anaerobic bacteria, exclusively anaerobic bacteria were found in nearly one-half of the cases of TOA.

On examination, the adnexal regions are very tender, and an adnexal or cul-de-sac mass is palpable. Ultrasonography is a particularly useful procedure for localization of pelvic abscess.

Rupture of a tubo-ovarian abscess causes severe pain referred to the site of involvement. Chills, fever, and signs of progressing peritonitis follow the onset of pain. Diarrhea may occur early but ceases as the peritonitis worsens. If large volumes of pus are released into the peritoneal cavity, infection may spread upward along the colonic gutters; subphrenic abscesses may form, causing pain in the shoulders.

Intravenous clindamycin, chloramphenicol, or metronidazole in combination with an aminoglycoside are suitable choices for therapy. If there is no clinical response after 48 to 72 hours or if the abscess enlarges, surgery is necessary, while antibiotic therapy is continued.

Surgery is also necessary with a tubo-ovarian abscess rupture. This is vital since the patient fatality rate approaches 90% with medical therapy alone. Rapid diagnosis of such an abscess is the keystone to a successful outcome.

REFERENCES

1. Smith, M. S., and Eschenbach, D. A. Pelvic inflammatory disease. A review. *Clin. Pediatr.* 19:791, 1980.

2. Forslin, L.; Falk, V.; and Danielson, D. Changes in the incidence of acute gonococcal and nongococcal salpingitis. *Br. J. Vener. Dis.* 54:247, 1978.

3. Gorbach, S. L. et al. Anaerobic microflora of the cervix in healthy women. *Am. J. Obstet. Gynecol.* 117:1053, 1973.

4. Chow, A. W.; Marshall, J. R.; and Guze, L. B. Anaerobic infections of the female genital tract—prospects and perspectives. *Obstet. Gynecol. Survey* 30:477, 1975.

5. Parker, R. T., and Jones, C. P. Anaerobic pelvic infections and developments in hyperbaric oxygen therapy. *Am. J. Obstet. Gynecol.* 96:645, 1966.

6. Swenson, R. M. et al. Anaerobic bacterial infections of the female genital tract. *Obstet. Gynecol.* 42:538, 1973.

7. Carter, B. et al. *Bacteroides* infections in obstetrics and gynecology. *Obstet. Gynecol.* 1:491, 1953.

8. Roberts, D. B., and Hester, L. L., Jr. Progressive synergistic bacterial gangrene arising from abscesses of the vulva and Bartholin's gland duct. *Am. J. Obstet. Gynecol.* 114:285, 1972.

9. Eschenbach, D. A., and Holmes, K. K. Acute pelvic inflammatory disease—current concepts of pathogenesis, etiology and management. *Clin. Obstet. Gynecol.* 18:35, 1975.

10. Carter, B. et al. A bacteriologic and clinical study of pyometra. *Am. J. Obstet. Gynecol.* 62:793, 1951.

11. Muram, D. et al. Pyometra. *Can. Med. Assoc. J.* 125:589, 1981.

12. Henriksen, E. Pyometra associated with malignant lesions of the cervix and the uterus. *Am. J. Obstet. Gynecol.* 72:884, 1956.

13. Eschenbach, D. A. et al. Polymicrobial etiology of pelvic inflammatory disease. *N. Engl. J. Med.* 293:166, 1975.

14. Cunningham, F. G. et al. Evaluation of tetracycline or penicillin and ampicillin for treatment of acute pelvic inflammatory disease. *N. Engl. J. Med.* 296:1380, 1977.

15. Trenharne, J. D. et al. Antibodies to chlamydia trachomatis in acute salpingitis. *Br. J. Vener. Dis.* 55:26, 1979.

16. Paavonen, J. et al. Chlamydia trachomatis in acute salpingitis. *Br. J. Vener. Dis.* 55:203, 1979.

17. Mardh, P. A., and Westrom, L. Tubal and cervical cultures in acute salpingitis with special reference to mycoplasma hominis and T-strain mycoplasma. *Br. J. Vener. Dis.* 46:179, 1970.

18. Finegold, S. M. Management of anaerobic infection. *Ann. Int. Med.* 83:375, 1975.

19. Taylor, E. S. et al. The intrauterine device and tubo-ovarian abscess. *Am. J. Obstet. Gynecol.* 123:338, 1975.

20. Thadepalli, H.; Gorbach, S. L.; and Keith, L. Anaerobic infections of the female genital tract: bacteriologic and therapeutic aspects. *Am. J. Obstet. Gynecol.* 117:1034, 1973.

CHAPTER 24

Skin and Soft Tissue Infections

Cutaneous Abscesses

Cutaneous abscesses are a commonly encountered infection in children. Subcutaneous and cutaneous abscesses can be caused by many aerobic and anaerobic pathogens, although treatment of these infections usually is surgical. Knowledge of the usual flora causing infection in certain anatomic loci should permit institution of therapy before the results of cultures are available.

Microbiology

The most common etiologic agents involved in skin and soft tissue infections in infants and children are *Staphylococcus aureus* and group A beta-hemolytic streptococci (GABHS).[1] These organisms frequently produce impetigo, furunculosis, cellulitis, and wound infections.[2]

Haemophilus influenzae is a rare cause of skin abscesses in infants.[3] Gram-negative rods such as *Escherichia coli* or *Klebsiella* organisms are occasional causes of mastitis in the nursing mother.[4] Gram-negative enteric bacteria also occasionally infect moist areas of the skin.

Anaerobic bacteria have not always been recognized as important in abscesses in children. Recent publications[5-7] have documented the isolation of anaerobes from abscesses in children, usually mixed with aerobes. Similar studies of adults[8] describe the isolation of anaerobes with a frequency comparable to aerobes in all nonperineal areas except the hand. In contrast, abscesses in the perineal region contained a greater variety and frequency of anaerobes.

In a recent study, specimens from 176 cutaneous abscesses in children were cultured for aerobic and anaerobic microorganisms.[9] Of these, 9 (5%) were sterile, and 46 (27.5%) yielded pure cultures predominantly of *S. aureus.* The rest of the abscesses yielded growth of two or more aerobic or anaerobic organisms. The data were organized according to these anatomic locations: head, neck, trunk, finger, hand, leg, buttocks, perirectal, and vulvovaginal areas. Aerobic bacteria only were present in 83 specimens (50%), anaerobes only were isolated in 43 (26%), and mixed aerobic and anaerobic bacteria were present in 41 abscesses (24%). A total of 351 isolates (202 anaerobes and 149 aerobes) were recovered (table 24.1), accounting for 2.0 isolates per specimen (1.2 anaerobes and 0.8 aerobes). The average number of isolates per abscess is reported by anatomic area in table 24.2. The presence of more than one anaerobe per abscess was obtained from the vulvovaginal, buttocks, perirectal, finger, and head areas. Aerobes were more prevalent in the neck, hand, leg, and trunk areas.

The predominant aerobes recovered were *S. aureus,* alpha- and nonhemolytic streptococci, GABHS, enterobacters, and *Escherichia coli* (table 24.1). The predominant anaerobes recovered were anaerobic Gram-positive cocci, *Bacteroides* species (including *Bacteroides fragilis* group and *Bacteroides melaninogenicus* group), and *Fusobacterium* species.

The most prevalent aerobe, *S. aureus,* was recovered from all areas where abscesses originate on skin surfaces. It was, however, recovered less often from the buttocks, perirectal, and vulvovaginal areas. These latter sites include abscesses that originated from adjacent mucous membranes rather than skin. Contrary to general clinical impression, *S. aureus* was isolated, except in the neck area, in only 50% or less of abscesses from each site. Usually it was found alone, infrequently with other aerobes, and, rarely, with anaerobes. This organism has a well-recognized propensity for abscess formation, both in local and in visceral infections resulting from hematogenous dissemination. In contrast to anaerobes,[10] its potential for abscess formation is not as dependent on synergistic bacterial mixtures.

Among Gram-negative aerobes, only enterobacters and *E. coli* were isolated frequently. Enterobacters were recovered mostly from the trunk and legs, while *E. coli* was recovered mainly from the vulvovaginal, buttocks, and perirectal areas. These Gram-negative rods were isolated in pure culture only once *(E. coli),* and in all other instances they were recovered mixed with other aerobic and anaerobic organisms.

Pathogenesis

Factors predisposing to the initiation of the infection include trauma, obstruction of drainage, ischemia, chemical irritation, hematoma formation, accumulation of fluid, foreign bodies, and stasis in the vascular system.

Table 24.1. Frequency of Isolation of Aerobic and Anaerobic Bacteria from 176 Specimens from Different Areas

	Head	Neck	Trunk	Finger	Hand	Leg	Buttocks	Peri-rectal	Vulvo-vaginal	Total Number of Isolates
Number of specimens	26	23	17	20	25	28	15	17	5	
Aerobes:										
Alpha- and non-hemolytic streptococci	2	1	3	4	2	1	2	1	2	18
Group A beta-hemolytic streptococci	1	5			4			2		12
Group B beta-hemolytic streptococci	3		1							4
Group D streptococci			1		1		2			4
S. aureus	9	14	8	9	16	14	1	5		76
S. epidermidis		1	1	1				1		4
N. gonorrhoeae	1									1
Proteus sp.				1			1	2		4
P. aeruginosa								2		2
E. coli							3	3	2	8
K. pneumoniae					2	1				3
Enterobacter sp.	1	1	2	1		3		1	1	10
H. parainfluenzae	2			1						3
Total number of aerobes	19	22	16	17	25	19	9	17	5	149

	Head	Neck	Trunk	Finger	Hand	Leg	Buttocks	Peri-rectal	Vulvo-vaginal	Total Number of Isolates
Anaerobes:										
Peptococcus sp.	3	2	1	2	1	3	7	8	4	31
Peptostreptococcus sp.	4		1	5	2	2	3	5	3	25
Veillonella sp.	2	1				1	1	1		6
Eubacterium sp.	2			1				2		5
Bifidobacterium sp.				1					2	3
Lactobacillus sp.	1		2	1					1	5
P. acnes	1		2		1	1	1			6
Clostridium sp.			3		1		1			5
Bacteroides sp.*	5			6	4	2	9	9	4	39
B. fragilis group†	2			3	2	2	8	9	3	29
B. melaninogenicus group	5		1	2	1	2	7	6		24
Fusobacterium sp.‡	5	1		6	2	2	3	4	1	24
Total number of anaerobes	30	4	10	27	14	15	40	44	18	202
Total number of isolates	26	26	26	44	39	34	49	61	23	351

SOURCE: Brook, I., and Finegold, S. M. Aerobic and anaerobic bacteriology of cutaneous abscesses in children. *Pediatrics* 67:891, 1981. Copyright 1981, American Academy of Pediatrics. Reprinted by permission.

Bacteroides sp. includes 8 *B. Corrodens*, 4 *B. oralis*, 2 *B. ruminicola*, ss. *brevis*.

†*B. fragilis* group includes 12 *B. fragilis*, 5 *B. distasonis*, 5 *B. thetaiotaomicron*, 4 *B. vulgatus*, and 3 *B. ovatus*.

‡*Fusobacterium* sp. includes 16 *F. nucleatum* and 1 *F. necrophorum*.

Table 24.2. Characterization of 176 Abscesses in Children (Outpatients)

Anatomic Area	Head	Neck	Trunk	Finger	Hand	Leg	Buttocks	Perirectal	Vulvo-vaginal
No. of abscesses	26	23	17	20	25	28	15	17	5
Percentage of total cultures	14.8	13	9.7	11.4	14.2	16	8.4	9.7	2.8
Type of bacterial growth									
No growth	0	9	6	5	8	11	0	0	0
Aerobes only	38	74	53	40	72	64	13	6	0
Anaerobes only	19	13	29	20	12	14	67	35	60
Aerobes and anaerobes	43	4	12	35	8	11	20	59	40
Bacterial sp. per abscess									
Aerobes	0.7	1.0	0.9	0.9	1.1	0.8	0.6	1.0	1.0
Anaerobes	1.3	0.2	0.6	1.4	0.6	0.6	2.7	2.6	3.6
Total	2.0	1.2	1.5	2.3	1.7	1.4	3.3	3.6	4.6

Source: Brook, I., and Finegold, S. M. Aerobic and anaerobic bacteriology of cutaneous abscesses in children. *Pediatrics* 67:891, 1981. Copyright 1981, American Academy of Pediatrics. Reprinted by permission.

Infection in some areas is more likely to be caused by certain organisms, and special features of the tissue reaction produced by some bacterial species make it possible to recognize infection by them with considerable accuracy. For example, staphylococci generally produce rapid necrosis and early suppuration with large amounts of creamy yellow pus. GABHS tend to spread rapidly through tissues, causing intense edema and erythema, while anaerobic bacteria may produce necrosis and profuse, brownish foul-smelling pus.

The location of the abscess is of paramount importance in identification of the organism that may be involved in the infection. Under appropriate conditions of lowered tissue resistance, almost any of the common bacteria can initiate an infectious process. Cultures from lesions frequently contain several bacterial species; as might be expected, the organisms found most frequently are the "normal flora" of these regions.

Aspirates from abscesses of the perineal and oral regions tend to yield organisms found in stool or mouth flora.[11] Conversely, pus obtained from abscesses in areas remote from the rectum or mouth contain primarily constituents of the microflora indigenous to the skin.[12] Multiple anaerobic organisms usually are recovered[9] from the perineal region, whereas only about one anaerobe per abscess is present at other sites. Anaerobes also are recovered alone, without aerobes, more often from the perineal area. Mixed aerobic and anaerobic infections are more prevalent in the perirectal, head, finger, and nailbed areas. The similarities in the rates of isolation of mixed aerobic and anaerobic flora and the high rate of recovery of anaerobes in these areas is of particular interest. This can be due, in the last two areas, to the introduction of mouth flora, which is predominantly anaerobic, onto the fingers by sucking, a common activity in children. This is parallel to the acquisition of infection following human bites and clenched fist injuries in which anaerobic mouth flora was the source of most bacterial isolates.[13]

Gram-positive anaerobic cocci are normal skin inhabitants and part of the normal fecal flora.[12] They also are isolated from intraabdominal abscesses.[14] They were isolated as frequently as *Bacteroides* species from abscesses of the perineal region and also were frequently isolated from nonperineal cutaneous abscesses.

Organisms belonging to the *B. fragilis* group, which predominate in the feces,[11, 15] were cultured most frequently from abscesses of the perirectal area. *B. melaninogenicus,* which occurs in stools as well as in the oral cavity,[11, 15] also was recovered from this site and from the head. Most strains of *B. fragilis* and many strains of *B. melaninogenicus* are resistant to penicillin.[16]

Diagnosis

Infection in soft tissue usually begins as a cellulitis, which is a diffuse acute inflammation with hyperemia, edema, and leukocytic infiltration but has little or no necrosis and suppuration. Some organisms will then cause necrosis, liquefaction, accumulation of leukocytes and debris, suppuration, loculation of the pus, and formation of one or more abscesses.

Infections of the skin and subcutaneous tissues produce the classic manifestations of redness, tenderness, heat, and swelling. Associating lymphangitis is characterized by the presence of reddish streaks extending proximally and associated with tender enlargement of regional lymph nodes. Systemic symptoms may be mild, and can include fever, malaise, and leukocytosis. The presence of fluctuation in the abscess indicates that the mass is ready for drainage. Laboratory findings include leukocytosis, rapid sedimentation rate, and often positive blood cultures. Certain organisms can cause bacteremia more frequently, and manipulation, including surgical incision, of the abscess may be followed by transient bacteremia.

Pus or fluid obtained by needle aspiration or incision should be Gram stained and examined directly, in addition to being cultured aerobically and anaerobically.

X-ray examinations may detect localized collections of pus when collections of gas are present or when abnormal tissue density is observed. Ultrasound and computerized axial tomography (CAT scan), angiography, and radionuclide scans may be helpful in demonstrating abscesses, especially in closed spaces.

Management

Surgical drainage is the treatment of choice for abscesses. Although antimicrobial drugs may prevent suppuration if given early or prevent spread of an existing abscess, they cannot be substituted for surgical drainage. Heat application can relieve the pain and speed suppuration and liquefaction. Elevation of the affected part reduces the edema and pain.

The early administration of antibiotics can abort the development of an abscess. Once the suppuration has appeared, however, drugs become incapable of eradicating the infecting organisms. Several antibiotics can be partially inactivated by the pus, while others can maintain their potency. Another factor that decreases the activity of antibiotics that are active only against multiplying organisms (penicillins and cephalosporins) is the failure of offending bacteria to multiply well in pus. Phagocytosis, which is essential to complete elimination of bacteria, is reduced in the abscess cavity. Because of the combination of these two factors, many abscesses are resistant to antimicrobial therapy.

Since anaerobic bacteria frequently are associated with cutaneous abscesses in pediatric patients, especially in areas adjacent to the mucosal surfaces, physicians should anticipate their presence if antimicrobial therapy is employed. Gram staining of aspirated pus and appropriate aerobic and anaerobic techniques can help the physician select proper therapy. Since some of the anaerobes are resistant to penicillin, therapy also should include appropriate coverage of these organisms in more serious infections. Therapy should consist of administration of either clindamycin, carbenicillin, ticarcillin, chloramphenicol, metronidazole, or cefoxitin.

Complications

The abscess may spread locally or systemically. The local spread of infection generally follows the path of least resistance along fascial planes. Lymphatic spread may lead to lymphangitis, lymphadenitis, or the formation of a bubo. Involvement of veins may lead to infective thrombophlebitis with resulting bacteremia, septic embolization, and systemic dissemination of infection. Staphylococci, streptococci, and *Bacteroides* organisms are notorious for the frequency with which they produce vascular lesions of this type.

Decubitus Ulcers

Decubiti and nonhealing wounds usually are produced by pressure or by circulatory dysfunction. In an area where the patient has no sensation the decubitus ulcer develops when pressure is placed on one site for a critical period of time, causing ischemia and then necrosis. Ulcers caused by circulatory dysfunction may result from large- or small-vessel disease or from venous stasis.

Patients who are bedridden, for whatever cause, are prone to decubitus ulcers. Poor nutrition, low serum albumin, anemia, and circulatory impairment add seriously to the hazard of this development.[17]

Sites of Formation of Decubitus Ulcers

Decubitus ulcers are rarely found in pediatric patients; however, they frequently occur in children who are brain-damaged or neurologically handicapped. Decubitus ulcers are common in bedridden adult patients, and most of the literature is based on data obtained from these patients.[18, 19]

Ninety-six percent of all pressure sores occur in the lower part of the body, 67% around the hips and buttocks and 29% on the lower limbs.[20] Any area that is subjected to pressure over a bony prominence is at risk, and ulcerations may occur on the ear, the occiput, the spinous processes of the vertebrae, the shoulder, iliac crest, the elbow, anterosuperior iliac spine, sacrum, trochanter, ischium, thigh, knee, Achilles tendon, lateral malleolus, heel, sole, medial malleolus, lateral edge of the foot, and the scrotum and penis.

Microbiology

Aerobic bacteria, Gram-negative enteric rods, *S. aureus,* and *Streptococcus faecalis* are the predominant organisms isolated from decubitus ulcers in adults.[21, 22] Anaerobic bacteria also have been recovered from decubitus ulcers when anaerobic methods were used.[23, 24] In studies that used methods adequate for isolation of anaerobes, many aerobic and anaerobic organisms have been isolated from infected decubitus ulcers. The aerobic organisms that were also capable of producing sepsis included *Proteus, E. coli,* enterobacters, *Pseudomonas aeruginosa, S. aureus,* streptococci, diphtheroids, and yeast. Anaerobic isolates include *Bacteroides* species (especially *B. fragilis*), fusobacteria, peptococci, peptostreptococci, microaerophilic streptococci, clostridia, and eubacteria.[18, 19, 23] It is obvious that bacteremia frequently is associated with infected decubitus ulcers and is commonly polymicrobial in nature with a predominance of many anaerobes, particularly *B. fragilis.*[18, 19, 23]

Brook recently studied 42 children with decubitus ulcers, using aerobic and anaerobic techniques.[25] As has been described in adults,[18, 19, 23] there were found in children polymicrobial, aerobic, and anaerobic flora in decubitus ulcers. Blood cultures, however, were not as valuable diagnostically in pediatric patients as in adults.[23]

Anaerobic bacteria were isolated in 21 (50%) of the children, 5 times as the only isolates and 16 times mixed with aerobes. Aerobes only were present in 20 (48%) of the patients. There were a total of 83 isolates, 46 aerobes and 37 anaerobes, with an average of two species per specimen (1.1 aerobes and 0.9 anaerobes) (table 24.3).

The most common aerobic isolates were *S. aureus,* GABHS, *H. influenzae,* and *Enterobacter agglomerans.* The predominant anaerobic isolates were Gram-positive cocci, *B. fragilis,* and *Fusobacterium nucleatum.*

Pathogenesis

An ulcer develops as a result of an active metabolic and inflammatory process that begins when sufficient pressure is applied on the skin, particularly over a bony prominence, to overcome the normal capillary pressure of 32 mm Hg at the arterial end,[26] with resultant tissue anoxia and cellular death.[27]

Table 24.3. Isolates of Bacteria in 42 Patients with Decubitus Ulcers

Isolates	No. of Bacteria Isolates
Aerobic bacteria	
S. aureus	23
Group D streptococcus	2
Group A beta-hemolytic streptococcus	6
E. agglomerans	5
E. coli	2
P. aeruginosa	3
H. influenzae	5
Total number of aerobic bacteria	46
Anaerobic bacteria	
Peptococcus sp.	6
Peptostreptococcus sp.	11
P. acnes	4
Eubacterium sp.	3
Veillonella sp.	1
B. fragilis	6
B. melaninogenicus	2
F. nucleatum	4
Total number of anaerobic bacteria	37
Total number of aerobic and anaerobic	83
Aerobes only	20
Anaerobes only	5
Mixed aerobic and anaerobic	16
No growth	1

SOURCE: Brook, I. Anaerobic and aerobic bacteriology of decubitus ulcers in children. *Am. Surg.* 46:624, 1980. Reprinted by permission.

The process initially is reversible on removal of pressure with the appearance of reactive hyperemia, which is due to active vasodilation. The anaerobes recovered from the decubitus ulcers are all part of the normal oral and fecal flora.[11] They may have contaminated the ulcer site by contact of the denuded area with oral or fecal excretions, or through contact with contaminated fomites.

When there are large areas of devitalized tissue, a variety of microorganisms will become implanted and will multiply in the superficial necrotic tissue. Such microbial growth may interfere with the normal healing process, and even more serious complications may arise if the micoorganisms penetrate surrounding tissue, or if they are capable of producing exotoxins, which can spread from the area of necrosis.

Diagnosis

The decubitus ulcer represents a loss of epidermis or dermis at a site where the pressure applied to the skin surface is too great for the area to sustain. Initially, there is a blanching erythema, which may become apparent within a few hours of tissue insult. This is decubital dermatitis. The lesion can progress to a nonblanching erythema or it can return to apparent normalcy. If the pressure continues, a vesicular eruption occurs, which may develop into a bulla. When it breaks, superficial ulcers are revealed. More extensive tissue destruction is manifested by a black eschar and a deep ulcer. In some instances, the area sloughs, leaving gangrenous remnants.

Patients with serious ulcers can present with fever, chills, hypotension, and tachycardia or tachypnea, or both.[23] There may be extensive tissue destruction with necrosis. Lesions may be foul-smelling with purulent drainage. Cultures for aerobic and anaerobic bacteria of the ulcer and the blood are essential.

Attempts to culture material will reveal a complex mixture of microorganisms that frequently changes from day to day. Semiquantitative estimates of the total bacterial load may be helpful in evaluating the results of such cultures, and qualitative identification of certain selected pathogens may be more useful.

Management

The most important treatment with this disease is surgical debridement. Morgan[28] has summarized the available topical therapy. The topical treatments include antibiotics, elements and simple compounds, hormones, foam sponges, plasma, ultrasound and electrotherapy, brine, enzymes, sugar, and tannic acid.

The care of an open wound consists of debridement of devitalized tissue, local and at times systemic control of infection, and coverage of the wound, primarily by skin grafting or flaps or secondarily by wound contraction. Grossly necrotic tissue is best removed by the surgeon, to the point of pain or bleeding, usually at the bedside. Additional debridement is best accomplished with frequent dressing changes with the use of coarse meshed gauze sponges, which absorb the debris and purulent discharge. The bacterial count can be decreased by choice of soft topically applied antibacterial agents. The most common ones are the organic synthetic iodide preparations, silver sulfadiazine, and mafenide cream. All of these compounds are absorbed through the open wound. General supportive measures, such as fluids given intravenously and vasopressor agents, are indicated.

Management also includes evaluation of the patient's condition and consideration of the decubitus ulcer as the source of sepsis. Initial antibiotic therapy should include an aminoglycoside, such as gentamicin, and should be administered to provide coverage for coliform organisms. Since some of the anaerobes, like *B. fragilis* and some strains of *B. melaninogenicus,* are resistant to penicillin, therapy also should include appropriate coverage for those organisms. These include antimicrobial agents such as clindamycin, chloramphenicol, carbencillin, cefoxitin, or ticarcillin. These agents are also effective against staphylococci and non-group D streptococci.

Complications

Osteomyelitis should be suspected in cases with extreme ulcers. Although sepsis associated with decubitis ulcers in children has not been reported, this has been shown to occur in adults.[23] Galpin and associates[23] documented bacteremia in 16 adults who had a 48% mortality. The bacteremia involved anaerobes in half of these patients and was polymicrobial in eight patients. When present, bacteremia tends to persist despite appropriate antimicrobial therapy, with a predominance of obligate anaerobes, particularly *B. fragilis.*

Paronychia

Paronychia is an inflammatory, infectious process of the structure surrounding the nails. Paronychia is common in housewives, cleaners, nurses, or others who often have their hands in water.[29] It is common also in children who suck their fingers or have poor skin hygiene.

Microbiology

The bacteriology of paronychia has been studied in the past[29-31]; however, the patients were primarily adults, and techniques for cultivation of anaerobic bacteria were not employed. These reports have described the isolation of *S. aureus, S. faecalis,* coliform organisms, *Proteus* species, *P. aeruginosa,* and *Candida albicans* from this infection.[29-31]

In a recent study,[32] pus specimens from 33 children with paronychia of the finger were cultured using aerobic and anaerobic techniques (see table 24.4). The study demonstrates the mixed aerobic and anaerobic bacteriology of paronychia in pediatric patients. Anaerobic organisms were isolated in pure culture from 9 patients (27%), aerobes only from 9 patients (27%), and mixed aerobic and anaerobic flora was present in 15 patients (46%). A total of 118 isolates were recovered,

Table 24.4. Organisms Isolated from 33 Pediatric Patients
with Paronychia

Anaerobic and Facultative Isolates	No. of Isolates	Anaerobic Isolates	No. of Isolates
Gram-positive cocci		Gram-positive cocci	
Alpha-hemolytic streptococci	4	*Peptococcus* sp.	3
		P. magnus	5
Gamma-hemolytic streptococci	7	*P. asaccharolyticus*	6
		Peptostreptococcus sp.	9
Group A beta-hemolytic streptococci	4	Gram-negative cocci	
Group D streptococci	3	*Veillonella* sp.	1
S. aureus	13	Gram-positive bacilli	
S. epidermidis	3	*Bifidobacterium* sp.	3
Gram-negative cocci		*Eubacterium* sp.	2
Neisseria sp.	2	Gram-negative bacilli	
Gram-negative bacilli		*Fusobacterium* sp.	4
K. pneumoniae	2	*F. nucleatum*	9
H. parainfluenzae	2	*F. necrophorum*	2
E. corrodens	4	*Bacteroides* sp.	9
A. calcoaceticus var. lwoffi	1	*B. melaninogenicus* ss. *melaninogenicus*	4
C. albicans	6	*B. melaninogenicus* ss. *intermedius*	3
		B. oralis	4
		B. ovatus	1
		B. corrodens	2
Total number of aerobes and facultatives	51	Total number of anaerobes	67

SOURCE: Brook, I. Bacteriology of paronychia in children. *Am. J. Surg.* 141:703, 1981. Reprinted by permission.

accounting for 3.6 isolates (2 anaerobes, 1.4 aerobes, and 0.2 *C. albicans*) per specimen. The predominant anaerobic organisms were *Bacteroides* species, Gram-positive anaerobic cocci, *Fusobacterium* species, and *Bifidobacterium* species. The predominant aerobic organisms were *S. aureus,* gamma-hemolytic streptococci, *Eikenella corrodens,* GABHS, alpha-hemolytic streptococci, *Klebsiella pneumoniae,* and *Haemophilus parainfluenzae. C. albicans* was recovered in six instances.

Seventeen beta-lactamase-producing organisms were recovered from 15 children (45%). These included all isolates of *S. aureus* (13) and *Bacteroides ovatus* (1), two of seven *B. melaninogenicus* and one of four isolates of *Bacteroides oralis.*

Pathogenesis

The role of anaerobic bacteria in paronychia in children was demonstrated clearly in the Brook study.[32] These organisms were the predominant isolates, outnumbering aerobes by a ratio of 3:2. Although *S. aureus* was recovered from 40% of patients, most of them had mixed aerobic and anaerobic bacteria recovered from their lesions. The anaerobic organisms isolated (fusobacteria, *B. melaninogenicus, B. oralis,* and Gram-positive anaerobic cocci) are part of normal oropharyngeal flora and may represent self-inoculation by the patient's own mouth flora onto the finger.

Nail biting and finger sucking are common in children. This predisposes to paronychia through direct inoculation of the fingers with flora of the mouth, where anaerobes outnumber aerobes in a ratio of 10:1.[12] This phenomenon is parallel to the acquisition of infection following human bites and clenched fist injuries. Studies that applied methodology for cultivation of aerobic organisms demonstrated the predominance of Gram-positive aerobic cocci (alpha-hemolytic streptococci, group A streptococci, and staphylococci) and mouth flora Gram-negative organisms (*Neisseria* species, *Haemophilus* species, and *Eikenella* species) in such infections.[33–35] A recent study,[13] however, also applied techniques for cultivation of anaerobes and showed that normal oral flora, rather than skin flora, are the source of most bacterial isolates. The predominant aerobic isolates were group A streptococci, *S. aureus,* and *E. corrodens.* Anaerobic organisms were recovered from 47% of the patients studied. The most common isolates were *Bacteroides* species, Gram-positive anaerobic cocci, and *F. nucleatum.*

Diagnosis

Paronychia may be acute or chronic. The acute form is manifested by erythema, temperature elevation, edema, and marked tenderness and is usually caused by bacteria. There is less erythema in chronic paronychia, with a cushionlike thickening of the paronychial tissue. The nail plates may be thickened and discolored, with pronounced transverse ridges.

This condition begins as a subcuticular or intracutaneous infection with exudate developing in a localized area, which eventually spreads under the base of the fingernail, elevating it from the nail matrix and eventually from the nail bed. Infection may follow the nail margin or may extend beneath the nail and suppurate. Rarely, the infection penetrates more deeply into the finger, causing necrosis of the tendons, and further extension along the sheaths may result. In rare instances osteomyelitis may develop. The chronically infected nail eventually becomes distorted.

When the exudate is purulent, a bacterial culture is indicated. Culture aspirates of the pus are important in establishing the diagnosis. A microscopic examination in potassium hydroxide and culture for *Candida* and dermatophytes are often helpful. A large amount of budding yeast on potassium hydroxide examination suggests that *Candida* may be of some etiologic significance. A positive culture for *Candida* in the absence of a positive potassium hydroxide examination and clinical signs suggestive of candidiasis would indicate that the organism is present only as a nonpathogen.

Management

An acute infection is treated with hot compresses or soaks and, if bacteria are present, with an appropriate systemic antibiotic. The accumulated debris is painful and should be drained. A purulent pocket should be opened cautiously with a scalpel. Infection extending along the tendon sheaths requires prompt surgical incision and drainage.

Chronic paronychia caused by dermatophytes that are sensitive to griseofulvin will respond readily to treatment with this agent. If *Candida* is present, nystatin or amphotericin B lotion may be incorporated with the steroid.

Since anaerobic bacteria play a role in the etiology of paronychia in children, the physician should consider their possible presence when selecting antimicrobial therapy. Although all but four of the anaerobes isolated[16] were susceptible to penicillin, growing numbers of *B. melaninogenicus* strains were reported to be resistant to that drug.

Special attention should also be given to *E. corrodens,* a capnophilic Gram-negative rod that is part of the normal oral flora and that was isolated from four of the patients studied. There are over 64 reported cases in which *E. corrodens* was isolated from human bite infections.[13] This is of note because of the unusual antibiotic sensitivity pattern of *E. corrodens.* It is susceptible to penicillin and ampicillin, but resistant to oxacillin, methicillin, nafcillin, and clindamycin.[36] Although many strains tested against cephalothin are reported to be susceptible, there are also isolates reported to be resistant.[36]

The patient should completely avoid water, detergents, and chemicals. The patient should take extreme care in drying fingernail areas after washing and should not mechanically irritate or manicure the nails. Sucking of fingers or nail biting should be avoided.

Perirectal Abscess

Perirectal abscess is encountered frequently in pediatric practice, but seldom has it been reported. A review of 3210 cases of pediatric proctologic disease from several institutions shows that perirectal abscess accounted for 2.5% of the patients seen.[37]

Perirectal abscess is seen most frequently in children younger than two years of age. Of 28 children seen with abscess and/or fistula-in-ano by Arminski and McLean,[38] 90% were newborns or infants. In the patients described by Enberg, Cox, and Burry,[39] 59% were younger than two years of age, and 45% of the patients seen were younger than two years.

There is a strong male predominance, particularly in infants. Arminski and McLean[38] reported 90% of the infants in their series were male.

Microbiology

The bacteriology of perirectal abscess in children has received little attention in the literature and has never been studied applying anaerobic and aerobic bacteriologic methods. Most of the data in the literature are derived from studies of adults.

Finegold[11] summarized the literature up to 1975, dealing with the bacteriology of perirectal abscesses in adults. Gram-negative enteric bacteria and anaerobic organisms generally accounted for more than 75% of the microorganisms isolated. The most frequent isolates reported were various *Bacteroides* species, including *B. fragilis, Fusobacterium* species, *Actinomyces* species, and *Clostridium* species.

In two reports on perirectal abscess in children, 29 patients were gathered in each study,[39, 40] and *S. aureus* and *E. coli* were the bacterial agents most frequently isolated from cultures of perirectal abscesses in both series. Kreiger and Chisid[40] recovered five *B. fragilis* and three *Peptostreptococcus* species from 29 patients. It is of interest, however, that no specific anaerobic bacteriology was used in the two studies, suggesting that if proper procedures are employed in the laboratory, many more anaerobes will be isolated from these types of specimens.

Brook and Martin[41] recently studied the bacteriology of perirectal abscess in children and were able to demonstrate that anaerobic organisms are the predominant isolates from these infections, outnumbering aerobes at a ratio of 2.8:1. In contrast to other investigators,[39, 40] Brook and Martin have not found *S. aureus* and *E. coli* to be the predominant isolates from this type of infection.

Table 24.5. Bacterial Isolates from 28 Pediatric Patients with Perirectal Abscesses

Aerobic and Faculative Isolates	No. of Isolates	Anaerobic Isolates	No. of Isolates
Gram-positive cocci		Gram-positive cocci	
S. pneumonia	1	*Peptococcus* sp.	10
Alpha-hemolytic streptococci	1	*Peptostreptococcus* sp.	5
Group A hemolytic streptococci	2	Gram-negative cocci	
		Veillonella sp.	2
Group D streptococci	1	Gram-positive bacilli	
S. aureus	6	*C. perfringens*	2
S. epidermidis	1	*Clostridium* sp.	1
Gram-negative bacilli		*P. acnes*	2
P. morganii	2	*Bifidobacterium* sp.	1
E. coli	6	*Eubacterium* sp.	3
K. pneumonia	1	Gram-negative bacilli	
P. aeruginosa	2	*Fusobacterium* sp.	2
		F. nucleatum	4
		Bacteroides sp.	7
		B. melaninogenicus	7
		B. ruminicola ss. *brevis*	1
		B. fragilis ⎫	8
		B. vulgatus ⎪	2
		B. distasonis ⎬ *B. fragilis* group	2
		B. thetaiota- omicron ⎭	2
		B. corrodens	3
Total	23	Total	64

Source: Brook, I., and Finegold, S. M. Aerobic and anaerobic bacteriology of cutaneous abscesses in children. *Pediatrics* 67:891, 1981. Copyright 1981, American Academy of Pediatrics. Reprinted by permission.

Brook and Martin[41] have obtained aspirates of pus from perirectal abscesses in 28 children studied (table 24.5). A total of 87 isolates (64 anaerobic and 23 aerobic) were recovered from the patients, an average of 2.3 anaerobes and 0.8 aerobes per specimen. Anaerobic organisms alone were recovered from 15 specimens (54%) and in nine specimens (32%) they were mixed with aerobic organisms (table 24.5). Aerobic organisms were recovered in pure culture from only four patients (14%). The predominant anaerobic organisms were *Bacteroides* species (including *B. fragilis* group and *B. melaninogenicus* group), Gram-positive anaerobic cocci, *Fusobacterium* species, and *Clostridium* species. The predominant aerobic organisms were *E. coli, S. aureus,* GABHS, *P. aeruginosa,* and *Proteus morganii.*

Pathogenesis

The isolation of anaerobic bacteria together with aerobic and facultative organisms from the perirectal site is not surprising since anaerobes are the predominant organisms in the gastrointestinal tract, where they outnumber aerobes at a ratio of 1000:1.[15]

The pathophysiology of the development of perirectal abscess in children is not well understood. It is believed that diarrheal or constipated stools abrade the anal canal and destroy the normal mucosal barrier, allowing bacteria to invade perianal tissues and anal glands. Invading bacteria may be stool flora, or, as in the case of many children, skin flora from the anal verge. When the anal glands become obstructed, abscess formation occurs. If untreated, the abscess may burrow along the rectal sphincter, exiting next to the anus on the buttock, forming a fistula-in-ano. Alternatively, it may burrow through the musculature of the perirectal sling into the deeper tissues, forming an ischiorectal abscess.

The presence of underlying disease can predispose patients to the development of perirectal abscess. In adults, the disease most commonly associated with perirectal abscess is ulcerative colitis.[42] In children, immunodeficiency, particularly neutropenia, seems to be a more important predisposing factor. Neutropenia may be primary or secondary to chemotherapy for a malignant neoplasm. The association between leukemia and perirectal infections is well established.[38]

Diagnosis

It is important to obtain aerobic as well as anaerobic cultures from the pus. Because of the association of bacteremia, blood cultures should be obtained.

There is generally elevated peripheral white blood cell count, except in patients with leukopenia.

Management

Surgery is the mainstay of the therapy of perirectal abscess. The abscess should be incised as soon as possible, since attempts to allow it to localize further may lead to the spread of infection to deeper tissue planes. Simple drainage is insufficient. The infected crypt must be probed and unroofed. Fistulous tracts must be opened and excised if necessary.

Early aspiration and Gram stain for presumptive bacteriologic diagnosis may be helpful if antimicrobial agents are to be used prior to surgical intervention.

The role of antibiotic therapy in the treatment of perirectal abscess and in the subsequent development of complications is unclear.

Enberg, Cox, and Burry[39] reported that fistula-in-ano developed in 24% of their patients with perirectal abscess. The outcome of infection was similar whether the children had received appropriate, inappropriate, or no antibiotic therapy in conjunction with surgery.

Kreiger and Chisid,[40] however, found a complication rate of 56% in their patients who had not received antibiotics, but in only 30% in those who had received some form of appropriate parenteral and/or oral antibiotic therapy around the time of surgery. Thus, it seemed that according to their data antibiotics may have reduced the overall rate of complications after surgery.

Although surgical drainage is still the therapy of choice, the predominance of anaerobic bacteria and enteric Gram-negative rods in perirectal abscess suggests a need for the administration of appropriate antimicrobial therapy. The presence of penicillin-resistant anaerobic bacteria such as *B. fragilis*[16, 43] may warrant the use of one or more of the following antimicrobial agents: clindamycin, chloramphenicol, cefoxitin, carbenicillin, ticarcillin, or metronidazole. Aminoglycoside therapy should provide adequate coverage for Gram-negative enteric rods.

Complications

Frequent complications include septicemia, development of fistula-in-ano, gangrene of the anus, and recurrence of the abscess. The complication rate is higher in children with neutropenia.

Pilonidal Abscess

Pilonidal sinus is encountered commonly in pediatric patients, especially in the adolescent age group. This is a dermal sinus, which is a small midline closure defect. The sinus is of importance primarily because it may be a site of collection of debris and subsequent inflammation, and when it is communicated with the subarachnoid space, it may be a route of entry of bacteria into the central nervous system.

Microbiology

Most of the microbiological data in the literature are derived from studies of adults.[11] Finegold[11] summarized 13 publications dealing with the bacteriologic characteristics of infected pilonidal cyst in adults. The most frequent isolates reported in those studies were various *Bacteroides* species, including *B. fragilis,* anaerobic Gram-positive cocci, and *Clostridium* species. A recent report[8] presented the bacteriologic features of pilonidal cyst abscess in 11 adults. Anaerobic organisms, such as *Bacteroides* species and Gram-positive anaerobic cocci, were the predominant isolates. Gram-negative enteric bacteria and *S. aureus* were not present.

Brook and associates[44] recently reported their experience in studying the microbiology of this infection in children. This study demonstrated that anaerobic organisms are the predominant isolates in these infections, outnumbering aerobes at a ratio of 5:1. In contrast to other investigators,[8, 45] Brook and co-workers[44] have been able to retrieve Gram-negative aerobic bacilli in seven instances. As in other investigations, *S. aureus* was not found to be a predominant isolate in this type of infection.

Table 24.6. Bacterial Isolates from 25 Pilonidal Cyst Abscesses in Children

Aerobic and Facultative Isolates	No. of Isolates	Anaerobic Isolates	No. of Isolates
Gram-positive cocci		Gram-positive cocci	
Alpha-hemolytic streptococci	2	*Peptococcus* sp.	11
		Peptostreptococcus sp.	5
Group D streptococci	2	Gram-negative cocci	
Non-hemolytic streptococci	1	*Veillonella* sp.	1
S. aureus	1	Gram-positive bacilli	
		C. perfringens	2
Gram-negative bacilli		*Clostridium* sp.	2
Proteus sp.	2	*P. acnes*	1
E. coli	4	Gram-negative bacilli	
K. pneumoniae	1	*Fusobacterium* sp.	3
		F. nucleatum	2
		Bacteroides sp.	9
		B. melaninogenicus	10
		B. ruminicola ss. *brevis*	2
		B. fragilis ⎫	5
		B. vulgatus ⎪	1
		B. distasonis ⎬ *B. fragilis* group	2
		B. thetaiotaomicron ⎪	2
		B. ovatus ⎭	2
		B. corrodens	3
Total	13	Total	63

SOURCE: Brook, I. et al. Aerobic and anaerobic bacteriology of pilonidal cyst abcess in children. *Am. J. Dis. Child.* 134:680, 1980. Copyright 1980, American Medical Association. Reprinted by permission.

This group[44] has studied aspirates of pus from pilonidal abscesses in 25 children. A total of 76 isolates (63 anaerobic and 13 aerobic) were recovered from the patients, accounting for 2.52 anaerobes and 0.52 aerobes per specimen (table 24.6). Anaerobic organisms were recovered from all the specimens, and in eight patients (32%) they were mixed with aerobic organisms. The predominant anaerobic organisms were *Bacteroides* species (including *B. fragilis* group and *B. melaninogenicus* group), Gram-positive anaerobic cocci, *Fusobacterium* species, and *Clostridium* species. The predominant aerobic organisms were *E. coli,* group D streptococci, alpha-hemolytic streptococci, and *Proteus* species.

Pathogenesis

The isolation of anaerobic bacteria mixed with aerobic and facultative organisms, such as enteric Gram-negative rods, at that site is not surprising. Anaerobes are the predominant organisms in the gastrointestinal tract, where they outnumber aerobes at a ratio of 1000:1.[15]

Diagnosis and Management

Since anaerobic bacteria frequently are associated with pilonidal abscess in pediatric patients, the physician should consider their presence if antimicrobial therapy is used. Gram staining of aspirated pus and appropriate aerobic and anaerobic techniques can help the physician select proper therapy. Since some of the anaerobes are resistant to penicillin, therapy should also include appropriate coverage of those organisms. Surgical drainage is still the therapy of choice; however, the presence of penicillin-resistant anaerobic bacteria, such as *B. fragilis*[16] and some strains of *B. melaninogenicus*,[16, 43] may warrant the administration of appropriate antimicrobial agents, such as clindamycin, chloramphenicol, cefoxitin, carbenicillin disodium, ticarcillin disodium, or metronidazole.

Aminoglycosides should be added if Gram-negative enteric rods are recovered from the infectious site.

REFERENCES

1. Marks, M. I. Common bacterial infection in infancy and childhood: a skin and wound infection. *Drugs* 16:202, 1978.

2. Maibach, H. I., and Hildick-Smith, G., eds. *Skin bacteria and their role in infection.* New York: McGraw-Hill, 1965.

3. Sanders, D. Y.; Russell, D. A.; and Gilliam, C. F. Isolation of *Haemophilus* species from abscesses of two children. *Pediatrics* 42:683, 1968.

4. Burry, V. F., and Beezley, M. Infant mastitis due to gram-negative organisms. *Am. J. Dis. Child.* 124:736, 1972.

5. Thirumoothi, M. C.; Keen, B. M.; and Dajani, A. S. Anaerobic infections in children: a prospective survey. *J. Clin. Microbiol.* 3:318, 1976.

6. Dunkle, L. M.; Brotherton, M. S.; and Feigin, R. D. Anaerobic infections in children. A prospective study. *Pediatrics* 57:311, 1976.

7. Brook, I. et al. The recovery of anaerobic bacteria from pediatric patients, a one-year experience. *Am. J. Dis. Child.* 133:1020, 1979.

8. Meislin, H. W. et al. Cutaneous abscesses. Anaerobic and aerobic bacteriology and outpatient management. *Ann. Intern. Med.* 97:145, 1977.

9. Brook, I., and Finegold, S. M. Aerobic and anaerobic bacteriology of cutaneous abscesses in children. *Pediatrics* 67:891, 1981.

10. Onderdonk, A. B. et al. Microbial synergy in experimental intra-abdominal abscesses. *Infect. Immun.* 13:22, 1976.

11. Finegold, S. M. *Anaerobic bacteria in human disease.* New York: Academic Press, 1977.

12. Gibbons, R. J. Aspects of the pathogenicity and ecology of the indigenous oral flora of man. In *Anaerobic bacteria: role in disease,* ed. A. Balows et al. Springfield, Ill.: Charles C Thomas, 1974, p. 267.

13. Goldstein, E. J. C. et al. Bacteriology of human and animal bite wounds. *J. Clin. Microbiol.* 8:667, 1978.

14. Moore, W. E. C.; Cato, E. P.; and Holdeman, L. V. Anaerobic bacteria of the gastrointestinal flora and their occurrence in clinical infections. *J. Infect. Dis.* 119:641, 1969.

15. Gorbach, S. L. Intestinal microflora. *Gastroenterology* 60:1110, 1971.

16. Sutter, V. L., and Finegold, S. M. Susceptibility of anaerobic bacteria to 23 antimicrobial agents. *Antimicrob. Agents Chemother.* 10:736, 1976.

17. Mooten, S. E. Bedsores in the chronically ill patient. *Arch. Phys. Med. Rehab.* 53:430, 1972.

18. Peromet, M. et al. Anaerobic bacteria isolated from decubitus ulcers. *Infection* 1:205, 1973.

19. Rissing, J. P. et al. *Bacteroides* bacteremia from decubitus ulcers. *South. Med. J.* 67:1179, 1974.

20. Peterson, N. C., and Bittman, S. The epidemiology of pressure sores. *Scand J. Plast. Reconstr. Surg.* 5:62, 1971.

21. Vasile, J., and Chaitin, H. Prognostic factors in decubitus ulcers of the aged. *Geriatrics* 27:126, 1972.

22. Alder, V. G., and Gillespie, W. A. Pressure sores and staphylococcal cross-infection: detection of sources by means of settleplates. *Lancet* 2:1356, 1964.

23. Galpin, J. E. et al. Sepsis associated with decubitus ulcers. *Am. J. Med.* 6:346, 1976.

24. Louie, T. J. et al. Aerobic and anaerobic bacteria in diabetic foot ulcers. *Ann. Intern. Med.* 85:461, 1976.

25. Brook, I. Anaerobic and aerobic bacteriology of decubitus ulcers in children. *Am. Surg.* 46:624, 1980.

26. Landis, E. Studies of capillary blood pressure in human skin. *Heart* 15:209, 1930.

27. Kosiak, M. Etiology and pathology of decubitus ulcers. *Arch. Phys. Med.* 40:62, 1959.

28. Morgan, E. J. Topical therapy of pressure sores. *Surg. Gynecol. Obstet.* 141:945, 1975.

29. Fleigelman, M. T., and Owen, L. G. How we treat paronychia. *Postgrad. Med.* 48:267, 1970.

30. Barlow, A. J. et al. Chronic paronychia. *Br. J. Dermatol.* 82:448, 1970.

31. Editorial. Chronic paronychia. *Br. Med. J.* 2:460, 1975.

32. Brook, I. Bacteriology of paronychia in children. *Am. J. Surg.* 141:703, 1981.

33. Chiunard, R. G., and D'Ambrosia, R. D. Human bite infections of the hand. *J. Bone Joint Surg.* 59A: 416, 1977.

34. Guba, A. M.; Mulliken, J. B.; and Hoopes, J. E. The selection of antibiotics for human bites of the hand. *Plast. Reconstr. Surg.* 56:538, 1975.

35. Weinstein, R. A. et al. Human bites. *J. Oral Surg.* 3:792, 1973.

36. Goldstein, E. J. C.; Sutter, V. L.; and Finegold, S. M. Susceptibility of *Eikenella corrodens* to ten cephalosporins. *Antimicrob. Agents Chemother.* 14:639, 1978.

37. Mentzer, C. G. Anorectal disease. *Pediatr. Clin. North Am.* 3:113, 1956.

38. Arminski, T. C., and McLean, D. W. Proctologic problems in children. *JAMA* 194:1195, 1965.

39. Enberg, R. N.; Cox, R. H.; and Burry, V. F. Perirectal abscess in children. *Am. J. Dis. Child.* 128:360, 1974.

40. Kreiger, R. W., and Chisid, M. J. Perirectal abscess in childhood: a review of 29 cases. *Am. J. Dis. Child.* 133:411, 1979.

41. Brook, I., and Martin, W. J. Aerobic and anaerobic bacteriology of perirectal abscess in children. *Pediatrics* 66:282, 1980.

42. Rawls, W. E. et al. Perianal abscess and anorectal fistula. *Minn. Med.* 46:327, 1963.

43. Murray, P. R., and Rosenblatt, J. E. Penicillin resistant and penicillinase production in clinical isolates of *Bacteroides melaninogenicus*. *Antimicrob. Agents Chemother.* 11:605, 1977.

44. Brook, I. et al. Aerobic and anaerobic bacteriology of pilonidal cyst abscess in children. *Am. J. Dis. Child.* 134:679, 1980.

45. Marrie, T. J. et al. Bacteriology of pilonidal cyst abscesses. *J. Clin. Pathol.* 31:909, 1978.

Wound and Subcutaneous Tissue Infections

Anaerobic infections of the skin and soft tissue frequently occur in areas of the body that have been compromised or injured by foreign body, trauma, ischemia, or surgery. Since the indigenous local microflora usually is responsible for these infections, anatomic sites that are subject to fecal or oral contamination are particularly at risk. These include wounds associated with surgery of the intestine or pelvic tract, human bites, decubitus ulcers in the perineal area, pilonidal cysts, omphalitis, and cellulitis around the fetal monitoring site.

Some of the clues to the anaerobic origin of such infections are putrid discharge, gas production, and extensive tissue necrosis with a tendency to burrow through subcutaneous and fascial planes.

Many wound and skin infections that complicate surgical operations or trauma are caused by mixed bacterial flora. Aerobic and anaerobic, Gram-negative and Gram-positive organisms, whose origins are most often lesions or perforations of the gastrointestinal, respiratory, or genitourinary tracts, may be present in such infections, and they may exist synergistically. All clinical manifestations can be seen: cellulitis, abscess formation, thrombosis, necrosis, gangrene, and crepitus.[1]

The majority of skin infections are associated with a mixed aerobic and anaerobic flora. There are, however, certain classic syndromes caused by specific anaerobes that have distinctive clinical presentations.

Crepitant Anaerobic Cellulitis

Crepitant cellulitis is an acute anaerobic infection of the soft tissue that is characterized by abundant connective tissue gas and minimal systemic toxicity. The condition usually occurs in patients with lower extremity vascular insufficiency and associated diabetes mellitus. It is sometimes known as clostridial cellulitis, but the clinical picture in the condition involving clostridia is not necessarily different from that involving non-spore-forming anaerobic bacteria.

Microbiology

The clostridial species generally present are *Clostridium perfringens* or *Clostridium septicum* and can be seen on Gram stain and culture. Other organisms that can be involved are *Bacteroides, Peptostreptococcus,* and coliforms.[2, 3]

Pathogenesis

The infection usually is found at the sites of dirty or inadequately debrided traumatic wounds, especially around the perineum, abdominal wall, buttocks, and lower extremities (i.e., areas contaminated with fecal flora).

Clinical Manifestation and Diagnosis

The lesion may spread rapidly. The process is necrotizing in nature and can involve the epifascial, retroperitoneal, or other connective tissues of the extremities, perineum, abdominal wall, buttocks, hip, or thorax. One can observe a dark, foul-smelling drainage, often containing fat globules. Frank crepitus seems to extend widely beyond the areas of active infection. Roentgenograms of soft tissue show abundant gas. The clinical presentation can vary from a well-localized "gas abscess" to extension of gas to areas far removed from the initial lesion.

Although the onset of anaerobic cellulitis is generally gradual with minimal systemic effects, spread of the infection may be rapid and extensive, and considerable morbidity or mortality may result if there is delay in initiating appropriate therapy. Crepitant cellulitis can be differentiated from gas gangrene and other more serious soft-tissue infections by the lack of marked systemic toxicity, gradual onset, pain, and the absence of muscle involvement.

Management

Initial antibiotic therapy should be based on the degree of tissue involvement by the primary infection, systemic signs, and results of the Gram stain of aspirated wound material. Since *B. fragilis* may be encountered, antimicrobial therapy should include coverage for this organism. Surgical therapy usually consists of local wound care with incision, drainage, and debridement as dictated by tissue infection but not by subcutaneous gas dissection.[4]

Necrotizing Fasciitis

The term *necrotizing fasciitis* originally described streptococcal gangrene or hospital gangrene. Currently, however, it denotes mixed bacterial infection. Although it is a rare infection, it is a serious one that requires prompt recognition.

Microbiology

A variety of organisms have been reported as predominant in these infections, including the aerobic organisms of beta-hemolytic streptococci, *Staphylococcus aureus,* and Gram-negative organisms; and anaerobic organisms of *Peptostreptococcus, Bacteroides,* and *Fusobacterium.* The latter two organisms invariably were found in combination with coliforms.[5, 6] Bacteremia is rarely demonstrable.

Pathogenesis

The infection is introduced through a break in the skin and occurs most frequently following minor trauma or surgery—subcutaneous or intravenous injection of illicit drugs, an incised wound, enterostomy, decubitus ulcer, perineal fistula, or diabetic foot.[5, 6] The highest incidence is seen in patients in whom extremity infections are most common: those with ischemic small vessel disease or who are drug addicts. In other patients, infections of the trunk, perineum, buttocks, and thighs represent spread of infection from previously infected sites (e.g., diabetic or decubitus ulcers) that had been ignored.

Infections of the scrotum and shaft of the penis have been described in children.[7]

Clinical Manifestations and Diagnosis

The course of necrotizing fasciitis is variable. Usually the portal of entry is obvious. It may remain an indolent undermining infection, or may suddenly become fulminant and rapidly progress to gangrene and death, in a manner similar to acute streptococcal gangrene.

In the progressive type of infection, cellulitis predominates. Multiple skin ulcers drain a thin, reddish-brown, foul-smelling fluid characterized as "dishwater pus." Multiple ulcerations are present that communicate beneath apparently normal, but undermined, skin. Crepitance in the soft tissues often can be felt, and sensation may range from exquisite local tenderness to anesthesia. The diagnosis may be made by passing a catheter or probing instrument through the area of necrosis and demonstrating that the tissue is undermined. Frank pus is unusual, despite widespread necrosis. The extent of the necrosis may be overlooked until sudden systemic toxicity supervenes.

Management

Initial management should consist of correction of fluid, electrolyte, and erythrocyte-mass deficiencies; treatment of hyperthermia; appropriate aerobic and anaerobic wound cultures; blood cultures; and a Gram stain of the wound exudate. Infections of the trunk, perineum, perirectal and periurethral areas, buttocks, and thighs frequently involve four types of organisms: Enterobacteriaceae, enterococci, anaerobic streptococci, and *Bacteroides* species. The initial antimicrobial therapy should cover all of these bacteria. Aminoglycosides would be adequate for the Enterobacteriaceae; penicillin would provide coverage for the enterococci, anaerobic cocci, and clostridia; and clindamycin or chloramphenicol would cover the penicillin-resistant *Bacteroides*.

Intravenous antibiotic therapy should begin shortly after cultures are obtained. The primary therapy of necrotizing fasciitis is prompt radical surgical incision and debridement of the affected areas. The incision should extend beyond the outermost extent of the fascial involvement in all planes.

Posteroperatively, the surgical wounds should be checked frequently to ascertain whether further dissection and extension of the surgical wound is required for adequate drainage. Repeated culturing of the wound is necessary, since secondary inoculation with *Pseudomonas, Serratia,* and *Candida* occurs. Mortality, which is significant (30%), is decreased by early recognition and prompt surgical therapy.[6]

Gas Gangrene

Microbiology

Gas gangrene is a rapidly progressive, life-threatening, toxemia caused by *Clostridium* infection of muscle. It usually follows the contamination by animal or human feces of severe crushing muscle injury. It may be part of clostridial cellulitis, but in its classical form, muscle is the principal site of involvement.[2, 3]

C. *perfringens* is isolated from most of the patients; other clostridial species that are less frequently isolated are *Clostridium novyi* and *C. septicum*. Other anaerobes and facultative organisms usually are isolated also, and more than one clostridial species can be recovered.[8] The clinical syndromes produced by all species are similar. All clostridia sporulate, producing potentially lethal organisms resistant to almost all physical and many chemical agents.

Pathogenesis

Gas gangrene results primarily as a complication of contaminated traumatic wounds. They are sometimes seen in wounds after large bowel or biliary tract surgery or in the presence of ischemic impairment of a muscular region, especially after amputations of the lower extremity for ischemic gangrene after penetrating wounds by foreign bodies.

Clinical Manifestations

The incubation period of gas gangrene is one to three days. The onset is acute accompanied with extreme local pain. The local lesion becomes rapidly edematous, cool, and tender. Swollen muscle may herniate through an open wound, and a serosanguineous, dirty-appearing discharge escapes that contains numerous organisms, but few leukocytes. The wound has a sweet-but-foul odor; gas bubbles may be visible in the discharge. The skin adjacent to the wound is swollen and pale, but rapidly becomes of yellow or bronze color. Tense blebs containing thick, dark fluid develop in the overlying skin, and areas of green-black cutaneous necrosis appear.

Toxemia is generally severe and the systemic signs are nonspecific. The patient is pale, sweaty, and apprehensive. Delirium may follow. Tachycardia, hypotension, shock, and renal failure appear in rapid succession. Fever generally is not too high. Hypothermia is associated with terminal shock, as is jaundice.[8]

Diagnosis

A Gram-stained smear of the wound exudate or an aspirate from one of the blebs reveals large Gram-positive bacilli with blunt ends. Other Gram-positive and Gram-negative bacteria may be present, particularly in grossly contaminated wounds, and the diagnosis may be overlooked if the physician depends solely on bacteriologic evidence; operative exploration is definitive.

Roentgenograms of the involved areas show extensive and progressive gaseous dissection of muscle and fascial planes.

Management

Prompt and early diagnosis and therapy are essential for successful management of clostridial myonecrosis. Surgery is the only therapeutic modality proved to be unequivocally effective.[2, 3, 9] Antimicrobial therapy should consist of high doses of intravenous penicillin G.[3] In patients with known severe penicillin allergy, chloramphenicol can be used. It should be remembered that a few strains of clostridia are resistant to clindamycin.

Surgical therapy consists of excision of all infected tissue. Muscular tissue will show varying degrees of necrosis, depending on the duration of illness. In certain cases, high amputation or radical excision and debridement of the abdominal wall or perineum may be required. The surgical wound should be examined for evidence of continued tissue destruction.

Supplementary hyperbaric oxygen therapy has been recommended.[10, 11] This technique may allow delay in excising tissue of questionable viability. Lack of availability of proper facilities often precludes the use of this modality. Mortality rates with and without hyperbaric oxygen therapy are comparable.[10, 11] The use of polyvalent gas gangrene antitoxin is thought to be desirable, especially in cases of hemolysis.[3]

Synergistic Necrotizing Gangrene

Progressive bacterial synergistic gangrene was described by Meleney[12] as an indolent, ulcerating infection of the skin and subcutaneous tissue with little systemic toxicity.

Microbiology

The classic etiology is the combination of a microaerophilic nonhemolytic *Streptococcus,* found primarily in the spreading periphery of the lesion, and *S. aureus* in the zone of gangrene. The predominate microaerophilic *Streptococcus* is *Streptococcus evolutus.* The *Streptococcus* can be an obligate anaerobe, and a wide variety of other organisms can be seen instead of or in addition to the *Staphylococcus* and *Streptococcus: Proteus, Enterobacter, Pseudomonas,* and *Clostridium* species have been isolated.[13]

Pathogenesis

The infection most often develops following abdominal or thoracic surgery or drainage of a peritoneal abscess or thoracic empyema. Sometimes it develops around a colostomy or ileostomy site, or following an accidental wound.

Clinical Manifestations

The major symptoms are severe pain and tenderness. The lesion first appears about two weeks after wounding in an area around a foreign body, suture, or wound closure. A purple central area of induration becomes surrounded by a zone of erythema and tenderness. As the lesion progresses, three zones become demarcated: the outer zone is very red; the middle is purple and tender; and the central portion becomes gangrenous, the color changing to a gray-brown or a yellow-green with a typical suede-leather appearance. As the lesion spreads outward, the inner margin of the gangrenous zone becomes undermined and melts away. Eventually, the center of the lesion becomes a granulating ulcer, and epithelium may generate here. The progression is slow but unremitting. Satellite lesions may emerge as the infection progresses under the fat layer. Fever is minimal, but anemia and malnutrition are common.

Management

The treatment of this infection requires wide excision of the involved tissues and high doses of systemic antibiotics.[4]

Synergistic Necrotizing Cellulitis

Synergistic necrotizing cellulitis is distinguished from Meleney's progressive synergistic gangrene by a rapid course, a high degree of systemic toxicity, and a different clinical setting.

Microbiology

The infection is caused by mixed infection between one or more species of Gram-negative aerobic bacteria such as *Klebsiella, Enterobacter,* and *Proteus* species; *Escherichia coli;* and at least one obligate anaerobe such as *Bacteroides, Peptostreptococcus,* or *Peptococcus* species.[13] Bacteremia is relatively common.

Pathogenesis

This infection generally occurs in the perineal area or lower extremities, and most of the patients have diabetes mellitus or other causes of impaired vascular supply or are malnourished.

Clinical Manifestations

There is rapidly spreading necrosis of the skin and epifascial connective tissues associated with a thin "dishwater" discharge, exquisite wound tenderness, and fever. A unique characteristic of this infection is discrete large skin areas of bluish gray necrosis separated by areas of normal skin. Patients appear to be in a toxic condition.

Management

Radical surgical debridement, drainage, and high dose systemic antibiotics are the prime mode of therapy.

REFERENCES

1. Dellinger, E. P. Severe necrotizing soft tissue infections: multiple disease entities requiring a common approach. *JAMA* 246:1717, 1981.

2. MacLennan, J. D. The histologic clostridial infections of man. *Bacteriological Reviews* 26:177, 1962.

3. Weinstein, L., and Barza, M. Gas gangrene. *N. Engl. J. Med.* 289:1129, 1973.

4. Baxter, C. R. Surgical management of soft tissue infection. *Surg. Clin. North Am.* 52:1483, 1972.

5. Crosthwait, R. W., Jr.; Crosthwait, R. W.; and Jordan, G. L., Jr. Necrotizing fasciitis. *J. Trauma* 4:149, 1964.

6. Rea, W. J., and Wyrick, W. J. Necrotizing faciitis. *Ann. Surg.* 172:957, 1970.

7. Yeldeman, J. J., and Weaver, R. G. The urologist: the urologist and necrotizing dermogenital infection. *J. Urol.* 100:74, 1909.

8. Finegold, S. M. *Anaerobic bacteria in human disease.* New York: Academic Press, 1977.

9. Altemeier, W. A. Diagnosis, classification and general management of gas-producing infections, particularly those produced by *Clostridium perfringens.* In *Proceedings of the Third International Conference on Hyperbaric Medicine,* eds. I. W. Brown, Jr. and B. G. Cox. Washington, D.C.: National Academy of Sciences, 1966, p. 481.

10. Brummelkamp, W. H. Treatment of clostridial infections. In *Anaerobic bacteria, role in disease,* eds. A. Balows et al. Springfield, Ill.: Charles C Thomas, 1974, p. 521.

11. Trippel, O. H. et al. Hyperbaric oxygenation in the management of gas gangrene. *Surg. Clin. North Am.* 47:17, 1967.

12. Meleney, F. L. *Clinical aspects and treatment of surgical infections.* Phildadelphia: W. B. Saunders, 1949.

13. Stone, H. H., and Martin, J. D. Synergistic necrotizing cellulitis. *Ann. Surg.* 175:702, 1972.

CHAPTER 26

Infections of Bones and Joints

Septic Arthritis

Septic arthritis is defined as a purulent infection in a joint cavity. The infection commonly reaches the joint in children either by hematogenous spread or by direct extension of pathogenic bacteria.

Microbiology

Staphylococcus aureus is a predominant etiologic agent of septic arthritis in all age groups, including the newborn. In the newborn, however, group B beta-hemolytic streptococci and Gram-negative enteric organisms are also involved. *Haemophilus influenzae* type B has become in recent years the most frequent etiologic agent in children between the ages of three months and five years.[1] Other organisms seen in that age group are staphylococci, streptococci, pneumococci, and meningococci. Gonococcal arthritis can occur in sexually active adolescents.

In heroin addicts, enteric bacteria such as *Pseudomonas aeruginosa* can cause septic arthritis, especially in the sternoclavicular joint and intervertebral disk space. Rare causes of septic arthritis include mycobacteria, *Mycoplasma pneumoniae*, and fungi[2, 3] (e.g., histoplasmosis and *Candida albicans*[4, 5]).

Anaerobes have rarely been reported as a cause of septic arthritis in children. Feigin and co-workers[6] reported two children with septic arthritis caused by clostridia.

Nelson and Koontz,[1, 7] who studied 219 cases of septic arthritis, reported three patients: one with *Clostridium novyi*, one with *Clostridium bifermentans*, and one with *Bacteroides funduliformis*. Sanders and Stevenson,[8] who reviewed the literature of *Bacteroides* infections in children up to 1968, reported five patients, of whom two were their patients, and three were reported by others.[9, 10] The patients of Sanders and Stevenson suffered also from agammaglobulinemia.

It is not clear whether cultures were performed for anaerobic bacteria or whether they were performed in proper fashion with adequate anaerobic transport. It is therefore possible that the lack of such measures accounts for the very few anaerobic bacteria recovered in these series.

A review of all the adult and pediatric literature by Finegold[11] revealed a total of 180 joint infections involving anaerobic bacteria. The majority of these cases were reported from the preantimicrobial era, and the most common anaerobe was *Fusobacterium necrophorum,* which accounted for a third of the anaerobes recovered from these patients.

Bacteroides species and other fusobacteria and Gram-positive anaerobic cocci were also recovered from many patients with septic arthritis involving anaerobes. The joints most frequently involved with anaerobic infection were the larger ones, especially the hip and knee, and less frequently the elbow and shoulder.

Most of the cases of anaerobic arthritis, in contrast to anaerobic osteomyelitis, involved a single isolate, and only about 8% involved mixed bacterial flora.

Pathogenesis

In the initial stages, there is an effusion in the joint cavity, and it rapidly becomes purulent. Destruction of cartilage occurs at areas of joint contact. Bone is not affected in the early stages, but the femoral and humeral heads, if involved, may undergo necrosis and subsequent fragmentation and pathologic dislocation. Epiphyses whose synchondroses are located within the joint capsule are at particularly high risk to be involved by infection and necrosis.

During the chronic phase of the disease and the phase of repair there is an organization of the exudate present in the joint, and granulation tissue appears and becomes fibrous. This may bind the joint surfaces together, causing a fibrous ankylosis. When motion is present, the synovial fluid tends to regenerate, but limitation of motion and associated pain generally remain as a result of the production of residual strong intrasynovial adhesions.

Most of the cases of anaerobic arthritis are secondary to hematogenous spread. Almost all of the isolates of anaerobic Gram-negative rods, including the fusobacteria and the Gram-positive anaerobic cocci that were reported in the literature, were also involved in a concomitant anaerobic sepsis. In contrast, arthritis secondary to penetrating wound or foreign body is associated with clostridia.[8]

The presence of multiple septic joints was commonly seen in cases of spread of the organisms from a primary site through the blood stream or in cases of endocarditis.[11] The ability of anaerobes to cause tissue destruction may be seen in the amount of damage they can inflict on the joints, cartilage, capsule, and adjacent periosteum.

Diagnosis

Severe systemic findings such as fever, malaise, and vomiting may be present. Pain may be severe; motion is limited, and the joint is splinted by muscular spasm. In infants this may produce a pseudoparalysis. An effusion occurs but may not be palpable at first. The overlying tissues become swollen, tender, and warm. As the infection proceeds, contractures and muscular atrophy may result. X-ray examination may reveal distention of the joint capsule and subsequent narrowing of the cartilage space, erosion of the subchondral bone, irregularity and fuzziness of the bone surfaces, bone destruction, and diffuse osteoporosis. Radiologic examination of the joint may also be useful in detecting unsuspected fracture or chronic bone or joint disease.

Other helpful tests include sedimentation rate, which may be elevated; peripheral white blood count, which is generally increased; and blood cultures, which may recover the causative organisms.

Arthrocentesis can provide a rapid diagnosis of suppurative arthritis. The joint fluid should be examined for glucose (which is generally reduced when compared to serum levels)[12] and white blood cells (which are generally elevated above 50,000 cells/mm^3). Gram stain should be done, and aerobic and anaerobic cultures should be done.

The joint fluid may have a foul odor in the case of anaerobic infection, and, rarely, there may be gas under pressure in the joint. Other clues to purulent arthritis involving anaerobes include failure to obtain organisms on routine culture, Gram stain of the joint fluid showing organisms with the unique morphology of anaerobes, and evidence of anaerobic infection elsewhere in the body.

The early and accurate diagnosis of septic arthritis is of great clinical importance. Differentiation of an infectious arthritis from a noninfectious inflammatory synovitis is a frequent diagnostic problem for physicians. Furthermore, synovial fluid analysis often fails to yield a diagnosis, despite careful bacteriologic examination and especially in partially treated cases.[12]

Brook and associates[13] have studied 84 patients with acute arthritis. Their data suggest that lactic acid measurements of joint fluid may clearly differentiate between septic arthritis, other than gonococcal arthritis, and other sterile inflammatory and noninflammatory conditions in the joints. Lactic acid levels higher than 65 mg/dl should be considered as highly suggestive of the presence of an inflammatory process.

The synovial fluid can also be studied for bacterial antigens by immunoelectrophoresis or gas liquid chromatography.[14, 15]

Management

Parenteral antibiotic therapy should be initiated immediately following aspiration of the joint, and the choice of therapy should be directed by Gram stain and bacterial cultures.

Therapy of anaerobic arthritis is not different from that required for arthritis caused by aerobes, including management of any underlying disease, appropriate drainage and debridement, temporary immobilization of the joint, and antimicrobial therapy pertinent to the bacteriology of the individual patient.

Beta-lactamase-resistant penicillin derivative should be administered to patients suspected of *S. aureus* infection. Ampicillin with chloramphenicol is administered for *H. influenzae* suppuration, until the antimicrobial susceptibility report is available. Clindamycin offers an alternative mode of therapy, affecting both *S. aureus* and most anaerobic bacteria.[1] The exact duration of antimicrobial therapy is not determined; however, it should be given for at least two to three weeks in mild cases.

Surgical drainage of the joint may be required when rapid reaccumulation of fluid occurs after the initial diagnostic drainage is performed. Drainage of pus may be by intermittent aspiration, or by open incision and drainage followed by continuous suction irrigation.

Osteomyelitis

Osteomyelitis is an inflammatory process that may involve all parts of a bone, although the initial focus is usually in the metaphysis of a bone. Acute osteomyelitis most often occurs in childhood between 3 and 12 years. The infection occurs twice as frequently in boys and requires early diagnosis and intensive therapy to achieve recovery.

Microbiology

S. aureus is the most common organism recovered from infected bones, accounting for more than half of the cases.[16–18] The proportion of infections caused by other organisms, particularly *H. influenzae* type B and Gram-negative enteric bacteria has been increasing in recent years.[17] Other causative agents are beta-hemolytic streptococci and

Streptococcus pneumoniae. Factors that predispose to the development of osteomyelitis include impetigo, furunculosis, burns, and direct trauma. Rare causes of osteomyelitis are mycobacteria, actinomycosis, and fungi.[19, 20]

Anaerobic bacteria have received increasing recognition in the bacteriology of osteomyelitis,[16, 21, 22] although the exact prevalence of anaerobes in this disease is unknown. Over 800 cases of bone infection involving anaerobic bacteria have been reported in the literature.[11] Undoubtedly, many of these cases occurred in children; however, specific details are not given to this age group in most of these studies. A few reports describe the recovery of anaerobic organisms from infected bones in children. Raff and Melo[22] reported the recovery of *S. aureus* mixed with *Eubacterium lentum* from osteomyelitis of the right femur of a 13-year-old child. Brook[23] recovered *Bacteroides fragilis, Bacteroides distasonis,* and *Bacteroides melaninogenius* from an infected occipital bone in a newborn who developed osteomyelitis and bacteremia following fetal monitoring.

Schubiner, Letourneau, and Murray[24] recovered fusobacteria from an infected tibia in a 7-year-old child with Gaucher's disease. Chandler and Breaks[25] reported the recovery of *Bacteroides* organisms from an osteomyelitis of the hip of a 12-year-old child. Brook has recovered *B. melaninogenicus* and anaerobic Gram-positive cocci from an infected metaphysis of a 14-year-old with paronychia,[26] and *Bacteroides* species from a 14-year-old with frontal osteomyelitis associated with pansinusitis.[27] Many anaerobes were recovered from children with infected mastoid bone (see chapter 18, section on mastoiditis).[28]

Finegold[11] reviewed the world literature on anaerobic osteomyelitis. He found that most of the cultures that yielded anaerobes also yielded aerobic or facultative organisms, except for infections involving actinomycetes. When anaerobes are present in combination with aerobic organisms, they may act synergistically in producing disease. Over one-third of the isolates were Gram-negative rods, mainly *Bacteroides* species and fusobacteria. Other frequently recovered anaerobes were anaerobic Gram-positive cocci, actinomycetes, and *F. necrophorum.* Infections of long bones involved mainly clostridia, and vertebral osteomyelitis involved actinomycetes. Anaerobic Gram-positive cocci were recovered mostly from small bones of the extremities.

Pathogenesis

Many patients with anaerobic organisms recovered from cases of osteomyelitis have evidence of anaerobic infection elsewhere in the body, which is the source of the organisms involved in osteomyelitis. Spread to bone is by contiguous infection extending to the bone or by infection that reaches the bone by way of the bloodstream during the course of sustained or intermittent bacteremia. This infection can be of any type, but often shows characteristic features of anaerobic infection such as abscess formation, septic thrombophlebitis, production of foul odor and gas, and tissue necrosis. Some of the patients with anaerobic osteomyelitis will also have arthritis involving anaerobic bacteria, usually in an adjacent joint. A certain number of patients will have positive blood cultures.

Diabetes mellitus and vascular insufficiency have been incriminated as predisposing factors in anaerobic infection.[29] Ischemia and necrotic tissue provide an optimum environment for invasion and proliferation of anaerobes.

Human bites frequently result in anaerobic osteomyelitis. Of patients with anaerobic osteomyelitis of the hand for whom a predisposing factor was given, more than two-thirds had sustained a human bite.[22]

Many other conditions may predispose to invasion of bone by anaerobic bacteria. These include chronic otitis media, decubitus ulcers, abscesses, and chronic sinusitis. The few reports of anaerobic osteomyelitis in children also show a direct extension of the anaerobic infection for an adjacent sinusitis,[27] or direct implantation of the organisms from the normal mouth[26] or vaginal flora.[23]

Diagnosis

Local inflammatory signs may be absent in the early stages. Later, there usually is localized erythema, warmth, tenderness, swelling, fever, elevated pulse, pain that is severe, constant, and throbbing over the end of the shaft; and limitation of joint motion. Laboratory findings may reveal leukocytosis. Blood cultures are generally positive early in the course. Smear of aspirated pus and aerobic and anaerobic cultures of aspirated pus are essential.

X-ray examination may show spotty rarefaction followed shortly by periosteal new bone formation, generally absent for the first 10 to 14 days of the disease. A considerable portion of bone usually is involved, and the bone is demineralized. Bone scintigraphy with technetium may be positive before body changes are present on the roentgenogram.

There were no significant clinical differences between the patients with and without anaerobes cultured from their bone infections.

There is a relative lack of systemic symptoms in the patients with bone infections involving anaerobes.[16] Foul odor may be noted in almost half of the patients.[21]

The importance of obtaining adequate specimens for Gram stain and culture cannot be overemphasized. Many cases of so-called "culture-negative" osteomyelitis may have been due to anaerobes that were not detected. Aliquots of bone obtained either by needle biopsy or as surgical specimens should be immediately placed in media under conditions appropriate for the isolation of obligate anaerobic pathogens.

Although the clinical presentation of anaerobic or mixed aerobic and anaerobic osteomyelitis may not differ markedly from that of aerobic osteomyelitis, anaerobic osteomyelitis should be suspected in particular clinical settings:

1. Hand infections occurring as a result of human bites.
2. Osteomyelitis of the pelvis or ilium following intraabdominal sepsis.
3. Sacral osteomyelitis following decubitus ulcers.
4. All patients with osteomyelitis of the skull and facial bones.
5. Chronic nonhealing indolent ulcers of the foot, particularly in diabetics or in patients with associated vascular insufficiency who have underlying foci of bony involvement.
6. When foul-smelling exudates are present.
7. When there is sloughing of necrotic tissue, gas in soft tissues, and/or black discharge from a wound.
8. When Gram stains of clinical material reveal multiple organisms having different morphologic characteristics.
9. When there is a failure to grow organisms from clinical specimens, particularly when the Gram stain has shown organisms, but also with negative Gram stains.
10. Presence of sequestra in the bone.
11. Presence of exacerbation of chronic osteomyelitis of long bones.

Management

Treatment of osteomyelitis includes symptomatic therapy, immobilization in some cases, adequate drainage of purulent material, and antibiotic therapy consisting of parenteral administration of antibiotics for at least 21 days. In some cases antibiotic therapy has been advocated for six weeks or longer.

Although antibiotic therapy most often is started before the results of cultures are available, treatment programs must be adjusted for the sensitivities of microorganisms recovered from bone cultures obtained by needle, surgery, or from blood cultures. Once cultures are obtained, the need to initiate therapy without delay cannot be overemphasized if treatment failures and structural complications are to be avoided.

In the choice of antibiotic, a number of factors are important. The least toxic agent should be given at doses that yield the optimal inhibitory concentration for a long enough period to inhibit all dormant organisms. Culture information is essential to this choice. In general, the penicillins, cephalosporins, and clindamycin have achieved clinically effective bone concentrations against staphylococci. Aminoglycosides should be used only when other agents would not be effective.

The most commonly encountered isolate is *S. aureus*. The drug of first choice is a penicillinase (beta-lactamase)-resistant penicillin. Alternatives are the cephalosporins, clindamycin, and vancomycin. Other Gram-positive organisms such as group A and B streptococci, *S. pneumoniae*, clostridia, actinomycetes, and Gram-positive anaerobic cocci usually are penicillin sensitive.

Gram-negative microorganisms should be treated with aminoglycosides. Penicillin G appears to be the drug of choice for most anaerobic infections other than those caused by *B. fragilis*.[11, 30]

If the anaerobic organism is *B. fragilis*, either clindamycin, lincomycin, or carbenicillin may be considered. Metronidazole is bactericidal for *B. fragilis*, and this may be a valuable feature in the treatment of osteomyelitis. Chloramphenicol is an alternative in patients who are unable to receive clindamycin because of its potential gastrointestinal toxicity or in those who cannot be given carbenicillin because of a hemorrhagic diathesis or the necessity to avoid sodium retention. Chloramphenicol may also be considered as a primary therapeutic agent, particularly in the presence of concomitant central nervous system infection.[31] It is a bacteriostatic compound, however, and many infectious disease specialists prefer a bactericidal compound in the treatment of osteomyelitis. If the anaerobic organism is other than *B. fragilis*, penicillin G remains the drug of choice in most instances.[11, 32]

Surgical intervention often is required to establish a diagnosis and to remove foreign material. Otherwise, surgery is limited therapeutically to a small number of cases where drainage of a subperiosteal collection or debridement of necrotic bone is necessary. Failure to respond to appropriate treatment, coupled with continued pain, swelling, fever, and elevated white cell count and sedimentation rate are all indications for surgery. In the case of vertebral osteomyelitis, neurologic compromise requires immediate surgical intervention to relieve cord compression. Surgery should also be used to drain a septic hip when it accompanies osteomyelitis.

Hyperbaric oxygen may also be considered as adjunctive therapy for anaerobic osteomyelitis. Slack, Thomas, and Perrins[33] treated five cases of chronic osteomyelitis caused by aerobic organisms and had encouraging results. Other authors[34, 35] have reported varying degrees of success in the treatment of wound infections caused by aerobic organisms and in experimental treatment of staphylococcal osteomyelitis.[36]

REFERENCES

1. Nelson, J. D. The bacterial etiology and antibiotic management of septic arthritis in infants and children. *Pediatrics* 50:437, 1972.

2. Lipscomb, P. R. Infection of synovial tissues by mycobacteria other than *Mycobacterium tuberculosis. J. Bone Joint Surg.* 49:1521, 1530, 1967.

3. Toone, E. C., Jr., and Kelly, J. Joint and bone diseases due to mycotic infections. *Am. J. Med. Sci.* 231:263, 1956.

4. Class, R. N., and Cascio, F. S. Histoplasmosis presenting as acute polyarthritis. *N. Engl. J. Med.* 287:1133, 1972.

5. Noble, H. B., and Lyne, E. D. *Candida* osteomyelitis and arthritis from hyperalimentation therapy. Case report. *J. Bone Joint Surg.* 56A:825, 1974.

6. Feigin, R. D. et al. Clindamycin treatment of osteomyelitis and septic arthritis in children. *Pediatrics* 55:213, 1975.

7. Nelson, J. D., and Koontz, W. C. Septic arthritis in infants and children: a review of 117 cases. *Pediatrics* 38:966, 1966.

8. Sanders, D. Y., and Stevenson, J. *Bacteroides* infection in children. *J. Pediatr.* 72:673, 1968.

9. Ament, M. E., and Gaal, S. A. *Bacteroides* arthritis. *Am. J. Dis. Child.* 114:427, 1967.

10. McVay, L. V., and Sprunt, D. H. *Bacteroides* infections. *Ann. Int. Med.* 36:56, 1952.

11. Finegold, S. M. *Anaerobic bacteria in human disease.* New York: Academic Press, 1977.

12. Ropes, M. W., and Bauer, W. *Synovial fluid changes in joint disease.* Cambridge, Mass.: Harvard University Press, 1953.

13. Brook, I. et al. Synovial fluid lactic acid: a diagnostic aid in septic arthritis. *Arthritis Rheum.* 21:774, 1978.

14. Brooks, J. B. et al. Gas chromatography as a potential means of diagnosing arthritis. I. Differentiation between staphylococcal, streptococcal, gonococcal, and traumatic arthritis. *J. Infect. Dis.* 129:660, 1974.

15. Feldman, S. A., and DuClos, T. Diagnosis of meningococcal arthritis by immunoelectrophoresis of synovial fluid. *Appl. Microbiol.* 25:1006, 1973.

16. Waldvogel, F. A.; Medoff, G.; and Swartz, M. N. Osteomyelitis: a review of clinical features, therapeutic considerations and unusual aspects. *N. Engl. J. Med.* 262:198, 260, 316, 1970.

17. Morse, T. S., and Pryles, C. V. Infections of the bone and joints in children. *N. Engl. J. Med.* 262:846, 1960.

18. Robertson, D. E. Primary acute and subacute localized osteomyelitis and osteochondritis in children. *Can. J. Surg.* 10:408, 1967.

19. Burch, K. H. et al. *Cryptococcus neoformans* as a cause of lytic bone lesions. *JAMA* 231:1057, 1975.

20. Rhangos, W. C., and Chick, E. W. Mycotic infections of bone. *South. Med. J.* 57:664, 1964.

21. Lewis, R. P.; Sutter, V. L.; and Finegold, S. M. Bone infections involving anaerobic bacteria. *Medicine* 57:279, 1978.

22. Raff, M. J., and Melo, J. C. Anaerobic osteomyelitis. *Medicine* 57:83, 1978.

23. Brook, I. Osteomyelitis and bacteremia caused by *Bacteroides fragilis.* A complication of fetal monitoring. *Clin. Pediatr.* 19:639, 1980.

24. Schubiner, H.; Letourneau, M.; and Murray, D. L. Pyogenic osteomyelitis versus pseudo-osteomyelitis in Gaucher's disease. Report of a case and review of the literature. *Clin. Pediatr.* 20:607, 1981.

25. Chandler, F. A., and Breaks, V. M. Osteomyelitis of femoral neck and head. *JAMA* 116:2390, 1941.

26. Brook, I. Bacteriology of paronychia in children. *Am. J. Surg.* 141:703, 1981.

27. Brook, I. et al. Complications of sinusitis in children. *Pediatrics* 66:586, 1980.

28. Brook, I. Aerobic and anaerobic bacteriology of chronic mastoiditis in children. *Am. J. Dis. Child.* 135:478, 1981.

29. Felner, J. M., and Dowell, V. R. Anaerobic bacterial endocarditis. *N. Engl. J. Med.* 283:1188, 1970.

30. Finegold, S. M. et al. Management of anaerobic infections. *Ann. Intern. Med.* 83:375, 1975.

31. Kelley, R. S.; Hunt, A. D., Jr.; and Tashman, S. G. Studies on the absorption and distribution of chloramphenicol. *Pediatrics* 8:362, 1951.

32. Gorbach, S. L., and Bartlett, J. G. Anaerobic infections. *N. Engl. J. Med.* 290:1177, 1974.

33. Slack, W. K.; Thomas, D. A.; and Perrins, D. Hyperbaric oxygenation in chronic osteomyelitis. *Lancet* 1:1093, 1965.

34. Irvin, T. T.; Norman, J. N.; and Suwanagel, A. Hyperbaric oxygen in the treatment of infections by aerobic microorganisms. *Lancet* 1:392, 1966.

35. McAllister, T. A. et al. Inhibitory effects of hyperbaric oxygen on bacteria and fungi. *Lancet* 2:1040, 1963.

36. Hambler, D. L. Hyperbaric oxygenation: its effects on experimental staphylococcal osteomyelitis in rats. *J. Bone Joint Surg.* 50A:1129, 1968.

CHAPTER 27

Pseudomembranous Colitis

The increased use of antibiotics in recent years has resulted in the potentially fatal complication of pseudomembranous enterocolitis. The clinical spectrum of this disease may range from a mild, nonspecific diarrhea to severe colitis with toxic megacolon, perforation, and death.[1] Discontinuation of antibiotics and supportive therapy usually lead to resolution of this disorder.[2] Pseudomembranous colitis may affect all age groups, although a lower incidence was noted in children.[3] Antimicrobial agents associated with the development of diarrhea and/ or colitis include penicillin G, ampicillin, amoxicillin, nafcillin, cephalexin, cephalothin, tetracycline, chloramphenicol, lincomycin, clindamycin, and metronidazole. Changes in fecal flora with elimination of many strains accompanying the administration of clindamycin to humans have been documented.[4] Several species of *Eubacterium* and *Clostridium* (*Clostridium difficile, Clostridium innocuum, Clostridium oroticum,* and *Clostridium ramosum*) were present in some patients in large numbers, along with *Candida* species and aerobic Gram-negative bacilli. Recent work[5, 6] has provided evidence to implicate *C. difficile* as an etiologic agent in most cases. Several reports have described infants[7] and adults[8, 9] with severe enterocolitis associated with *C. difficile* toxin in the stools and without previous antibiotic exposure.

Microbiology and Pathogenesis

Staphylococcus aureus was considered for many years to be associated with pseudomembranous colitis.[10, 11] The recovery of many patients from the disease when treated with oral vancomycin reinforced the impression that the pathogen was indeed *S. aureus*.

In recent years, however, many studies failed to recover *S. aureus* from stools of patients with colitis or enterocolitis. A renewed interest in the disease occurred following an increased incidence in the last decade.

Clindamycin, ampicillin, and the cephalosporins are the drugs most frequently associated with development of pseudomembranous colitis at present, although nearly all antimicrobials with an antibacterial spectrum have been implicated as causes of diarrhea and colitis. The resistance of some clostridia to clindamycin led several workers to speculate that clostridia might play a role in clindamycin-associated colitis. Data presented by Bartlett and colleagues[12] established that a toxigenic strain of *C. difficile* is a major cause of clindamycin-associated colitis in hamsters. Several groups[13, 14] have isolated toxin-producing strains of *C. difficile* from patients with clindamycin- and ampicillin-associated pseudomembranous colitis. These data are supported by the finding of high-level clindamycin resistance of the *Clostridium* species isolated from the hamster (MIC = 128 µg/ml), protection afforded by pretreatment with vancomycin, and protection achieved by prior incubation of sterile filtrates of cecal material with polyvalent clostridial gas-gangrene antitoxin. Rifkin and co-workers[15] also noted the induction of colitis in hamsters by clindamycin and the protection afforded by pretreatment with vancomycin, heating of cecal contents, and prior incubation of cecal contents with polyvalent gas-gangrene antitoxin.

Stools from approximately 98% of patients with antibiotic-associated pseudomembranous colitis contain the cytotoxin, and bacterial cultures of these specimens almost invariably yield *C. difficile*.[16] Studies[16, 17] of stool specimens from healthy adults have not shown this cytotoxin, and the carrier rate for *C. difficile* is believed to be below 3%; however, recent studies suggest the patient rendered susceptible by antibiotic exposure may acquire the organism from an environmental source. It is of interest that this organism was described initially as a component of the fecal flora of healthy neonates.[18] Nearly 30% of healthy neonates harbor *C. difficile,* and some also have the toxin without clinically apparent consequences.[5, 19] Carrier rates for *C. difficile* in stool decrease with age, and this microbe is rarely found in flora analyses in children more than one year of age.

Recent work has indicated that *C. difficile* can be spread in a neonatal nursery by fomites, but significant clinical disease has not been associated with the carriage of *C. difficile* in neonates.[20]

The ability of *C. difficile* to produce disease almost solely in the presence of antibiotic exposure is explained by the organism's ability to flourish in an environment in which there is reduced bacterial competition. Animal studies support this hypothesis. There are only three models in which disease is produced by colonizing animals with *C. difficile:* the newborn animal, which has a sterile intestine; the gnotobiotic animal, which has no competing flora; and the animal that has been given an antibiotic that suppresses the normal flora.

In humans, the only host risk factor other than antibiotic exposure implicated to date is age; the incidence of antibiotic-associated diarrhea and colitis seems to rise with increasing age. The entity has been documented in children as well, although with less frequency.

The mechanisms by which *C. difficile* causes the pathology have been investigated. It has been found that *C. difficile* can produce two toxins.[21] The cytotoxin is potent in tissue culture assays and is a relatively sensitive and specific marker for *C. difficile*-induced disease, whereas toxin A is considerably more potent in biologic assays of enteric toxins when animal models are used, and it may be more important in the clinical expression of gastrointestinal complications.

These differences may explain some of the conflicts between clinical observations and the results of tissue culture assays: the lack of correlation between the severity of the disease and cytotoxicity titers, the occasional patient with documented pseudomembranous colitis and negative toxin assays but positive cultures, the occasional adult with positive toxin assays but no symptoms, the prolonged carriage of the cytotoxin following recovery noted in some patients, and the high incidence of positive toxin assays in healthy neonates. These phenomena may be attributable to interrelationships between the two toxins, of which little is known.

Pseudomembranous enterocolitis recently has been described in the neonatal periods. Adler, Chandrika, and Berman[22] described a 12-week-old infant with pseudomembranous colitis. No prior antibiotics were administered, although the child had received dicyclomine hydrochloride. *C. difficile* and its toxin were detected in the child's stool. Severe disseminated intravascular coagulopathy developed; the patient required total colectomy but eventually recovered.

Donta, Stuppy, and Myers[23] have reported a 10-day-old infant with *C. difficile* colitis associated with administration of penicillin that was given for the treatment of group B streptococcal sepsis. Recently, Kim, Dupont, and Pickering[24] recovered *C. difficile* and its toxin from children who suffered from diarrhea and attended the same day care center. This report is of particular interest because it implicates *C. difficile* in acute diarrheal epidemic in children.

The toxin of *C. difficile* has not generally been implicated in the pathogenesis of necrotizing enterocolitis, although it has been identified in the stools of healthy infants. Rietra and associates[25] found that 17 of 121 stools (14%) from infants zero to five months of age caused cytotoxicity in tissue culture that was consistent with the effect of *C. difficile* toxin. No toxin was identified in stools from 24 patients with necrotizing enterocolitis examined by Bartlett and colleagues[26] or from 18 patients with necrotizing enterocolitis studied by Chang and Areson.[27] Cashore and co-workers[28] found toxin in five infants with necrotizing enterocolitis, which suggests a role for clostridial toxin in some cases of this disease. Hypoxia and circulatory disturbances in small premature infants at risk for necrotizing enterocolitis may lead to ischemic segments of bowel, in which multiplication of clostridia antitoxin production may result in bowel ulceration, infarction, pneumatosis, and the clinical picture of enterocolitis.

Incidence

The occurrence of pseudomembranous enterocolitis remains unusual in the pediatric age group. A review of the literature revealed 14 deaths in children with that disease; the cases reported involved patients with serious coexistent illness, infection, or congenital defects. Antibiotics were given in most instances and usually were administered parenterally. Two deaths have been reported in children with pseudomembranous enterocolitis following parenteral administration of ampicillin alone. Fee and associates[29] and Lazar and colleagues[30] implicate intravenously administered ampicillin as the cause of death in two children, but numerous other antimicrobial agents also were used in these patients. Oral ampicillin therapy is implicated in three childhood cases.[31] There was complete recovery after discontinuation of medication in two, and one child died.

It is noteworthy that many of these children, as in the present series, had received antimicrobial agents for clinical conditions in which the value of such treatment is questionable. The reports reviewed did not include data concerning the more recent work with tissue cultures of stool and bacterial cultures of *C. difficile.*

Brook[32] recently isolated toxin-producing *C. difficile* from two children who developed diarrhea following oxacillin and dicloxacillin therapy. The diarrhea ceased, and *C. difficile* was not recovered again following discontinuation of the antimicrobial agents. These findings suggest a possible role for these organisms in diarrhea following administration of antimicrobial agents in children.

Schussheim and Goldstein[33] described two siblings who presented with penicillin-associated pseudomembranous colitis. Viscidi and Bartlett[34] recently presented 10 cases of antibiotic-associated pseudomembranous colitis in children. The ages ranged from 4 years to 17 years; the most frequently implicated antimicrobial agents were penicillins in six children and clindamycin in two. Stool assays of specimens taken from all ten patients yielded a cytopathic toxin. Bacterial cultures of nine specimens uniformly yielded *C. difficile* with a median concentration of $10^{5.4}$ organisms per gram of wet weight. All nine isolates of *C. difficile* showed in vitro production of a cytopathic toxin.

Clinical Presentation

The clinical expression of *C. difficile*-induced gastrointestinal disease varies. Diarrhea is found in almost all patients with antibiotic-associated colitis. About one-half to two-thirds of patients develop diarrhea during the course of antibiotic administration; in the rest, diarrhea does not develop until up to four to six weeks after cessation of antibiotic therapy. It should be emphasized that most patients with antibiotic-associated diarrhea do not have colitis; *C. difficile* is implicated in only 15% to 25% of these "benign diarrheas," and the etiologic mechanism in the majority is unknown. The average duration of diarrhea when considering all cases is 8 to 10 days after the implicating drug is discontinued, but in some patients diarrhea can persist for four weeks or longer; in several cases, there may be as many as 30 stools daily.

Patients with antibiotic-associated colitis may present with only diarrhea, but most will have abdominal cramps, abdominal tenderness, leukocytosis from 10,000 to 20,000/mm^3 and fever up to 106°F.

Diagnosis

The diagnostic test of choice to detect the presence of *C. difficile* toxin is a tissue culture assay to demonstrate a cytopathic toxin that may be neutralized by clostridial antitoxin.[5, 6, 35] Two alternative methods to detect *C. difficile* toxin are the enzyme-linked immunoabsorbent assay (ELISA) and the counterimmunoelectrophoresis (CIE). Potential advantages of these methods are that the required technology is readily available in most hospitals, results are available within one to two hours, and special storage conditions are not necessary.

Stool cultures for *C. difficile* should be attempted, although the isolation of the organism should be accompanied by a reliable toxin assay.

Endoscopy is used to detect the typical plaquelike lesions of the pseudomembrane. Sigmoidoscopy may be sufficient in many cases because the distal colon is usually the involved site, but pseudomembranes occasionally will be restricted to the right colon, necessitating colonoscopy. Endoscopic findings in patients who have antibiotic-associated diarrhea range from a normal mucosa through a spectrum of changes including erythema and edema, friability, ulceration, and hemorrhage, as well as pseudomembranous colitis. The most useful x-ray study is air-contrast barium enema, but its findings are often nonspecific, and care must be exercised to avoid complications. It should be emphasized that the demonstration of pseudomembranous colitis by either x-rays or endoscopy provides an anatomic, not an etiologic, diagnosis.

Management

Patients with mild diarrhea and no systemic complications may need only supportive therapy. A child with severe symptoms or persistent diarrhea caused by *C. difficile* is a candidate for more aggressive treatment. Vancomycin, which is almost universally effective, however, has three disadvantages: high expense, bad taste, and a 20% relapse rate. The cause of relapses may be reacquisition of the organism or the persistence of spores in the colon. Fortunately, patients with a relapse will respond to the same treatment, but occasionally patients will have multiple recurrences.[36]

An alternative to vancomycin is cholestyramine, which is an anion exchange resin that binds both *C. difficile* toxins. Although cholestyramine is more likely to result in primary treatment failure than is vancomycin, it is less likely to be followed by relapse. This drug has the theoretic advantage of avoiding antibiotic treatment of an antibiotic complication. If the patient is seriously ill or fails to respond to cholestyramine, the clinician is advised to use vancomycin.[37] Another antibiotic that has been used to treat patients with disease induced by *C. difficile* is bacitracin. Preliminary results with bacitracin suggest response rates and relapses comparable to those associated with vancomycin. Another drug reported to produce a good response is metronidazole, although metronidazole has been implicated as a cause of pseudomembranous colitis in a few cases.[37]

Complications

Severe complications include dehydration, electrolyte imbalance, hypotension, hypoalbuminemia with anasarca, and toxic megacolon. With the identification of the microbial pathogen and the availability of specific treatment modalities, mortality today is virtually nil.

Oral vancomycin therapy has been associated with a relapse rate of 15% to 20%.[36] The mechanism of relapse has not been defined, but theoretical considerations include reacquisition of the organism from an environmental source or failure to eradicate the organism because of sporulation.

Prevention

It is recommended that clinicians become cautious about administering drugs that have been associated with pseudomembranous colitis to patients with intestinal disease. In patients with idiopathic inflammatory bowel disease, it might be wise to avoid ampicillin, clindamycin, and cephalosporins, the drugs most frequently associated with pseudomembranous colitis, because if the patient developed diarrhea, it would be difficult to ascertain whether the underlying disease was responsible or another had been superimposed, with the possibility of more devastating consequences.

Because of the risk of acquiring enterocolitis, antibiotic therapy should be limited to patients who unequivocally need the drugs, and prudent use of antimicrobials should be avoided. Patients who receive antimicrobial agents, and especially those known to cause colitis, should be warned about this complication and should be told to contact their physician as soon as symptoms of the disease occur.

There are two means by which a human might acquire antibiotic-associated pseudomembranous colitis. The first, in which a host is susceptible by virtue of being a carrier of the microbe, would account for sporadic cases, particularly community-acquired cases. The second, in which a noncarrier takes an antibiotic and is then exposed to the microbe from an environmental source, would account for outbreaks.

Nosocomial spread of the disease in hospitals has been known for years. Reports of clustering of cases of pseudomembranous colitis[38] suggest that *C. difficile* is readily transmittable among hospital patients. Rogers and colleagues[39] reported the spread of this organism among leukemic children receiving oral nonabsorbable antibiotics to suppress their commensal bowel flora. Transmission of the organism in hospitals has been documented to occur through fomites and the hands of asymptomatic personnel. In an attempt to prevent spread of this organism in a susceptible population, isolation techniques and enteric isolation precautions are recommended, with special attention to cleansing of hands and potentially contaminated surfaces.[37]

Patients with *C. difficile* diarrhea should be isolated until they are no longer excreting the organism, and their hospital rooms should be decontaminated with mechanical cleansing and germicides upon discharge from the hospital. Sigmoidoscopes and colonoscopes used to examine such patients should be decontaminated to avoid possible transmission of the disease to other patients.

REFERENCES

1. Brown, C. H.; Ferrante, W. A.; and David, W. D. Toxic dilation of the colon complicating pseudomembranous enterocolitis. *Am. J. Dig. Dis.* 13:813, 1968.

2. Tedesco, F. J.; Barton, R. W.; and Alpers, D. H. Clindamycin-associated colitis: a prospective study. *Ann. Intern. Med.* 81:429, 1974.

3. Keefe, E. B. et al. Pseudomembranous enterocolitis. Resurgence related to newer antibiotic therapy. *West. J. Med.* 121:462, 1974.

4. Sutter, V. L., and Finegold, S. M. The effect of antimicrobial agents on human fecal flora: studies with cephalexin, cyclacillin, and clindamycin. In *The normal microbial flora of man*, eds. F. A. Skinner and J. G. Carr. London: Academic Press, 1974, p. 229.

5. Larson, H. E. et al. *Clostridium difficile* and the aetiology of pseudomembranous colitis. *Lancet* 1:1063, 1978.

6. Bartlett, J. G. Antibiotic associated pseudomembranous colitis. *Rev. Infect. Dis.* 1:123, 1979.

7. Hyams, J. S.; Berman, M. M.; and Helgason, H. Nonantibiotic-associated enterocolitis caused by *Clostridium difficile* in an infant. *J. Pediatr.* 99:750, 1981.

8. Larton, H. E., and Price, A. B. Pseudomembranous colitis: presence of clostridial toxin. *Lancet* 2:1312, 1977.

9. Wald, A.; Mendelow, H.; and Bartlee, J. G. Non-antibiotic-associated pseudomembranous colitis due to toxin-producing clostridia. *Ann. Intern. Med.* 92:798, 1980.

10. Altemeier, W. A.; Hummel, R. P.; and Hill, E. O. Staphylococcal enterocolitis following antibiotic therapy. *Ann. Surg.* 157:847, 1963.

11. Tan, T. L. et al. The experimental development of pseudomembranous colitis. *Surg. Gynecol. Obstet.* 108:415, 1959.

12. Bartlett, J. G. et al. Clindamycin-associated colitis due to a toxin producing species of *Clostridium* in hamster. *J. Infect. Dis.* 136:701, 1978.

13. Bartlett, J. G. et al. Antibiotic-associated pseudomembranous colitis due to toxin-producing clostridia. *N. Engl. J. Med.* 298:531, 1978.

14. George, W. L. et al. Aetiology of antimicrobial-agent-associated colitis. *Lancet* 1:802, 1978.

15. Rifkin, G. D. et al. Antibiotic-induced colitis. Implication of a toxin neutralized by *Clostridium sordellii* antitoxin. *Lancet* 2:1103, 1977.

16. Willey, S., and Bartlett, J. G. Cultures for *Clostridium difficile* in stools containing a cytotoxin neutralized by *Clostridium sordellii* antitoxin. *J. Clin. Microbiol.* 10:880, 1979.

17. George, W. L.; Sutter, V. L.; and Finegold, S. M. Toxicity and antimicrobial susceptibility of *Clostridium difficile*. A cause of antimicrobial agent-associated colitis. *Curr. Microbiol.* 1:55, 1978.

18. Hall, J. C., and O'Toole, E. Intestinal flora in newborn infants with description of a new pathogenic anaerobe, *Bacillus difficilis*. *Am. J. Dis. Child.* 49:390, 1935.

19. Snyder, M. L. Further studies on *Bacillus difficilis*. *J. Infect. Dis.* 60:223, 1937.

20. DePasse, B. M., and Siegel, J. D. Nosocomial spread of *Clostridium difficile* in the neonatal nursery (abstr. 708). *Proceedings,* 21st Interscience Conference on Antimicrobial Agents and Chemotherapy. Chicago, 1981.

21. Bartlett, J. G. et al. Clinical and laboratory observations in *Clostridium difficile* colitis. *Am. J. Clin. Nutr.* 33:2521, 1960.

22. Adler, S. P.; Chandrika, T.; and Berman, W. F. *Clostridium difficile* associated with pseudomembranous colitis. Occurrence in a 12-week-old infant without prior antibiotic therapy. *Am. J. Dis. Child.* 135:820, 1981.

23. Donta, S. T.; Stuppy, M. S.; and Myers, M. G. Neonatal antibiotic associated colitis. *Am. J. Dis. Child.* 135:181, 1981.

24. Kim, K.; Dupont, H. L.; and Pickering, L. K. *Clostridium difficile* in children attending day care centers (abstr. C179). *Proceedings,* 82nd Annual Meeting of the American Society for Microbiology, Atlanta, Ga., 1982, p. 301.

25. Rietra, P. J. G. M. et al. Clostridia toxin in feces of healthy infants. *Lancet* 2:319, 1978.

26. Bartlett, J. G. et al. Role of *Clostridium difficile* in antibiotic-associated pseudomembranous colitis. *Gastroenterology* 75:778, 1978.

27. Chang, T. W., and Areson, P. Neonatal necrotizing enterocolitis: absence of enteric bacterial toxins. *N. Engl. J. Med.* 299:424, 1978.

28. Cashore, W. J. et al. Clostridia colonization and clostridial toxin in neonatal necrotizing enterocolitis. *J. Pediatr.* 98:308, 1981.

29. Fee, H. J. et al. Fatal outcome in a child with pseudomembranous colitis. *J. Pediatr. Surg.* 10:959, 1975.

30. Lazar, H. L. et al. Pseudomembranous colitis associated with antibiotic therapy in a child: report of a case and review of the literature. *J. Pediatr. Surg.* 13:488, 1978.

31. Auritt, W.; Hervada, A. R.; and Fendrick, G. Fatal pseudomembranous enterocolitis following oral ampicillin therapy. *J. Pediatr.* 93:882, 1978.

32. Brook, I. Isolation of toxin producing *Clostridium difficile* from two children with oxacillin and dicloxacillin associated diarrhea. *Pediatrics* 65:1154, 1980.

33. Schussheim, A., and Goldstein, J. C. Antibiotic-associated pseudomembranous colitis in siblings. *Pediatrics* 66:932, 1980.

34. Viscidi, R. P., and Bartlett, J. G. Antibiotic-associated pseudomembranous colitis in children. *Pediatrics* 67:381, 1981.

35. Chang, T. W.; Lauermann, M.; and Bartlett, J. G. Cytotoxicity assay in antibiotic-associated colitis. *J. Infect. Dis.* 140:765, 1979.

36. Bartlett, J. G. et al. Relapse following oral vancomycin therapy of antibiotic associated pseudomembranous colitis. *Gastroenterology* 78:431, 1979.

37. George, W. L.; Rolfe, R. D.; and Finegold, S. M. Treatment and presentation of antimicrobial agents-induced colitis and diarrhea. *Gastroenterology* 79:366, 1980.

38. Fekety, R. et al. Epidemiology of antibiotic associated colitis. *Am. J. Med.* 70:906, 1981.

39. Rogers, T. R. et al. Spread of *Clostridium difficile* among patients receiving nonabsorbable antibiotics for gut decontamination *Br. Med. J.* 283:408, 1981.

Other Types
of Anaerobic
Infections

CHAPTER 28

Anaerobic Bacteremia

Although anaerobes have been reported to account for 8% to 11% of episodes of bacteremia in adults,[1] anaerobic organisms rarely have been isolated from blood cultures of pediatric patients. These microbes represent a small percentage of the total number of positive blood cultures recovered from children. This may be due partly to the difficulty in isolating and identifying these organisms. There is, however, a growing awareness of the role of anaerobic organisms in bacteremia.[2-6]

Incidence

In a survey of anaerobic infections in children, blood cultures have been found to be the second most frequent source of anaerobic organisms.[2, 4] In one of these reviews of the recovery of anaerobes from children over one year in a university hospital,[4] 13 blood cultures were positive and contained 14 anaerobes. In a large prospective study during a one-year period, only 0.3% of blood cultures contained anaerobic bacteria that were involved in the pathogenesis of the patient's disease.[3] In contrast, pathogenic aerobes were recovered from 9% of the cultures done during that period. Anaerobes accounted for 5.8% of all bacteremic episodes (8.7% in the newborn period and 4.8% in children over one year of age). It should be noted that 10% of the newborns with clinical bacteremia had only anaerobes recovered from their blood cultures.

Microbiology

Anaerobic bacteremia has rarely been described in pediatric patients.[7, 8] Sanders and Stevenson[6] in a review of the literature summarized 11 cases of *Bacteroides* bacteremias in children. In one study, anaerobic organisms were recovered from 6 of 34 children who required general

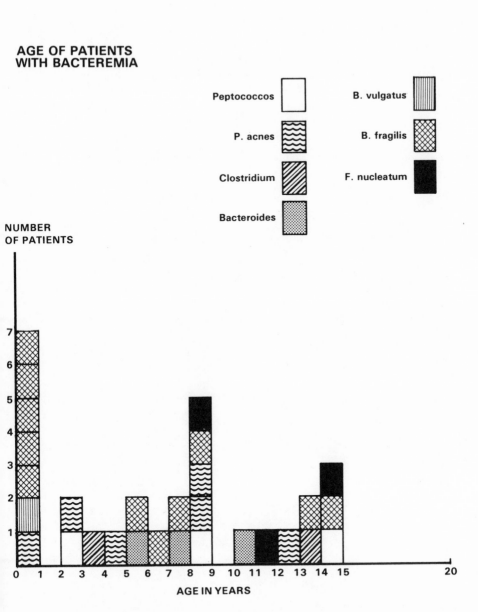

Figure 28.1. Age distribution of patients with anaerobic bacteremia. (Brook, I. et al. Recovery of anaerobic bacteria from pediatric patients: a one-year experience. *Am. J. Dis. Child.* 133:1020–1024, 1979. Copyright 1979, American Medical Association. Reprinted by permission.)

Table 28.1 Clinical Data on 28 Patients With Bacteremia Caused by Anaerobic Bacteria

Organism	No. of Cases	Probable Source	Underlying Conditions	Other Complications	Antimicrobial Therapy	Results	Other Infectious Sites With Similar Bacteria
Peptococcus sp.	3	Abscesses (2),* sinusitis (1)	None (3)	Subdural empyema (1); meningitis (1)	Penicillin G potassium (1); ampicillin sodium (1); oxacillin sodium (1)	Cured (3)	Subdural empyema and sinus (1); abscess (1)
P. acnes	4	Cardiovascular shunts (3); periorbital cellulitis (1)	Hydrocephalus (1)	Meningitis (2)	Penicillin (2); methicillin (1); ampicillin (1)	Cured (3); died (1)	CSF (2)
Clostridium sp.	4	Gastrointestinal (GI) tract (4)	Sickle cell disease (2)	None (4)	Penicillin (2); ampicillin (2)	Cured (4)	None (4)
Bacteroides sp.	3	Perforation viscus (2); ileus (1)	Acute lymphocytic leukemia (1)	Peritonitis (1)	Clindamycin hydrochloride (2); carbenicillin disodium (1)	Cured (3)	Peritoneal fluid (2)
B. fragilis group	11	Perforated appendix (3); pneumonia (3); abscesses (3); GI tract (1); necrotizing enterocolitis (1)	Mental retardation (2); acute lymphocytic leukemia (1); selective IgG deficiency (1); prematurity (1); recent hip surgery (1)	Meningitis (2); peritonitis (2); septic shock (1); empyema (1)	Clindamycin (6); penicillin (3); chloramphenicol sodium succinate (2); ampicillin (2); carbenicillin (1)	Cured (7); died (4)	Abscess (3); tracheopulmonary aspiration (2); peritoneal fluid (2); CSF (1)
F. nucleatum†	3	Sinusitis (2); perforated appendix (1)	Chronic otitis media (1)	Subdural empyema (1); periorbital cellulitis (1)	Chloramphenicol (2); clindamycin (1)	Cured (3)	Sinuses (2)

SOURCE: Brook, I. et al. Recovery of anaerobic bacteria from pediatric patients: a one-year experience. *Am. J. Dis. Child.* 133:1020–1024, 1979. Copyright 1979, American Medical Association. Reprinted by permission.

*Number of cases in parentheses.

†In one case, *Peptococcus* sp. was also recovered in the blood culture.

anesthesia and nasotracheal intubation for dental repair.[9] Another study documented bacteremia in 28 children who were undergoing dental manipulations.[10] Among the 28 isolates recovered, 21 were anaerobes (*Propionibacterium* species, nine; *Veillonella alcalescens,* five; *Bacteroides melaninogenicus,* three; *Peptostreptococcus* species, two; and *Eubacterium* species and *Fusobacterium* species, one each).

Dunkle, Brotherton, and Feigin[2] recovered 14 anaerobes from blood cultures over a one-year study. The anaerobes recovered were *Clostridium* species (four species), *Fusobacterium nucleatus* (three species), Gram-positive cocci (three species), and *Bacteroides fragilis* (two species). Although 27 isolates of *Propionibacterium acnes* were recovered, only three were associated with clinical infection.

Thirmuoothi, Keen, and Dajani[3] reviewed their experience over a period of 18 months, and reported 35 isolates from 34 blood cultures. The predominant isolates were four each of Gram-positive cocci and *Bacteroides* species and two isolates each of *Fusobacterium* species, *Bifidobacterium* species, and *Clostridium* species. Although *Propionibacterium* species were recovered in 18 instances there was no apparent relationship between their recovery from the blood and the 18 patients' clinical illness. Brook and colleagues[11] recently summarized their experience in the diagnosis of anaerobic bacteremia noted in 28 children. Twenty-nine anaerobic isolates were recovered from 28 patients ranging in age from 1 week to 15 years (table 28.1, fig. 28.1): of these, 14 were *Bacteroides* species (11 of which belonged to the *B. fragilis* group); four were *Clostridium* species; four were anaerobic Gram-positive cocci; four were *P. acnes;* and three were *Fusobacterium* species. Although the predominant isolate from blood cultures (56% to 65%) is *P. acnes,*[2, 3] a normal inhabitant of the skin, many of these isolates may reflect contamination of the blood cultures by the skin flora. *P. acnes* can cause bacteremia, however, especially in association with shunt infections.[12] All of the patients with *P. acnes* bacteremia included in this study had clinical infection, and all but one responded to antimicrobial therapy. Furthermore, two patients had meningitis caused by this organism after installation of cardiovascular shunts.

Pathogenesis

Source of Entry

As reported for adults,[7] the strain of anaerobic organisms recovered depended to a large extent on the portal of entry and the underlying disease. The probable portals of entry for the blood culture isolates in the 28 patients studied by Brook and associates[11] are given in table 28.2. The gastrointestinal (GI) tract predominated (13 patients), followed by the respiratory tract (ear, sinus, and oropharynx, seven), the

Table 28.2. Probable Sites of Source of Bacteremia According to Anaerobic Bacteria (Number of Cases)

Bacteria	Ear, Sinus, Oropharynx	Skin, Soft Tissue	Shunts	Gastrointestinal Tract	Lower Respiratory Tract	Total
Peptococcus sp.	4*					4
P. acnes	1		3			4
Clostridium sp.				4		4
Bacteroides sp.				3		3
B. vulgatus					1	1
B. fragilis		3		5	2	10
F. nucleatum	2*			1		3
Total	7	3	3	13	3	29*

SOURCE: Brook, I. et al. Recovery of anaerobic bacteria from pediatric patients: a one-year experience. Am. J. Dis. Child. 133:1020–1024, 1979. Copyright 1979, American Medical Association. Reprinted by permission.

*Represents a mixed infection with Peptococcus sp. and F. nucleatum lower respiratory tract (three), cardiovascular shunts and neurologic shunts (three), and skin and soft tissue (three). When the GI tract was the probable portal of entry, *Bacteroides* species (eight isolates, including five of the *B. fragilis* group) and *Clostridium* species (four isolates) were the organisms most frequently recovered from blood. The predominant anaerobic organisms recovered in association with infections of the ear, sinus, and oropharynx were *Peptococcus* species (from four patients) and *F. nucleatum* (from two patients). *P. acnes* was grown in cultures taken from four patients, three of whom had artificial cardiac valves or ventriculoatrial shunts. Two of these patients also were initially observed to have meningitis caused by a similar organism. All lower respiratory tract infections that served as a probable source of bacteremia were due to isolates belonging to the *B. fragilis* group.

No obvious focus of infection was noted in six patients; however, it is of interest that all of these patients had some GI problem that might have served as a source of the bacteremia. It is of interest also that four of these patients had bacteremia caused by *Clostridium* species.

These findings support, therefore, previous studies of adults[13, 14] and children[6, 8] that report that *Bacteroides* species, including the *B. fragilis* group, were the predominant isolates from patients in whom the GI tract was the probable portal of entry. As summarized by Sanders and Stevenson,[6] however, *Bacteroides* species caused bacteremia in children with otitis media and abscesses.

The ear, sinus, and oropharynx were found to be possible portals of entry that predisposed patients to bacteremia with *Peptococcus* species and *Fusobacterium* species. This is not surprising since these organisms are part of the normal flora of such anatomic sites and can be involved in local infections.[7]

Three patients developed pneumonia subsequent to bacteremia with organisms belonging to the *B. fragilis* group. This has also been noted in adults[1] and newborns.[5] Although *Bacteroides* accounted for the majority of the episodes of bacteremia in this study, other studies have shown relatively infrequent isolation of these organisms from children,[1] except during the neonatal period.[5]

Predisposing Factors

B. fragilis, anaerobic Gram-positive cocci, and *Fusobacterium* species were the other anaerobic organisms most commonly isolated from blood cultures in three recent studies.[2–4] Most of the patients described in these studies were over six weeks of age and suffered from chronic debilitating disorders such as malignant neoplasms, immunodeficiencies, or chronic renal insufficiency, and carried a poor prognosis. *Bacteroides* species were also isolated frequently after perforation of viscus and appendicitis.[15, 16]

Predisposing factors to anaerobic bacteremia in adults include malignant neoplasms,[17, 18] hematologic disorders,[19] transplantation of organs,[20] recent GI or obstetric gynecologic surgery,[18, 19, 21] intestinal obstruction,[22] diabetes mellitus,[18] postsplenectomy,[20] use of cytotoxic agents or corticosteroids,[18] and use of prophylactic antimicrobial agents for bowel preparation prior to surgery.[18, 21]

Predisposing conditions were noted also in pediatric patients.[11] Two patients had malignant neoplasms, two suffered from hematologic abnormalities, and one had an immune deficiency. It is of interest that 82% of the bacteremias in this series of patients[11] occurred in children who had no immunosuppression or malignant neoplasms. This is in contrast to another study[8] in which anaerobic bacteremia occurred more frequently in children with these predisposing factors.

Diagnosis and Clinical Features

The clinical features of anaerobic bacteremia in these patients were not much different from other types of bacteremia in children; however, a relatively longer period was needed before an etiologic diagnosis could be made. This can be a result of the smaller volume of blood drawn from children for culture inoculation and the longer time needed for growth and identification of anaerobic organisms.

Management

Prolonged therapy with antimicrobial agents alone apparently is adequate for most patients. The average duration of therapy in the patients who recovered was 20 days (range, 7 to 72 days), and the duration of therapy was related to the presence and severity of other infectious sites and complications (table 28.2). Therapy was longest in the treatment of meningitis, wound abscess, sinusitis, and empyema. When anaerobes resistant to penicillin, such as the *B. fragilis* group, are suspected or isolated, alternative medication such as clindamycin, chloramphenicol, carbenicillin, or ticarcillin disodium should be administered. Surgical drainage is essential when pus has collected. Organisms identical to those causing anaerobic bacteremia often can be recovered from other infected sites (as in 15, or 58%, of patients in the study by Brook and co-workers).[11] No doubt these extravascular sites may have served as a source of persistent bacteremia in some cases; however, the majority of patients will recover completely when prompt treatment with appropriate antimicrobial agents is instituted before any complications develop. The early recognition of anaerobic bacteremia and administration of appropriate antimicrobial and surgical therapy play a significant role in preventing mortality and morbidity in pediatric patients.

Complications

Certain other serious concomitant complications can be present in children. The most frequent complication noted was meningitis, which occurred in five patients. Peritonitis occurred in three patients, subdural empyema in two, and septic shock in one. Although many of the children were seriously ill, most responded well to therapy.

The mortality following anaerobic bacteremia was 18%[11] (five patients) and depended on such factors as age of the patient, underlying disease, nature of the organism, speed with which the diagnosis was made, and surgical or medical therapy instituted. This mortality rate was similar to that reported in adults.[7] Of the three infants who died, two were newborns and one was eight months old. Four patients were infected with organisms of the *B. fragilis* group that were resistant to penicillin; inappropriate antimicrobial therapy was administered to two of these patients, owing to the length of time needed for identification of the organisms; and the other two patients had underlying disorders that further aggravated their conditions. The fifth child who died had a ventriculoatrial shunt that was infected with *P. acnes,* along with severe hydrocephalus and mental retardation. Other sites of infections can be present in children with anaerobic bacteremia.

Meningitis

In five (18%) of the children included in the report by Brook and co-workers,[11] meningitis occurred that was associated with *B. fragilis* (two patients), *P. acnes* (two), and *Peptococcus* species (one) (tables 28.1, 28.2). A direct extension of the organism from an infection site to the meninges might have occurred in two of these children, both of whom had surgical drainage of their local collection of pus. One of these patients had pansinusitis and required a Caldwell-Luc procedure, where a direct extension of the inflammation to the subdural space through the cribriform plate was demonstrated. Ethmoid drainage and frontal craniotomy yielded pus from the sinus as well as from the subdural space. The child with pilonidal sinus had surgical drainage and subsequent removal of the sinus tract.

Extravascular Infection

Anaerobic organisms recovered from blood were isolated also from other infected sites in 16 (57%) of the patients reported.[11] In 8 of the 16 patients, anaerobic bacteria were mixed with other anaerobic and/or with aerobic organisms (two to five bacteria per specimen of pus). Extravascular sites from which anaerobic organisms were recovered included abscesses (four patients), cerebrospinal fluid (three), peritoneal fluid (four), tracheopulmonary aspiration (two), sinuses (two), and sinus and subdural empyema (one). Seven of the eight children who had soft-tissue abscesses or local collections of pus required surgical drainage. Some of these patients had recurrent or persistent bacteremia until proper surgical drainage was performed. Four patients also had extravascular collections of pus; however, anaerobic organisms were not recovered from these sites either because anaerobic cultures were not obtained or because the specimens were inappropriately transported.

Neonatal Bacteremia

Although this topic is addressed in a separate chapter (see chapter 9), a short review is warranted. A recent report[5] described anaerobic bacteremia in 23 newborns and reviewed 57 additional cases from the literature. The yield of anaerobic bacteria in 23 newborns seen over a period of 3.5 years represented 1.8 cases per 1000 live births and accounted for 26% of all instances of neonatal bacteremia at that hospital. The bacteremia episodes were associated with prolonged labor, premature rupture of membranes, maternal amnionitis, prematurity, fetal distress, and respiratory difficulty. In that series, the patients with neonatal anaerobic bacteremia had better prognoses than did newborns with bacteremia caused by facultative bacteria. Only one patient of the 23 (4%) died; however, the mortality from the cases of anaerobic bacteremia reviewed from the literature was 26%. Neonatal sepsis from facultative organisms has been reported to range from 30% to 44%.[23, 24]

The isolation of nonhistotoxic *Clostridium* species from 18 newborns with bacteremia has been described.[25] Bacteremia was also found to be associated with necrotizing enterocolitis of the newborn. *Clostridium butyricum* recently was isolated from blood cultures obtained from 12 newborns with that disease.[26]

Bacteremia in newborns has also been attributed to *Bacteroides* species[27–29] and *F. nucleatum*,[30] organisms that can be acquired during the infant's passage through the birth canal. Moreover, six episodes of *B. fragilis* bacteremia associated with perinatal pneumonia were reported recently.[2, 31] The two newborns in the series by Brook and colleagues[11] died within four days of therapy. These patients were infected by organisms of the *B. fragilis* group and received inappropriate antimicrobial therapy. Although the occurrence of bacteremia in newborns is infrequent, experience indicates the need for proper antibiotic coverage of the newborn against *B. fragilis*.

REFERENCES

1. Chow, A. W., and Guse, L. B. Bacteroidaceae bacteremia: clinical experience with 112 patients. *Medicine* 53:93, 1974.

2. Dunkle, L. M.; Brotherton, M. S.; and Feigin, R. D. Anaerobic infections in children. A prospective study. *Pediatrics* 57:311, 1976.

3. Thirmuoothi, M. C.; Keen, B. M.; and Dajani, A. S. Anaerobic infections in children: a prospective study. *J. Clin. Microbiol.* 3:318, 1976.

4. Brook, I. et al. Recovery of anaerobic bacteria from pediatric patients: a one-year experience. *Am. J. Dis. Child.* 133:1020, 1979.

5. Chow, A. W. et al. The significance of anaerobes in neonatal bacteremia: analysis of 23 cases and review of the literature. *Pediatrics* 54:736, 1974.

6. Sanders, D. U., and Stevenson, J. *Bacteroides* infections in children. *J. Pediatr.* 72:673, 1968.

7. Finegold, S. M. *Anaerobic bacteria in human disease.* New York: Academic Press, 1977, pp. 182, 456.

8. Echeverria, P., and Smith, A. L. Anaerobic bacteremia observed in a children's hospital. *Clin. Pediatr.* 9:688, 1978.

9. Berry, F. A., Jr. et al. Transient bacteremia during dental manipulation in children. *Pediatrics* 51:476, 1973.

10. DeLeo, A. A. et al. The incidence of bacteremia following oral prophylaxis on pediatric patients. *Oral Surg.* 37:36, 1974.

11. Brook, I. et al. Anaerobic bacteremia in children. *Am. J. Dis. Child.* 134:1052, 1980.

12. Beeler, B. A. et al. *Proprionibacterium acnes:* pathogen in central nervous system infection. *Am. J. Med.* 61:935, 1976.

13. Mederios, A. A. *Bacteroides* bacillemia. *Arch. Surg.* 105:819, 1972.

14. Washington, J. A., II. Relative frequency of anaerobes. *Ann. Intern. Med.* 83:908, 1975.

15. Marchildon, M. B., and Dudgeon, D. L. Perforating appendicitis: a current experience in Children's Hospital. *Ann. Surg.* 185:84, 1977.

16. Stone, J. H. Bacterial flora of appendicitis in children. *J. Pediatr. Surg.* 11:37, 1976.

17. Donaldson, S. S. et al. Characterization of postsplenectomy bacteremia among patients with and without lymphoma. *N. Engl. J. Med.* 287:69, 1972.

18. Goodman, J. S. *Bacteroides* sepsis, diagnosis and therapy. *Hosp. Pract.* 6:121, 1971.

19. Alpern, R. J., and Dowell, V. R., Jr. *Clostridium septicum* infections and malignancy. *JAMA* 209:385, 1969.

20. Myerowitz, R. L.; Medeiros, A. A.; and O'Brien, T. F. Bacterial infection in renal homotransplant recipients: a study of 53 bacteremic episodes. *Am. J. Med.* 53:308, 1972.

21. Wilson, W. F. et al. Anaerobic bacteremia. *Mayo Clin. Proc.* 47:639, 1972.

22. Felner, J. M., and Dowell, V. R., Jr. *Bacteroides* bacteremia. *Am. J. Med.* 50:787, 1970.

23. Alvack, L.; Wood, H. F.; Fousek, H. D. Septicemia of the newborn. *Pediatr. Clin. North Am.* 13:1131, 1966.

24. Buetow, K. C.; Klein, S. W.; and Lane, R. B. Septicemia in premature infants: the characteristics, treatment, and prevention of septicemia in premature infants. *Am. J. Dis. Child.* 110:29, 1965.

25. Alpern, R. J., and Dowell, V. R., Jr. Nonhistotoxic clostridial bacteremia. *Am. J. Clin. Pathol.* 55:717, 1971.

26. Howard, M. F. et al. Outbreak of necrotizing enterocolitis caused by *Clostridium bu-tyricum. Lancet* 2:1099, 1977.

27. Pearson, H. E., and Anderson, G. V. Perinatal deaths associated with *Bacteroides* infections. *Obstet. Gynecol.* 30:486, 1967.

28. Tynes, B. S., and Frommeyer, W. B., Jr. *Bacteroides* septicemia: cultural, clinical, and therapeutic features in a series of 25 patients. *Ann. Intern. Med.* 56:12, 1962.

29. Harrod, J. R., and Sevens, D. A. Anaerobic infections in the newborn infant. *J. Pediatr.* 85:399, 1974.

30. Robinow, M., and Simonelli, F. A. *Fusobacterium* bacteremia in the newborn. *Am. J. Dis. Child.* 110:92, 1965.

31. Brook, I.; Martin, W. J.; and Finegold, S. M. Bacteriology of tracheal aspirates in intubated newborns. *Chest* 78:875, 1980.

CHAPTER 29

Botulism

Botulism is an intoxication manifested by neuromuscular disturbances after ingesting food containing a toxin elaborated by *Clostridium botulinum*. There are three forms: food-borne botulism, wound botulism, and infant botulism. Symptoms and pathologic findings relate to the toxin's effects on the nervous system and are characterized by neuromuscular dysfunction and resultant flaccid paralysis of muscles.

Food-Borne Botulism

Epidemiology

Food-borne botulism, the most common form of botulism, usually occurs in small sporadic outbreaks.[1] An average of 9.4 outbreaks involving 24.2 cases occur annually in the United States. Children acquire the disease less often than adults, perhaps reflecting protection or more fastidious eating habits. The disease occurs throughout the United States. In the West, type A intoxications predominate; in the Mississippi valley and Atlantic coast regions, type B intoxications are more common. The toxin is ingested in the preformed state along with food that has become contaminated with *C. botulinum* during canning or other preparatory process.[2]

C. *botulinum* spores are highly heat-resistant; they may survive several hours at 100°C; however, exposure to moist heat at 120°C for 30 minutes will kill the spores. The toxins, on the other hand, are readily destroyed by heat, and cooking food at 80°C for 30 minutes safeguards against botulism.[2] In the United States, preserved foods in which the toxin is most commonly found are string beans, corn, mushrooms, spinach, olives, beets, asparagus, seafood, pork products, and beef.[1,3] Improperly smoked or canned fish is the source of type E intoxications.

Etiology and Pathophysiology

The causative agent is one of several types of exotoxin elaborated by the sporulating, anaerobic bacillus *C. botulinum*. Human poisoning is usually caused by type A, B, or E toxin, rarely by type C, D, or F. Type A and B toxins are highly poisonous proteins resistant to digestion by gastrointestinal enzymes. Following absorption, the toxins give rise to neurologic symptoms by interfering with the release of acetylcholine from the terminal endings of cholinergic nerve fibers.[4,5] The disease almost always follows ingestion of improperly preserved food in which the toxin has been produced during the growth of the causative organism.

Clinical Findings

The onset of this disease is abrupt, usually 18 to 36 hours after ingestion of the toxin, although the incubation period may vary from four hours to eight days. Following a short period of lassitude and fatigue, visual disturbances develop. These may include diplopia, diminished visual acuity, blepharoptosis, loss of accommodation, and diminished or total loss of pupillary light reflex. Vomiting and diarrhea are typically absent, but may occur in about a third of cases, probably from ingestion of spoiled food rather than from botulinus toxin. Outbreaks caused by type E strains in contaminated commercially canned fish have been associated with early nausea and vomiting. Symptoms of bulbar paresis (dysarthria, dysphagia, nasal regurgitation) develop. Difficulty in swallowing may lead to aspiration pneumonia. The muscles of the extremities and trunk become weak. There are no sensory disturbances and the sensorium characteristically remains clear until shortly before death. The temperature remains normal or subnormal unless intercurrent infection develops. Routine studies of the blood, urine, and cerebrospinal fluid usually are normal.[4,6]

In summary, there are four cardinal clinical features of botulism:

1. Symmetric and descending neurologic manifestations.
2. Mental processes are intact.
3. No sensory disturbances, although vision may be impaired because of involvement of the extraocular muscles.
4. Absence of fever unless secondary infectious complications occur.

Diagnosis

Diagnosis is suggested by the pattern of neuromuscular disturbances and a likely food source. The simultaneous occurrence of two or more cases following ingestion of the same food simplifies the diagnosis. Diagnosis is confirmed by demonstration of botulinus toxin or *C. botulinum* in suspected food, and, occasionally, of toxin in the circulating blood. Electromyography is helpful in the diagnosis of botulism. The isolated muscle action potential is reduced, but repetitive nerve stimulation results in facilitation of the action potentials. Suggestive confirmatory evidence may be derived from the recovery of *C. botulinum* from vomitus, feces, intestinal contents, and, rarely, from viscera. Pets that have eaten the same contaminated food may also develop botulism.[6]

Botulism may be confused with poliomyelitis, viral encephalitis, myasthenia gravis, Guillain-Barré syndrome, tick paralysis, and atropine or mushroom poisoning.

Management

Prevention of the disease is of utmost importance. Proper home and commercial canning and adequate heating of food before serving are essential. Food showing any evidence of spoilage should be discarded.

Hospitalization is essential in the management of the acute phase. Airway control and management of adequate ventilation is of great importance. Endotracheal intubation may be required in serious cases. Supportive care includes proper oxygenation and management of secondary infections.

Oral or parenteral antimicrobial agents such as penicillin have limited value but may destroy some viable *C. botulinum* organisms. Bowel purges have been suggested as a mode of eliminating unabsorbed toxin from the intestine. The administration of appropriate antitoxin is recommended.

Several forms of equine botulism antitoxin are available: monovalent type E, bivalent AB, trivalent ABE, and polyvalent ABCDEF. The trivalent ABE preparation seems to be the most available one through the Center for Disease Control in Atlanta, Georgia. If the causative toxigenic type is unknown, or if type-specific antitoxin is not available, the trivalent ABE preparation should be used. Monovalent antitoxins should be used only for type established disease. The polyvalent ABCDEF preparation is reserved for established cases of C, D, or F disease.[6, 7]

If hypersensitivity to horse serum is not demonstrated, the antitoxin can be given intravenously at a dose of one vial every four hours for a total of four or five vials. If toxin is still detectable in subsequent serum samples, additional antitoxin may be given after repeat skin testing. Occasionally, toxin is still demonstrable in serum up to several weeks after the onset of illness.

Wound Botulism

Epidemiology

Wound botulism is rare in the United States. Only 21 cases have been reported,[1, 8-21] ten of them in children less than 16 years of age. Thus, far, all cases have involved wounds located on an extremity, and four patients have died.

Predisposing Conditions

Wound botulism has been associated with compound fractures, severe trauma, lacerations, puncture wound, and hematoma. Of the pediatric cases in the United States, more than half have been associated with compound fracture.[8, 10, 11, 14, 15, 17, 18, 20] The disease has occurred primarily in young males during March through November, the period of maximum outdoor activity.

Etiology

The pathogenesis and etiology of wound botulism are similar to the food-borne disease. Most wound cases have been associated with type A toxin-producing organism, although some cases have been associated with type B.

Clinical Signs and Diagnosis

Since wound botulism symptoms result from infection with *C. botulinum* organisms and subsequent in vivo production of toxin, the incubation period is longer (4 to 18 days) than for food-borne illness (six hours to eight days).[7] The clinical manifestations are similar to those of food-borne botulism except for the lack of early gastrointestinal symptoms. Early symptoms can include appearance of lethargy owing to muscle weakness, ptosis, blurred or double vision, and dry, sore throat.[7] Fever, which usually is absent in food-borne botulism, may be present in wound botulism.

The diagnosis of wound botulism is suggested by clinical findings and the presence of an apparent wound source. Confirmation of the diagnosis is made by demonstration of toxin in serum or by isolation of *C. botulinum* and/or toxin from the wound in association with appropriate clinical findings. Electromyogram can be helpful in diagnosis when lowered amplitude action potentials following low-frequency stimulation and posttetanic facilitation of the muscle action potential can be demonstrated.

Differential diagnosis in a child without a suggestive food ingestion history and sudden onset of neurologic symptoms includes Guillain-Barré syndrome, myasthenia gravis, cerebrovascular accident, tick paralysis, intoxications, and infectious diseases of the central nervous system.

Management

Treatment of wound botulism must include debridement, drainage, and irrigation of the wound. Good supportive care, primarily respiratory support, is also an important aspect of management for patients with botulism. Although antitoxin will not improve paralysis from toxin already bound at the neuromuscular junction, antitoxin will bind circulating toxin.

Recent evidence on infant botulism has suggested a potentiation of neuromuscular weakness by aminoglycosides.[22] Subsequent data in a mouse model also have suggested potentiation by gentamicin of the neuromuscular block produced by botulinus toxin.[23] Aminoglycosides should be avoided if possible in a patient with botulism. The role of guanidine hydrochloride therapy in the treatment of botulism is controversial.[4, 24–26] In some patients there was no improvement,[25] and toxic effects were observed,[26] but in others improvement of muscle function has been observed.[4, 24] Unfortunately, extraocular muscles and skeletal muscles have been more responsive to therapy than respiratory muscles.[4, 24]

The efficacy of treatment with systemic antimicrobics is unclear; moreover, antimicrobics have not prevented the development of wound botulism in several cases.

REFERENCES

1. Black, R. E., and Arnon, S. S. Botulism in the United States, 1976. *J. Infect. Dis.* 136:829, 1977.
2. Petty, C. S. Botulism: the disease and the toxin. *Am. J. Med. Sci.* 249:345, 1965.

3. Dolman, C. E. Human botulism in Canada, 1919–1973. *Can. Med. Assoc. J.* 110:191, 1974.

4. Cherington, M. Botulism: ten–year experience. *Arch. Neurol.* 30:432, 1974.

5. Koenig, M. G. et al. Type B botulism in man. *Am. J. Med.* 42:208, 1967.

6. Donadio, J. A.; Gangarosa, E. J.; and Faich, G. A. Diagnosis and treatment of botulism. *J. Infect. Dis.* 124:108, 1971.

7. Werner, S. B., and Chin, J. Botulism. Diagnosis, management and public health considerations. *Calif. Med.* 118:84, 1973.

8. Wound botulism: Texas, California, Washington. *Morbidity and Mortality Weekly Report* 29:34, 1980.

9. Charington, M., and Ginsburg, S. Wound botulism. *Arch. Surg.* 110:436, 1975.

10. Davis, J. B.; Mattman, L. H.; and Wiley, M. *Clostridium botulinum* in a fatal wound infection. *JAMA* 146:646, 1951.

11. DeJesus, P. V. et al. Neuromuscular physiology of wound botulism. *Arch. Neurol.* 29:425, 1973.

12. Grizzle, C. O. Botulism from a puncture wound. *Rocky Mt. Med. J.* 69:47, 1972.

13. Hampson, C. R. A case of probable botulism due to wound infection. *J. Bacteriol.* 61:647, 1952.

14. Hansen, N., and Tolo, V. Wound botulism complicating an open fracture: a case report and review of the literature. *J. Bone Joint Surg.* 61:312, 1979.

15. Kennedy, T. L., and Merson, M. H. An infected wound as a cause of botulism in a 12-year-old boy: debridement, medical management, and intensive respiratory support resulted in complete recovery. *Clin. Pediatr.* 16:151, 1977.

16. Lewis, S. W. et al. Prolonged respiratory paralysis in wound botulism. *Chest* 75:59, 1979.

17. Merson, M. H., and Dowell, V. R. Epidemiologic clinical and laboratory aspects of wound botulism. *N. Engl. J. Med.* 289:1005, 1973.

18. MacCracken, B. B. Wound botulism. In *Morbidity and mortality, reportable diseases.* County of Los Angeles, Department of Health Services, December 1974.

19. Miller, N. R., and Moses, H. Ocular involvement in wound botulism. *Arch. Ophthalmol.* 95:1788, 1977.

20. Thomas, C. G.; Keleher, M. F.; and McKee, A. P. Botulism, a complication of *Clostridium botulinum* wound infection. *Arch. Pathol. Lab. Med.* 51:623, 1951.

21. Wapen, B. D., and Gutmann, L. Wound botulism: a case report. *JAMA* 227:1416, 1974.

22. L'Hommedieu, C. et al. Potentiation of neuromuscular weakness in infant botulism by aminoglycosides. *J. Pediatr.* 95:1065, 1979.

23. Swensen, P.; Santos, J. I.; and Glasgow, L. A. Potentiation of *Clostridium botulinum* toxin by gentamicin (abstr.). *Clin. Res.* 28:113, 1980.

24. Puggiari, M., and Cherington, M. Botulism and guanidine: ten years later. *JAMA* 240:2276, 1978.

25. Kaplan, J. E. et al. Botulism, type A, and treatment with guanidine. *Ann. Neurol.* 6:69, 1979.

26. Faich, G. A.; Graebner, R. W.; and Sato, S. Failure of guanidine therapy in botulism A. *N. Engl. J. Med.* 285:773, 1971.

CHAPTER 30

Tetanus

Tetanus is an acute toxemic illness with a high fatality rate resulting from *Clostridium tetani* infections at a break in the skin or laceration. Since *C. tetani* organisms are disseminated worldwide in soils and animal feces, agricultural workers suffer a higher incidence of infection than others. Tetanus may also complicate burns, puerperal infections, infections of the umbilical stump (tetanus neonatorum), and certain surgical operations in which the source of infection may be contaminated sutures, dressings, or plaster.

Tetanus is an intoxication manifested primarily by neuromusuclar dysfunction. It is caused by tetanal exotoxin (tetanospasmin), an extraordinarily potent exotoxin elaborated by *Clostridium tetani*. The illness begins with tonic spasms of the skeletal muscles and is followed by paroxysmal contractions. The muscle stiffness involves the jaw (lockjaw) and neck first and later becomes generalized. The disease can be prevented by immunization with tetanal toxoid.

Epidemiology

The organisms are worldwide in distribution and have been isolated from several sites including soil, feces, ordinary house dust, and contaminated heroin. Since tetanus affects individuals and does not cause outbreaks, it is less noticed than certain other infectious diseases. Nevertheless, despite the availability of simple benign protective measures, tetanus ranks high among the infectious diseases as a cause of death throughout the world, and in developing countries it is an important cause of neonatal death.

In the United States, less than 200 cases of tetanus have been reported annually since 1968,[1] but this figure probably is not accurate. From 1950 to 1966 in the United States there has been a reduction of about one-half in incidence of tetanus; however, the case fatality rates have remained unchanged at between 50% and 65% for the past two decades. On a national basis, the incidence is approximately one case per million per year. The annual incidence rate for neonatal tetanus in the United States declined significantly from 0.73 cases per 100,000 live births in 1965–1967 to 0.19 in 1968–1969 and to 0.14 in 1970–1971.[2] About two-thirds of the cases in the United States occur between May and November. This is probably a function of greater outdoor activity and exposure to soil in the spring and summer; the highest incidence is in the southern states. Factors contributing to the geographic distribution may include climate, the prevalence of spores of *C. tetani* in the soil, and immunization levels in selected population groups. The incidence of tetanus in the United States is higher in newborn infants than in older children; however, in recent years, the number of reported cases has been greatest in children between one and five years of age.[3]

Beyond the neonatal period the attack rate and age related mortality rate is higher in males.

Etiology

The tetanus bacillus is a slender, Gram-positive, anaerobic rod that may develop a terminal spore, giving it a drumstick appearance. The spores are very resistant to heat and the usual antiseptics. They may persist in tissues for many months in a viable although dormant state. They can survive in soil for years if not exposed to sunlight. They may be found in house dust, soil, salt and fresh water, and the feces of many animal species. Both spores and vegetative organisms may be found in the intestinal contents of humans.[4]

The organism is not able to invade tissue of its own accord, and the spores are unable to germinate in tissues with normal oxygen tension. Therefore, the role of other pathogens and necrotic tissue in producing a favorable environment for germination and toxin formation becomes evident. The toxins are produced by only the vegetative form of the organism.

Two toxins are produced, tetanolysin and tetanospasmin. Tetanolysin is responsible for the hemolysis of red blood cells in vitro but does not appear to exert this effect in humans. Tetanospasmin affects the neuromuscular end plates and the motor nuclei of the central nervous system and thereby produces skeletal muscle spasm and convulsions.[5-8]

The toxin in tetanus, tetanospasmin, is extremely potent. As little as 130 µg of purified tetanospasmin may be lethal in humans. The neurotoxin elaborated by *C. tetani*, tetanospasmin, is a relatively simple protein with a molecular weight of approximately 67,000.[5, 6] The toxin is extermely potent; each milligram may contain as many as 75 million times the lethal dose for a mouse. The toxin has a high affinity for neural tissue. The toxin binds to, and has an effect on, several areas of the nervous system. Tetanospasmin may reach the central nervous system by absorption at myoneural junctions, followed by migration through perineural tissue spaces of nerve trunks, or by transfer by the lymphocytes to blood and then to the central nervous system. There is considerable debate regarding the modes of spread; both mechanisms probably are important.

Tetanospasmin becomes bound to gangliosides within the central nervous system. The physiologic action of tetanospasmin is similar to that of strychnine, suppressing inhibitory influences on the motor neurons and interneurons without directly enhancing synaptic excitatory action. Additional actions of tetanospasmin are evident in the neuro-circulatory, neuroendocrine, and vegetative nervous systems. It has also been postulated that the toxin directly affects electrolyte flux in the sarcotubular system of muscles and synaptic transmission at myoneural junctions.[7]

The toxin also acts at an unknown site in the central nervous system. This site of action probably is responsible for cardiac arrhythmias, tachycardia, fluctuating blood pressure, hectic fevers, and diaphoresis.[9] Once bound to tissue, toxin cannot be dissociated or neutralized by tetanus antitoxin. Antitoxin may prevent binding in the central nervous system if binding has occurred only in the periphery. Antitoxin has no effect upon the germination of the spores of *C. tetani* or multiplication of its vegetative organisms in tissues.

The portal of entry is usually the site of minor puncture wounds or scratches. About two-thirds of all injuries leading to tetanus occur in the home, and about 20% take place on farms and in gardens. Deep puncture wounds, burns, crushing, and other injuries that promote favorable conditions for the growth of anaerobic organisms may be followed by tetanus. Occasionally, no apparent portal of entry can be found. Under these circumstances it is conceivable that the site of infection may have been the alimentary tract. Sources of infection that have been incriminated are tonsils, ear lesions, and infected vaccines, sera, and catgut.

Clinical Manifestation

A wound may or may not be present when manifestations of infection first appear. The incubation period for tetanus varies from 1 to at least 54 days, but is usually 6 to 15 days, with a median of 7 or 8 days.[9] Poor prognosis is directly proportionate to rapidity of onset of the clinical syndrome. Both the length of time from inoculation to onset of first symptoms as well as the length of time from first symptoms to the onset of the first generalized spasm are good parameters of the severity of the disease.

Early symptoms and signs often consist of irritability, restlessness, headache, and low-grade fever. Patients remain alert. The presentations of tetanus have been classified as to both the extent of involvement (localized or generalized) and the severity of the disease (mild, moderately severe, or severe). Patients with mild tetanus may present with mild generalized stiffness or with findings compatible with local tetanus.[8]

Localized, relatively benign forms of the disease may occur rarely. Thus, the disease may be limited to a wounded extremity, particularly in a partially immunized individual. *Localized tetanus* produces pain and continuous rigidity and spasm of muscles in proximity to the site of injury. The symptoms may persist for weeks and disappear without sequelae. Occasionally, this form of the disease precedes the development of the generalized disorder. The fatality rate of localized tetanus is about 1%. The manifestations in *cephalic tetanus*[8] are limited to the head. Cephalic tetanus is characterized by a short incubation period, facial paralysis, and dysphagia (there may be dysfunction of cranial nerves III, IV, VII, IX, X, and XII) associated with infection on the face or head. Cases following otitis media have occasionally been reported.[10, 11] Rarely, disease may be limited to the trunk (thoracoabdominal tetanus). It is important to recognize, however, that evidence of muscle spasm in the region of a wound may be the earliest manifestations of generalized tetanus.

Generalized tetanus is the most common form of the disease. The onset may be insidious (with progressively increasing stiffness of the voluntary muscles), but trismus is the presenting symptom in over 50% of patients. Spasm of the masseter muscle may be associated with stiffness of the muscles in the neck and with difficulty in swallowing. Restlessness, irritability, and headache also are early findings.[8, 12] Within 24 to 48 hours after the onset of the disease, rigidity may be fully developed and may spread rapidly to involve the trunk and extremities. With spasm of the jaw muscles, trismus (lockjaw) develops. The wrinkling of the forehead and the distortion of the eyebrows and the angles of the mouth produce a peculiar facial appearance: *risus sardonicus* (sardonic grin). The neck and back become stiff and arched, a condition called *opisthotonos*. The abdominal wall is boardlike. The extremities are usually stiff and extended.

Spasms of the muscles of the trunk and extremities may be widespread and may result in opisthotonos and boardlike rigidity of the abdomen and other portions of the body. In patients with moderate to severe degrees of generalized tetanus, there are acute, paroxysmal, uncoordinated widespread spasms of muscles. These tonic convulsions occur intermittently and unpredictably, lasting for a few seconds to several minutes. As these continue, they become severe and painful and exhaust the patient. Such paroxysms may occur spontaneously, but are often precipitated by various stimuli such as drafts of cold air, minor noises, turning the light on in the room, attempting to drink, and attempting to move or turn the patient. They may also be precipitated by such conditions as a distended bowel or bladder, or mucous plugs in the bronchi. Spasms of the pharyngeal and laryngeal musculature may lead to difficulty in swallowing, cyanosis, and even sudden death from respiratory arrest. Dysuria or urinary retention may develop secondary to spasms of the bladder sphincter. Alternatively, involuntary defecation and urination may be noted. The forcefulness of the contractions may produce compression fractures of the spine and hemorrhage into muscle.

During the illness, the patient's sensorium is usually clear. The fever is generally low grade or absent, but temperatures of 40°C have been noted owing to the intense output of energy that accompanies tetanic seizures. Patients with severe tetanus also may develop labile hypertension and tachycardia, irregularities of cardiac rhythm, peripheral vascular constriction, fever, increased carbon dioxide output, increased urinary catecholamine excretion, and, at times, the late development of hypotension.[9, 13]

Complications in patients with severe tetanus include atelectasis, aspiration, pneumonia, pulmonary emboli, ventilation-perfusion problems,[14] sepsis, gastric ulcer, fecal impaction, urinary retention or infection, decubitus ulcers, compression fractures, deformities or subluxation of vertebrae (particularly in thoracic vertebrae and in children), and spontaneous rupture of muscles and intramuscular hematoma.

Signs and symptoms increase over a period of three to seven days, plateau during the course of the second week, and then abate gradually. Complete recovery takes place in two to six weeks.[12]

Diagnosis

The diagnosis is easily made on clinical grounds in the typical, fully developed case. Most cases occur in individuals who are unimmunized or in infants of unimmunized mothers. The vast majority have evidence of a wound or a trauma that has occurred within the previous two weeks. In addition to trismus, a physical examination may reveal marked hypertonicity of muscles, hyperactive deep tendon reflexes, clear mentation, low-grade fever, and the absence of sensory involvement. Local or general paroxysmal spasms may be observed.

Laboratory studies are not particularly helpful. The cerebrospinal fluid is normal in patients with tetanus, although spinal fluid pressure may be elevated because of muscular contractions. There is usually a moderate leukocytosis in the peripheral blood. Neither electroencephalography nor electromyography is helpful. Wound cultures are positive for *C. tetani* in only about one-third of patients with this dis-

ease. Heating a specimen to 80°C for 15 minutes to get rid of other
organisms that are not spore formers in mixed cultures may facilitate
recovery of *C. tetani*. The fluorescent antibody technique may be useful
in identifying the organism as well. Diagnosing tetanus in individuals
with reliable histories of having two or more injections of tetanus toxoid in the past is very unusual. In this situation, serum should be obtained for assay of antitoxin level. The presence of 0.01 IU antitoxin
per milliliter of serum generally is considered protective.[15]

Differential Diagnosis

Tetanus must be differentiated from other local and systemic diseases.
Trismus may be associated with alveolar, parapharyngeal, or retropharyngeal abscesses. These conditions can be differentiated from tetanus by careful history, physical examination, and appropriate roentgenographic studies. Phenothiazine reactions may cause trismus, but
the associated tremors, asthetoid movements, and torticollis should
alert one to this possibility. Administration of diphenhydramine hydrochloride will cause subsidence of the tetanuslike reaction to phenothiazine drugs.

A history of ingestion of poisons containing strychnine is helpful
in distinguishing this intoxication from tetanus. Trismus is rare and,
when it occurs, develops after the onset of generalized tonic activity.
Usually, there is complete relaxation between convulsions.

Purulent meningitis can be excluded by an examination of the
cerebrospinal fluid. Encephalitis occasionally is associated with trismus
and muscle spasms; however, the sensorium of such patients is
clouded. The muscular spasms of rabies occur early in the course of
the disease, and they involve the muscles of respiration and degluti-
tion. Trismus is not present, and the spinal fluid may be pleocytotic.
The history of an animal bite is not diagnostic of rabies, for tetanus
also occurs after bites. The incubation period of rabies is much longer
than that of tetanus. Abdominal rigidity in tetanus may suggest an
acute intraabdominal process requiring surgery. Although physical examination should reveal early trismus and rigidity of the neck, tetanus
occasionally results from obstructions and perforations of the intestinal
tract. Hysterical conversion reactions and phenothiazine reactions also
need to be considered.

Management

Therapy

Management of patients with tetanus can be a particularly difficult
problem. Several distinct goals of therapy can be identified: the provi-

sion of supportive care until the toxin fixed to nervous tissue has been metabolized, the neutralization of circulating toxin, and the removal of the source of the toxin.

The neutralization of tetanus toxin can be achieved by the use of tetanus immune globulin (TIG) of human origin. A total dose of 3000 U to 10,000 U injected as three equal portions into three sites intramuscularly is recommended. It is desirable to give TIG in the proximal portion of an extremity where the inciting wound is located when this is feasible. This preparation must not be given intravenously. Analysis of accumulated data in two recent reports[16, 17] showed a significantly lower case fatality ratio for those patients treated with tetanus antitoxin. Intrathecal administration of the toxin has been tried with some success, but this is still experimental. TIG has no effect on toxin that is already fixed to neural tissue and does not penetrate the blood-cerebrospinal fluid barrier, but it can neutralize circulating or uncombined tetanospasmin. If TIG is not available and skin testing shows no hypersensitivity, tetanus antitoxin (TAT) can be given in a single dose of 50,000 to 100,000 units. This antitoxin is divided equally; half the dose is given intramuscularly and half intravenously, with careful observation of the precautions detailed in the package insert. Active immunization should be started at the same time. Intramuscularly injected toxoid does not interfere with efficacy of TIG, and TIG does not nullify the immunogenicity of the toxoid.[8, 12]

The toxin can be eliminated further by aggressive debridement of the causative wound and removal of foreign bodies that may facilitate growth of the organism. If necrotic tissue is present, wide excision of involved tissue may be advisable. Amputation should be considered in tetanus arising from a gangrenous lesion. Surgical efforts should be delayed until the patient has been sedated and antitoxin has been administered. Antimicrobial agents are of doubtful value in the therapy of tetanus. Any situation in the body that is suitable for the growth of *C. tetani* must be devoid of an adequate blood supply, and, therefore, antimicrobics penetrate poorly into sites of tetanal toxin production. Nevertheless, antimicrobics usually are given. *C. tetani*, like all species of *Clostridium*, is susceptible to penicillin G. Large doses should be given in an effort to favor the diffusion of penicillin into devitalized areas. Penicillin G (200,000 units/kg/24 hr) may be used intravenously in six divided doses for 10 days. Tetracycline is an alternative drug for patients allergic to penicillin; dosage is 25 mg/kg/day in four divided doses (no more than 2 gm) for children (over age eight years).

Supportive Care

Meticulous nursing care is imperative. The patient should be placed in a quiet environment and every effort made to control or eliminate auditory and visual stimuli. A respirator, oxygen, suction, and equipment for tracheostomy should be available. An important aspect of the supportive care of the tetanus patient is management of the airway. Virtually all patients with generalized tetanus will require tracheostomy; however, the decision of when to perform tracheostomy must be individualized. In patients with rapid onset and progression of symptoms, and predisposition to severe disease, early tracheostomy is advisable. Tracheostomy can protect the patient in the event of laryngospasm; can be of great value in the management of pulmonary secretions; and may assist in preventing aspiration.

Pulmonary complications are the most common cause of death in tetanus patients; therefore, careful attention must be paid to the development of atelectasis, pulmonary infiltrates, aspiration syndromes, or pulmonary embolism. The patient must be monitored with serial chest radiographs and objective measurements of ventilatory mechanics and gas exchange. Criteria for initiating ventilatory assistance include increased partial pressure of carbon dioxide in arterial blood, decreased vital capacity, and diminished inspiratory effort.

Control of Muscular Spasms

Diazepam can effectively control muscular rigidity and spasms in many cases, and has the advantages of being rapidly metabolized and offering sedation as well as spasm reduction. Large doses are required; occasionally spasms are refractory and require adjunctive therapy by neuromuscular blockade. Since large doses of diazepam may depress respiration, patients receiving high-dose diazepam therapy must be monitored.

The phenothiazines (particularly chlorpromazine) and the barbiturates, which may assist in sedating the patient, may be valuable as adjunctive therapy. Meprobamate may also be of value. Combinations of any or all of these agents occasionally may fail to control spasms; in such cases, paralysis with neuromuscular blocking agents may be required.

Neuromuscular blocking agents such as D-tubocurarine or gallamine have been used either to control seizures while sparing respiration or to produce complete respiratory paralysis that is then managed by artificial ventilation. The latter technique has produced the best survival rates but can be applied only in centers where continuous intensive care and highly trained respiratory care teams are available.

Meprobamate and diazepam serve as tranquilizers and sedatives, as well as to abolish muscle spasm. The effect of both of these agents may be prolonged by addition of small doses of phenobarbital. Milder cases usually can be managed with supportive care and a combination of muscle relaxants and sedatives.

Infants may receive 50 to 100 mg/dose of meprobamate. Children two to five years of age can be given 100 to 200 mg every three to four hours. Children older than six years and adults may receive 400 mg of meprobamate intramuscularly every two to four hours. Trismus, abdominal rigidity, and opisthotonos diminish or disappear within 10 minutes after dosage. During convalescence, smaller oral doses of meprobamate every four hours are usually sufficient initially, and they are reduced as the patient improves.

Diazepam is a suitable alternative to meprobamate. In mild cases in adults, oral doses may be repeated as needed. In moderate and severe cases, diazepam is best given by continuous intravenous drip. The drug may also be administered through a nasogastric or gastrostomy tube.

Prevention

Since many cases of tetanus follow minor abrasions and lacerations that are ignored, control of the disease can be best achieved by active immunization with toxoid *before* exposure. All infants should be routinely immunized with tetanus toxoid that is incorporated with diphtheria toxoid and pertussis vaccine. The usual basic series of the triple antigen is given at four- to eight-week intervals for three doses beginning at one to three months of age. Booster doses are given approximately one and four years later and at 10-year intervals thereafter.[18] If a previously immunized patient acquires a "dirty" wound more than five years after immunization, he or she should receive a new immunization; a protective antitoxin level usually is achieved within one week.

All breaks of the skin surface are potential portals of entry for *C. tetani.* Certain trauma are more prone to allow exposure to the organism; including compound fractures, gunshot wounds, burns, crush injuries, wounds with retained foreign bodies, deep puncture wounds, wounds contaminated with soil or feces, wounds untended for more than 24 hours, wounds infected with other microorganisms, wounds with devitalized or avascular tissue, and induced abortions. Immediate, thorough surgical treatment of wounds is imperative; this is the single most important maneuver in tetanus prophylaxis.[19]

The prophylactic administration of a single 250-unit dose of TIG should be reserved for patients with tetanus-prone wounds who have had no previous immunization,[20] only one dose of tetanus toxoid, or unreliable histories of immunization. In severe wounds 500 units may be indicated. Although effective, TIG does not guarantee protection; nearly 5% of cases seen in the United States occur in persons given TIG at the time of injury.

When wound contamination and tissue destruction have been very great, for example, in cases of extensive third-degree burns, both active and passive immunization at the time of injury may be beneficial, even if the patients have received active immunization previously. In such cases, tetanus may develop more rapidly than in the four to seven days that are required to obtain maximal response to a booster dose of tetanus toxoid.[21] Recovery from tetanus does not confer immunity. For this reason, active immunization of the patient following recovery is imperative.

Tetanus Neonatorum

Most cases in the United States of newborns with neonatal tetanus have been delivered outside a hospital to unimmunized mothers when unsterile techniques were used during delivery or in cutting and tying of the umbilical cord, the usual portal of entry.[22] Neonatal tetanus is frequent in many developing countries, especially where the local birthing practice in rural areas includes application of soil or animal stool to the umbilical stump.[23]

Neonatal tetanus can be prevented entirely by providing at least two doses of tetanus toxoid to pregnant women, training midwives in aseptic techniques, and administering TIG to infants born under unsterile conditions outside of the hospital to unimmunized mothers. Unimmunized or incompletely immunized mothers should receive TIG intramuscularly immediately before or at the time of delivery. This is especially important if they are not delivered in the hospital. Immunization with tetanus toxoid can be started or continued at this same time by using separate syringes and different extremities for injection.[24]

The organism gains entrance into the newborn's body by way of the stump of the umbilical cord that has been cut by an unsterile instrument or covered with an unclean dressing. Rarely, a vaccination wound produced by an unclean instrument or upon contaminated skin imperfectly cleansed constitutes a portal of entry.[22, 23]

Tetanus neonatorum usually begins when the newborn infant is 3 to 10 days old. The onset is generalized in nature and is manifested by difficulty in suckling and by excessive crying. The baby's jaw becomes too stiff for sucking and swallowing is difficult. Thereafter, stiffness of the body develops, and intermittent jerking spasms may ensue. The temperature often rises to 104°F and 106°F. Variable degrees of trismus, risus sardonicus, generalized muscle contraction, and spasms or convulsions occur. The spasms can occur frequently or rarely, spontaneously or in response to stimuli. The fists are held tightly clenched and the toes rigidly fanned. Characteristic are the opisthotonic spasms plus clonic jerkings that follow sudden stimulation by touch or by loud noise. Deep tendon reflex activity may be increased, or may show no response because of constant stiffness. Opisthotonos may be so extreme that the head almost touches the heels. The infant's cry varies from a repeated, short, mildly hoarse cry to a strangled voiceless noise. The child's color can vary from normal to slate-blue cyanosis to pale from poor aeration and impending shock. The severe spasms may be followed by anoxia, gray discoloration, flaccidity, and exhaustion.[22, 23]

The infant may die within the first week after onset from respiratory arrest during a convulsive episode. If the child does not die, improvement will generally come within three to seven days by gradual decline of temperature, decrease in the number of episodes of spasm, and slow resolution of rigidity. Complete disappearance of all signs of illness may take as long as six weeks.[22, 23, 25]

The newborn can present special problems relating to ventilation, hydration, and sedation. Therapy should be aggressive and include tracheostomy, neuromuscular blocking agents, and assisted ventilation. Where facilities are not available, sedatives and muscle relaxants may be given orally. Syrup of chlorpromazine (3 mg every six hours), elixir of phenobarbital (10 to 20 mg every six hours), or elixir of mephenesin (130 to 160 mg every six hours) may be used. Diazepam may be given intravenously in a dose of 0.3 mg/kg and repeated as needed to control severe spasms. In an attempt to eliminate toxin, omphalectomy has also been used successfully.

Tetany of the newborn should never be confused with tetanus. Infants with tetany appear well between their convulsive episodes. Tetany may be characterized by carpopedal spasm and laryngospasm, but trismus is rare. The diagnosis is confirmed by a low serum calcium concentration.

The infant who is generally rigid from birth trauma has shown evidences of brain injury from birth, before the first sign of tetanus could possibly appear. Extraocular palsies commonly are present and abdominal rigidity absent. Response to stimulation is depressed rather than increased.

REFERENCES

1. Furste, W. Tetanus statistics. *JAMA* 228:28, 1974.

2. Blake, P. A., and Feldman, R. A. Tetanus in the United States, 1970–1971. CDC news. *J. Infect. Dis.* 131:745, 1975.

3. Alfery, D. D., and Rauscher, L. A. Tetanus: a review. *Crit. Care Med.* 7:176, 1979.

4. LaForce, F. M.; Young, L. S.; and Bennett, J. V. Tetanus in the United States (1965–1966): epidemiologic and clinical features. *N. Engl. J. Med.* 280:569, 1969.

5. Brooks, V. B., and Asanuma, H. Action of tetanus toxin in the cerebral cortex. *Science* 137:674, 1962.

6. Brooks, V. B.; Curtis, D. R.; and Eccles, J. C. Mode of action of tetanus toxin. *Nature* (London) 175:120, 1955.

7. Kaeser, H. E., and Sauer, A. Tetanus toxin: a neuromuscular blocking agent. *Nature* (London) 223:842, 1969.

8. Weinstein, L. Tetanus. *N. Engl. J. Med.* 289:1293, 1973.

9. Kerr, J. H. et al. Involvement of the sympathetic nervous system in tetanus: studies on 82 cases. *Lancet* 2:236, 1968.

10. Fischer, M. G. W.; Sunakorn, P.; and Duangman, C. Otogenous tetanus: a sequelae of chronic ear infections. *Am. J. Dis. Child.* 131:445, 1977.

11. Nourmand, A. Clinical studies on tetanus: notes on 42 cures in southern Iran with special emphasis on portal of entry. *Clin. Pediatr.* 12:652, 1973.

12. Henderson, D. K. et al. Infectious disease emergencies: the clostridial syndromes. *West. J. Med.* 129:101, 1978.

13. Tseuda, K.; Oliver, P. B.; and Richter, R. W. Cardio-vascular manifestations of tetanus. *Anesthesiology* 40:588, 1974.

14. Femi-Pearse, D. Blood gas tensions, acid-base status, and spirometry in tetanus. *Am. Rev. Respir. Dis.* 110:390, 1974.

15. Rothstein, R. J., and Baker, F. J. II. Tetanus. Prevention and treatment. *JAMA* 260:675, 1978.

16. Buchanan, R. M. et al. Tetanus in the United States, 1968 and 1969. *J. Infect. Dis.* 122:564, 1970.

17. Blake, P. A. et al. Serologic therapy of tetanus in the United States, 1965–1971. *JAMA* 235:42, 1976.

18. Centers for Disease Control. Diphtheria and tetanus toxoids and pertussis vaccine. *Morbidity and Mortality Weekly Report* 26:401, 1977.

19. Blake, P. A. et al. Serologic therapy of tetanus in the United States, 1965–1971. *JAMA* 235:42, 1976.

20. McCracken, G. H., Jr.; Dowell, D. L.; and Marshall, F. N. Double-blind trial of equine antitoxin and human immune globulin in tetanus neonatorum. *Lancet* 1:1145, 1971.

21. Furste, W. Four keys to 100 percent success in tetanus prophylaxis. *Am J. Surg.* 128:616, 1974.

22. Klingler, H. Tetanus of the newborn. *JAMA* 218:1437, 1971.

23. Harvin, J. R.; Hastings, W. D., Jr.; and Baker, C. R. F. Tetanus neonatorum. *J. Pediatr.* 32:561, 1948.

24. Stanfield, J. P.; Gall, D.; and Bracken, P. M. Single-dose antenatal tetanus immunization. *Lancet* 1:214, 1973.

25. Marshall, F. N. Tetanus of the newborn with special references to experiences in Haiti, W. I. *Adv. Pediatr.* 15:65, 1968.

Burn Infections

Burn wounds are a common form of injury during childhood. Fortunately, most burns are minor and are easily treated by cleansing and applying protective creams and dressings. Each year, however, a large number of children are seriously burned and require hospitalization and comprehensive treatment.

Burn injuries are the second leading cause of death in childhood. Of the 300,000 individuals hospitalized for burn therapy and the 8000 who die from burn injuries in the United States each year, one-third are children.[1] The most serious and common complication of burns is infection. A third-degree burn is more likely to be associated with severe infection than is a partial thickness burn. Infection may be localized to the site of the burn or may be manifested as an overwhelming general sepsis.

Burn wound sepsis is a major cause of death among patients of all ages.[2] Sepsis is characterized by progressive bacterial proliferation within the burned tissue, invasion into adjacent tissue, and systemic dissemination.[3]

The surface of every burn wound is contaminated to some degree by bacteria.[2] Therefore, most burn centers routinely monitor surface bacterial growth, allowing the determination of the effect of therapy and prediction of the bacterial strains that may be involved in sepsis.

Microbiology

Microorganisms usually gain access to burns directly because microbiota are normally present on the skin, and the skin is the interface with the outside world. Soon after a burn injury, surface cultures may reveal multiple organisms. Within three to five days, the wound will become colonized by one or two specific organisms that have survived the competition with other microorganisms or have proven particularly resistant to burn wound therapy.

The progression of invasion by various organisms in the individual burn patient may parallel the course of the historical progression of predominance and control of various bacteria: during the 1940s and 1950s, beta-hemolytic streptococcus was the predominant pathogen. With development of sulfonamides and penicillin, the threat of this organism was obviated. Subsequently, the infectious threat became penicillin-resistant *Staphylococcus aureus*. The eventual development of the penicillinase-resistant synthetic penicillins and the cephalosporins permitted control of penicillinase-producing *S. aureus*. During the late 1950s, however, Gram-negative facultative anaerobes (*Pseudomonas aeruginosa*, *Proteus* species, and *Klebsiella* species) emerged as the dominant pathogens and today constitute the greatest septic threat to the burn patient.[3] The problem is further complicated by the emergence of fungal organisms such as *Candida albicans* and *Candida tropicalis* in response to control of Gram-negative species by antibacterial agents.

A recent report[5] summarized data obtained from a prospective study of the flora of burn surfaces in children, applying aerobic and, for the first time, anaerobic microbiological methodology. The data reflected a longitudinal evaluation of the mode of colonization at different anatomic sites and described the effect of antimicrobial agents administered to these children.

Aerobic and anaerobic bacterial flora of burn sites in 180 children were monitored. Specimens were obtained twice a week; each patient had between 1 and 21 cultures taken (mean 2.4). A total of 392 specimens were collected over a period of 2 years. Aerobic bacteria alone were present in 225 specimens (71%), and anaerobic bacteria alone were present in 26 (8%). Mixed aerobic and anaerobic bacteria were present in 68 burn specimens (21%).

A total of 551 isolates (419 aerobes and 132 anaerobes) were recovered, accounting for 1.7 isolates per specimen (1.3 aerobes and 0.4 anaerobes). The predominant aerobic isolates were *Staphylococcus epidermidis*, *S. aureus*, alpha-hemolytic streptococcus, *Pseudomonas* species and group D streptococci. The predominant anaerobic isolates were: *Propionibacterium acnes*, anaerobic Gram-positive cocci and *Bacteroides* species (including *Bacteroides melaninogenicus* and *Bacteroides fragilis*).

Blood cultures were drawn from 45 children. Four of these children showed bacterial growth of one of each of the following isolates: *S. aureus*, *Escherichia coli*, *Peptococcus asaccharolyticus*, and *B. fragilis*.

The number of isolates per specimen was higher in the oral and anal areas (3.2 and 2.8) than in the extremities and trunk (1.8 and 0.9). Gram-negative enteric rods and group D streptococci were recovered more frequently from the anal area. *S. aureus*, *S. epidermidis*, and *P. acnes* were more frequently recovered from extremities. *Bacteroides* sp. and *Fusobacterum nucleatum* were more frequently recovered from the anal and oral areas. Specimens from burns of the anal and oral region tended to yield organisms found in the stool or mouth flora.[6, 7] Specimens obtained from burns in areas remote from the rectum or mouth grew primarily the microflora indigenous to the skin. With the exception of *P. acnes,* multiple anaerobic organisms usually were recovered from the anal and oral areas, whereas fewer anaerobic organisms were present at other sites. Anaerobes were most frequently found in the anal and oral areas. The high rate of recovery of anaerobes in these areas is of particular interest and could be due to the introduction of mouth and stool flora, which is predominantly anaerobic at the burn site.

All children were treated with local application of Silvadene cream and antimicrobial therapy was administered to 128 children. Statistical analysis showed no correlation between the bacteria isolated and the administration of antimicrobial agents.

Thus, with the incorporation of the data about the recovery of anaerobes in the burn patient, the progression of dominant infectious organisms can be anticipated: beta-hemolytic streptococci and then *S. aureus* may be early controllable threats. As the burn wound becomes chronic (after the first week postinjury), there is an increasing frequency of colonization by Gram-negative organisms. The site of the burn can also affect the colonizing bacteria, whereas anaerobes belonging to the *Bacteroides* and *Fusobacterium* species can be found in burns in the oral and anal areas. Later in the course of recovery (three to four weeks postinjury), the wound may become colonized by fungal organisms, most often by *C. albicans.* Frequently, a synergistic colonization of the wound may occur, with two organisms existing apparently to mutual benefit. The combination could be between different aerobes as well as between aerobes and anaerobes. A frequently occurring combination is that of a *Pseudomonas* and enterococcus (*Streptococcus faecalis*). The combination appears to have a greater invasive potential than *Pseudomonas* alone.

Pathogenesis

The burn wound itself creates the most obvious defect in the body's defense against infection. The protective barrier of skin, the body's first line of defense, is damaged or destroyed, and a point of entry for bacteria is established. The larger the burn wound, the greater is the incidence of sepsis and mortality. The threat of septicemia persists until the burn wound is entirely healed, and the skin resumes its protective function.

Unfortunately, the burn victim's humoral and cellular defense systems are diminished. Deficiencies in the inflammatory response include diminished chemotaxis, diminished ability of the neutrophils to phagocytose and thereby kill offending bacteria, and a decrease in opsonin, an antibody that renders the bacteria susceptible to phagocytosis.

With a full-thickness eschar of necrotic tissue serving as the culture medium, the concentration of bacteria may increase above 10^5 microorganisms per gram viable tissue; at this point the local resistance factors are overwhelmed and systemic invasion occurs, with perivascular infiltration and lymphatic spread.

Although the source of contamination of the burn wound in most instances proves to be endogenous flora, the potential of cross-patient contamination exists, and preventive measures should be carefully followed. The most common sources of cross-contamination are the hands of hospital personnel, the hydrotherapy unit, parenteral catheter, and urinary catheter.

The failure to use anaerobic methodology may account for the lack of recovery of anaerobes in previous studies of the flora of burns. The recovery of these organisms from burns is not surprising, since anaerobes are part of the normal flora of the mucous membranes and skin of each individual[6-8] and participate in many of the infectious processes adjacent to those areas.

P. acnes, the predominant anaerobic isolate, is a normal inhabitant of the skin. It can on occasion cause bacteremia or shunt infections,[8, 9] however. Gram-positive anaerobic cocci are normal skin inhabitants and part of the normal fecal flora.[7, 8] They have also been isolated from intraabdominal abscesses.[10] They were isolated as frequently from abscesses of the perineal region as *Bacteroides* species, and were also frequently isolated from nonperineal cutaneous abscesses.

B. fragilis, a predominant anaerobe in the feces,[8] was cultured most frequently from burns of the anal area. *B. melaninogenicus,* which occurs in stool as well as in the oral cavity,[8] was most frequently recovered from the oral region. Most strains of *B. fragilis* and growing numbers of *B. melaninogenicus* are resistant to penicillin.[11]

The data presented by Brook and Randolph[5] demonstrate that anaerobes can colonize burn wounds, although no evidence is available so far to prove their pathogenicity. Two patients in this study, however, experienced a bacteremic episode associated with anaerobic organisms, and the ability of anaerobes to cause bacteremia associated with decubitus ulcer has been shown.[12]

Diagnosis

The signs of infection in a burn may be minimal, especially in the early stages. Local infection is recognized only by frequent inspection. An area of purulence or inflammation at the edge of the eschar may be the only sign. Systemic manifestations of sepsis include fever, tachycardia, acute respiratory distress, adynamic ileus, gastrointestinal hemorrhage, cardiovascular changes including septic shock, petechiae, and occasionally, evidence of other metastatic foci of infection. Deterioration of the patient's mental faculties may accompany a worsening of the vital signs.

The diagnosis of infection in a burn wound depends on an awareness of the real possibility of this complication. Approaches to diagnosis should include frequent inspection of the site of the burn for purulent exudate, cracks in the eschar, evidences of cellulitis, and cultures of blood, the wound, and any exudates. The surface of every burn wound is contaminated to some degree by bacteria[4] and because of this, most burn centers continually monitor surface growth. Monitoring enables the physician to determine the effect and predict the bacterial strains that may be involved in wound sepsis. The burn wound can be the primary focal point for subsequent invasive infection of incipient bacteremia. Monitoring bacterial growth is a significant part of the overall treatment of the severely burned patient. Without topical antibacterials, the progress of burn wound infection from simple colonization to general invasive infection may be rapid.

The presence of organisms in the burn wound does not always indicate sepsis. Burn wound sepsis occurs only with the invasion of viable tissue. If surface cultures obtained with wet swab indicate colonization of the wound by any pathogenic organisms, wound biopsies may be done for quantitative culture or histologic examination. Either a growth of greater than 10^5 microorganisms per gram of tissue or the demonstration of organisms within viable tissue is diagnostic of invasive sepsis.

With the demonstration of invasive sepsis, sensitivities to antibiotics should be determined for all organisms cultured. These sensitivities will dictate the selection of antibiotic, and therapy can be initiated prior to the onset of systemic signs and symptoms of septicemia. Treatment of positive cultures with specific antibiotics during wound colonization does *not* guarantee the prevention of sepsis but may merely provide for the emergence of resistant organisms.

Management

Prevention

A primary objective in the management of burns and prevention of wound sepsis is construction of a barrier between the burned area and the environment. Bacterial wound invasion takes 48 hours in young children, probably because of their thin skin. The 0.5% silver nitrate soaks used with great benefit in the past have been largely replaced by topical creams, which are easier to use and do not require dressings.[13] Silver nitrate soaks are very effective against *Pseudomonas* and a variety of other oganisms as well. Ten percent mafenide hydrochloride cream is effective against *Pseudomonas* organisms but causes pain and an acidosis related to carbonic anhydrase inhibition. Mafenide acetate cream is used currently to minimize the problem of acidosis, and it is effective in diminishing mortality from burn wound sepsis in children.[14] Although mafenide application causes severe local pain, it appears to be the best drug for patients with extensive burns involving thick eschar, since mafenide penetrates eschar to a greater degree than other topical agents. Silver sulfadiazine was found to be very effective against *Pseudomonas* without producing pain or significant metabolic toxicity.[15] Povidone-iodine ointment is a useful agent. It diffuses well through the eschar, is nontoxic and has a wide spectrum. It is important to remember that despite the effectiveness of the various topical antibacterial agents, invasive burn wound sepsis still occurs, particularly in patients with large burn injuries.

General Supportive Measures

The survival of patients with major burns depends upon appropriate resuscitation for burn shock, maintenance of nutrition, adequate pulmonary care, and the ability to control infection. In patients with wound sepsis, general supportive measures are essential to maintain vital organ functions until the sepsis is controlled. The goals of the supportive measures are to prevent respiratory insufficiency and cardiovascular collapse and to alleviate the adynamic ileus.

Systemic Antibiotics

Streptococcal cellulitus was in the past a frequent early complication of burn injury and, therefore, intravenous penicillin was recommended to be given on a prophylactic basis for the first three to five days postburn.[16] Recent studies, however, question the value of prophylactic penicillin therapy and suggest that the use of early prophylactic penicillin may be harmful from the standpoint of sensitivity and the establishment of resistant flora.[17] It is, therefore, recommended that systemic antimicrobial agents should be administered on the basis of information gained from bacteriologic cultures and should be given for five days with either penicillin G or beta-lactamase-resistant penicillin. Since anaerobic bacteria frequently are associated with burns in pediatric patients, especially in areas adjacent to the mucous membrane surfaces, the physician should consider their presence if antimicrobial therapy is employed. Using appropriate aerobic and anaerobic microbiological techniques in monitoring the bacterial colonization of burns can help the physician select proper therapy if complications occur. The presence of penicillin-resistant anaerobic bacteria may warrant the administration of appropriate antimicrobials for the organisms, including such agents as clindamycin, chloramphenicol, cefoxitin, carbenicillin, ticarcillin, or metronidazole. Local debridement of the wound should be done with application of local therapy of silver sulfadiazine 1%, mafenide acetate, or aqueous silver nitrate 0.5%.

In cases of invasive burn wound sepsis or septicemia, the wound should be examined, and a meticulous search made for subeschar abscesses. If no abscesses are found, multiple incisions through the eschar are made, to provide open drainage and to allow the antibacterial cream access to the deeper tissues.

General supportive measures should include evaluation of other sources of invasion (urinary tract infection, thrombophlebitis, pneumonia, etc.) as indications for intravenous fluid therapy and ventilatory assistance.

Broad-spectrum antibiotics should be administered parenterally until culture reports are available. This includes an aminoglycoside for coverage of enteric Gram-negative rods and a synthetic penicillin or cephalosporin for coverage of beta-hemolytic streptococci, enterococci, and *S. aureus*. If anaerobes are suspected, adequate coverage should include one of the agents previously mentioned.

Patients who are not immunized against tetanus should have both active and passive immunization.

REFERENCES

1. Artz, C. P.; Moncrief, J. A.; and Pruitt, B. A. *Burns: a team approach.* Philadelphia: W. B. Saunders, 1973.

2. Pruitt, B. A., Jr., and Foley, F. D. The use of biopsies in burn patient care. *Surgery* 98:292, 1969.

3. Teplitz, C. et al. *Pseudomonas* burn wound sepsis. I. Pathogenesis of experimental *Pseudomonas* burn wound sepsis. *J. Surg. Res.* 4:200, 1964.

4. Lawrence, J. C., and Lilly, H. A. A quantitative method for investigating the bacteriology of skin: its application to burns. *Br. J. Exp. Pathol.* 50:550, 1972.

5. Brook, I., and Randolph, J. G. Aerobic and anaerobic bacterial flora of burns in children. *J. Trauma* 21:313, 1981.

6. Gibbons, R. J. et al. Studies of the predominant cultivable microbiota of dental plaque. *Arch. Oral Biol.* 9:365, 1964.

7. Gorbach, S. L. Intestinal microflora. *Gastroenterology* 60:1110, 1971.

8. Finegold, S. M. *Anaerobic bacteria in human disease.* New York: Academic Press, 1977.

9. Everett, E. D.; Eickhoff, T. C.; and Simon, R. H. Cerebrospinal fluid of shunt infections with anaerobic diphtheroids (*Propionibacterium* species). *J. Neurosurg.* 44:580, 1976.

10. Moore, W. E. C.; Cato, E. P.; and Holdeman, L. V. Anaerobic bacteria of the gastrointestinal flora and their occurrence in clinical infections. *J. Infect. Dis.* 119:641, 1969.

11. Sutter, V. L., and Finegold, S. M. Susceptibility of anaerobic bacteria to 23 antimicrobial agents. *Antimicrob. Agents Chemother.* 10:736, 1976.

12. Rissing, J. P. et al. *Bacteroides* bacteremia from decubitus ulcers. *South. Med. J.* 67:1179, 1974.

13. Moyer, C. A. et al. Treatment of large human burns with 0.5 per cent silver nitrate solution. *Arch. Surg.* 90:812, 1965.

14. Moncrief, J. A. Topical therapy for control of bacteria in the burn wound. *World J. Surg.* 2:151, 1978.

15. Fox, C. L.; Roppole, B. W.; and Stanford, W. Control of *Pseudomonas* infection in burns by silver sulfadiazine. *Surg. Gynecol. Obstet.* 128:1021, 1969.

16. Leidberg, N. et al. Infection in burns: the problem and evaluation of therapy. *Surg. Gynecol. Obstet.* 98:535, 1954.

17. Larkin, J. M., and Moylan, J. A. The role of prophylactic antibiotics in burn care. *Am. Surg.* 42:247, 1976.

CHAPTER

32

Bite Wounds

Human bites and other orally contaminated wounds are relatively common. According to the United States Public Health Service, more than 1 million animal bites occur in the United States each year that require medical attention.[1] Although they may look innocuous initially, they frequently lead to serious complications.[2, 3]

Dog bite is an extremely common problem in the United States. The annual incidence appears to be rising, and at least 1 million persons per year are bitten.[1] Dogs account for 80% to 90% of all animal bites requiring medical care[4] and almost 1% of emergency department visits. Although half of all bites are trivial in nature, at least 10% require suturing and follow-up visits, and 1% to 2% require hospitalization.[5]

Children are especially prone to animal bites. A sample of 1869 dog bites reported to the New York City Health Department showed that the majority were inflicted on individuals less than 20 years of age.[6]

Microbiology

Human Bites

Earlier studies noted alpha-hemolytic streptococci and *Staphylococcus aureus* to be the most common organisms isolated.[7, 8] The presence of anaerobic spirochetes and fusiform bacilli were noted to correlate with a less favorable prognosis.

Most studies that did not employ anaerobic methodology have reported *S. aureus* to be the most frequent organism isolated, recovered from 62% to 80% of wounds and the one most often correlated with severity of and complications from human bite infection.[2, 9] Penicillin-resistant Gram-negative rods alone or in mixed culture have been reported in 24% to 43% of bite wounds cultured.[3, 9, 10]

A recent study that employed anaerobic methodologies[11] reported the recovery of anaerobic bacteria in 18 of 34 human bite wounds and clenched-fist injuries. A total of 42 strains of anaerobic bacteria were isolated. *Bacteroides* species were the most frequent isolates (21 isolates), none of which were *Bacteroides fragilis*. The predominant *Bacteroides* species recovered belonged to the *Bacteroides melaninogenicus* group (11 isolates). There were four strains of *Fusobacterium nucleatum* and 10 anaerobic Gram-positive cocci. The predominant aerobes recovered were *S. aureus* (10 strains), group A beta-hemolytic streptococci (9 strains), and *Eikenella corrodens* (4 strains).

The results of this study show the normal oral flora, rather than the skin flora, to be the source of most bacteria isolated from human bite wound cultures.

Animal Bites

Most studies of animal bite wounds and infections have focused on the isolation of *Pasteurella multocida*[12, 13] and disregarded the role of anaerobes. More recently, studies of the gingival canine flora, with an effort to correlate it with bite wound bacteriology,[14, 15] have been reported.

Using optimal aerobic and anaerobic cultural methods, Goldstein, Citron, and Finegold[16] studied 27 dog bite wounds and recovered 109 organisms, of which 87 were aerobes and 22 were anaerobes. All positive cultures yielded multiple organisms, most of which were potential pathogens. *P. multocida* was isolated from 7 of 27 wounds (26%), and the most common aerobic isolates were the alpha-hemolytic streptococci (12 strains) and *S. aureus* (5 strains). Anaerobic pathogens were present in 41% of wounds. These included *Bacteroides* species (5 strains, all but one belonging to the *B. melaninogenicus* group) and *Fusobacterium* species (5 strains). These authors and others[11] studied other animal bites (cats, squirrels, other rodents, and rattlesnakes) and had similar data.

Pathogenesis

The potential for infection of human or animal bites is great. For example, a dog's teeth are not very sharp, but can exert a pressure of 200 to 450 psi[17]; this pressure is strong enough to perforate sheet metal. The result is a crush injury with much devitalized tissue, rather than a laceration. The average dog mouth harbors more than 64 species of bacteria, including *S. aureus*, *P. multocida*, anaerobic bacteria (especially of the *B. melaninogenicus* group), and CDC types IIj and EF-4—all known human pathogens.[11, 15] Since anaerobes predominate in the normal oral flora of humans and various animals, it follows that they have an important role in oral contamination of bite wounds.

A number of risk factors determining likelihood of wound infection have been identified and define the patient likely to develop this complication.[18] An important risk factor is delay of more than 24 hours in seeking treatment. Puncture wounds are much more likely than other types to become infected. Facial wounds show an infection rate of only 4% regardless of treatment, while hand wounds have a rate of 28%.[18]

Diagnosis

The symptoms following a bite depend on the animal species inflicting the injury. Immediate local or systemic symptoms can be severe following venomous animals (snake, lizard, spider, etc.). Human or dog bites do not generally cause immediate symptoms different from those of a laceration injury. Because of the direct introduction of oral and skin flora into the wound, however, an infection when it occurs develops quite rapidly. The signs of infection can include redness, swelling, and clear or pussy discharge. The adjacent lymph nodes may be enlarged, and reduction in range of movement of an extremity can be present. In severe cases, there may be a peripheral leukocytosis of 15,000 to 30,000 cells per cubic millimeter.

Human bites generally are more severe than those of animals. This is particularly true in clenched fist injury when the skin over the knuckles is penetrated after striking the teeth of another person. The teeth may cause a deep laceration that implant oral and skin organisms into the joint capsules or dorsal tendons, thus causing septic arthritis or osteomyelitis. Radiographs of hands injured by teeth are recommended.[19]

Not all bites cause infection. About 2% to 5% of all typical dog bite wounds seen in emergency departments become infected.[5, 18] This figure includes, however, many trivial surface abrasions. Wounds that fully penetrated the skin have an infection rate of 6% to 13%, depending on location.[18] In comparison, the infection rate of clean lacerations of all types repaired in the emergency department is about 5%.[20]

Human and animal bite wounds should be cultured for both aerobes and anaerobes. The use of Gram stain as an indicator of the presence of pathogens in the wound can be of assistance.

Management

The rules governing the management of any laceration apply as well to animal bites: cleanse, explore, irrigate, debride, drain, and possibly suture.

Bite wounds should be washed vigorously with soap or a quaternary ammononium compound and water. The physician should explore for damage to tissues caused by crushing or tearing and search for damaged tendons, blood vessels, joints, and bones. X-ray examination for fractures and foreign bodies should be done when feasible. The wound should be irrigated through a 19-gauge needle with 150 ml or more of sterile normal saline or lactated Ringer's solution. Devitalized tissues should be debrided. Drainage of the wound, when necessary, can be done in customary fashion or with gentle suction using a 19-gauge scalp vein tubing connected to a vacuum blood collecting tube.[21]

Margins of puncture wounds should be excised and left open after irrigation. Margins of other wounds should be carefully excised and primary closure carried out, with or without drainage.[21]

Bites of the hand are at high risk of deep damage and severe infection because sharp teeth may penetrate tendon sheaths or the midpalmar space. Nardi and Zuidema[22] recommend that human bites be treated by opening the wound widely, debriding, and irrigating thoroughly. Primary closure and tendon nerve repair should be delayed. Following debridement and irrigation, dog bites can be considered clean, and primary closure can be carried out. Hospitalization for several days is recommended, with immobilization by splinting or bulky dressings and elevation.

Bites to the face, especially of children, require meticulous management. Nearly all facial bite victims do well with careful debridement, ample irrigation and cleansing, and loose closure by suture. Close follow-up for five days or longer is required. Subsequent plastic reconstruction may be considered, and consultation with a plastic surgeon at the time of initial repair may be helpful.

Early treatment of all human bites, especially those to the hand, must be thorough and aggressive. Unfortunately, the injury sometimes is seen only after severe infection has occurred.

Rabies prevention should be instituted after dog bites that indicate such measures.[23] This includes hyperimmune serum and active immunization.

A tetanus toxoid booster should be administered if the patient has been immunized previously. Tetanus immune globulin (human) is required if tetanus immunization has not taken place.

The infectious complications of dog bites make the concept of prophylactic antibiotics attractive. The use of antibiotics may be helpful, particularly in high-risk wounds such as those of the hand.

The choice of a particular antibiotic for prophylaxis and/or treatment must be based on bacteriology. Unfortunately, no one antibiotic can be expected to effectively treat infections caused by all the organisms that can be present in an infected bite.

Antimicrobial therapy should be administered for all bite wounds, with the exception of those patients who present 24 hours or more after injury and have no clinical signs of infection. Antimicrobial therapy of bite wounds is not usually prophylactic, but rather therapeutic, intervention. Penicillin is adequate as initial empiric therapy. If *S. aureus* infection is suspected (from Gram stain), a penicillinase-resistant penicillin should be added.

E. corrodens, a capnophilic Gram-negative rod that is part of the normal oral flora[7] can be isolated from 25% of human bite wounds.[11] This is of note because of the unusual antibiotic sensitivity pattern of *E. corrodens*. It is susceptible to penicillin and ampicillin, but resistant to oxacillin, methicillin, nafcillin, and clindamycin, and some strains are resistant to cephalosporins.[7] Therefore, when isolated, *E. corrodens* should have susceptibility testing if cephalosporin therapy is to be considered.

When antibiotics are used in this manner and combined with good wound toilet, most bite wounds may be sutured with good results and an acceptable infection rate.

Complications

Hand wounds present a special problem, as 30% or more become infected.[17, 18] Because of the presence of avascular tendon and sheath spaces, the propensity for spread of infection, and disastrous results of such infection on function, the threat of complications following bite wounds must be addressed. In addition to local wound infection, known complications include lymphangitis, osteomyelitis,[19] meningitis,[24] brain abscess,[25] and sepsis with disseminated intravascular coagulation.[26] Rabies must also be considered; its prophylaxis entails considerable expense and morbidity.[22]

REFERENCES

1. United States Public Health Service. Annual summary, 1976, Publication No. CDC 77-8241, *Morbidity and Mortality Weekly Report* 25:34, 1977.

2. Farmer, C. B., and Mann, R. J. Human bite infections of the hand. *South. Med. J.* 59:515, 1966.

3. Mann, R. J.; Hoffeld, T. A.; and Farmer, C. B. Human bites of the hand: twenty years of experience. *J. Hand Surg.* 2:97, 1977.

4. Thomson, H. G., and Svitek, V. Small animal bites: the role of primary closure. *J. Trauma* 13:20, 1973.

5. Kizer, K. W. Epidemiologic and clinical aspects of animal bite injuries. *JACEP* 8:134, 1979.

6. Harris, D.; Imperato, P. J.: and Oken, B. Dog bites: an unrecognized epidemic. *Bull. NY Acad. Med.* 50:981, 1974.

7. Manson, M. L., and Koch, S. L. Human bite infections of the hand. *Surg. Gynecol. Obstet.* 51:591, 1930.

8. Welch, C. E. Human bite infection of the hand. *N. Engl. J. Med.* 215:901, 1936.

9. Guba, A. M.; Mulliken, J. B.; and Hoopes, J. E. The selection of antibiotics for human bites of the hand. *Plast. Reconstr. Surg.* 56:538, 1975.

10. Shields, C. et al. Hand infections secondary to human bites. *J. Trauma* 15:235, 1975.

11. Goldstein, J. C. et al. Bacteriology of human and animal bite wounds. *J. Clin. Microbiol.* 8:667, 1978.

12. Francis, D. P.; Holmes, M. A.; and Brandon, G. *Pasteurella multocida* infections after domestic animal bites and scratches. *JAMA* 233:42, 1975.

13. Hawkins, L. G. Local *Pasteurella multocida* infections. *J. Bone Joint Surg.* 51:363, 1965.

14. Laphir, D. A., and Carter, G. R. Gingival flora of the dog with special reference to bacteria associated with bites. *J. Clin. Microbiol.* 3:344, 1976.

15. Baile, W. E.; Stowe, E. C.; and Schmitt, A. M. Aerobic bacterial flora of oral and nasal fluids of canines with reference to bacteria associated with bites. *J. Clin. Microbiol.* 7:223, 1978.

16. Goldstein, E. J. C.; Citron, D. M.; and Finegold, S. M. Dog bite wounds and infection: a prospective clinical study. *Ann. Emerg. Med.* 9:508, 1980.

17. Chambers, G., and Payne, J. Treatment of dog bite wounds. *Minn. Med.* 52:427, 1969.

18. Callaham, M. Treatment of common dog bites: infection risk factors. *JACEP* 7:83, 1978.

19. Szalay, G. C., and Sommerstein, A. Inoculation osteomyelitis secondary to animal bites. *Clin Pediatr.* 11:687, 1972.

20. Galvin, J. R., and DeSimone, D. Infection rate of simple suturing. *JACEP* 5:332, 1976.

21. Graham, W. P. III; Calabretta, A. M.; and Miller, S. H. Dog bites. *Am. Fam. Physician* 15:132, 1977.

22. Nardi, G. L., and Zuidema, G. D., eds. *Surgery: a concise guide to clinical practice,* 3rd edition. Boston: Little, Brown, 1972.

23. Center for Disease Control. Rabies prevention. *Morbidity and Mortality Weekly Report* 29:265, 1980.

24. Bracis, R.; Seibers, K.; and Jullien, R. M. Meningitis caused by IIJ following a dog bite. *West. J. Med.* 131:438, 1979.

25. Klein, D. M., and Cohen, M. E. *Pasteurella multocida* brain abscess following perforating cranial dog bite. *J. Pediatr.* 92:588, 1978.

26. Check, W. An odd link between dog bites, splenectomy. *JAMA* 241:225, 1979.

PART V

Principles of Management

Treatment of Anaerobic Infections

The recovery of a child from an anaerobic infection depends on prompt and proper management. The strategy for therapy of anaerobic infections consists of surgical drainage of pus, debridement of any necrotic tissue, and appropriate antibiotics. Certain types of adjunct therapy such as hyperbaric oxygen may also be useful. Antimicrobial therapy is in many patients the only form of therapy required, whereas in others it is an important adjunct to a surgical approach.

Surgical therapy may be the only therapy required in some cases, as for localized abscesses or decubitus ulcers without signs of systemic involvement. In treatment of such lesions, antibiotics are indicated whenever systemic manifestations of infection are present or when suppuration has either extended or threatened to spread into surrounding tissue. Antibiotics are needed in the majority of cases, however. Selection of antimicrobial agents is simplified when culture result of a reliable specimen is available. This may be particularly difficult in anaerobic infections because of the problems encountered in obtaining appropriate specimens. Because of this difficulty, many patients are treated empirically on the basis of suspected, rather than established, pathogens. Fortunately, the types of anaerobes involved in many anaerobic infections and their antimicrobial susceptibility patterns tend to be predictable. Some anaerobic bacteria have become resistant to antimicrobial agents, however, and many can become resistant while a patient is receiving therapy.[1]

Aside from susceptibility patterns, other factors influencing the choice of antimicrobial therapy include the pharmacologic characteristics of the various drugs, their toxicity, their effect on the normal flora, and bactericidal activity.[2] Although identification of the infecting organisms and their antimicrobial susceptibility may be needed for selection of optimal therapy, the clinical setting and Gram stain preparation of the specimen may indicate the types of anaerobes present in the infection as well as the nature of the infectious process.

Since anaerobic bacteria generally are recovered mixed with aerobic organisms, selection of proper therapy becomes more complicated. In the treatment of mixed infection the choice of the appropriate antimicrobial agents should provide for adequate coverage of most of the pathogens. Some broad spectrum antibacterial agents possess such qualities, while for some organisms additional agents should be added to the therapeutic regimen.

This chapter reviews the various antimicrobial agents used for the treatment of anaerobic infections, alone or in combination, and the clinical significance of the production of beta-lactamase by *Bacteroides* species.

Effective Antimicrobial Agents

Penicillin G

Penicillin G is the drug of choice when the infecting strains are susceptible to this drug in vitro. This includes the vast majority of strains other than those belonging to the *Bacteroides fragilis* group.[1] Only about 42% of clinical isolates of the *B. fragilis* group are susceptible to 16 units/ml penicillin G, and 10% require up to 256 units/ml for inhibition of growth.[1] Therefore, penicillin G should not be used for the treatment of infections by the *B. fragilis* group. Other strains that may show resistance to penicillins are growing numbers of *Bacteroides,* such as the *Bacteroides melaninogenicus* group and *Bacteroides oralis,* strains of clostridia, *Fusobacterium* species (*Fusobacterium varium* and *Fusobacterium mortiferum*), and microaerophilic streptococci. Some of these strains show minimal inhibitory concentration (MIC) in dosages of 8 to 32 units/ml of penicillin G. In these instances, administration of very high dosages of penicillin G may eradicate the infection. Clinical experience with penicillin G in the management of susceptible anaerobic bacterial infections has been good. Ampicillin and amoxacillin and penicillin generally are equally active, but the semisynthetic penicillins are less active than the parent compound. Methicillin, nafcillin, and the isoxazolyl penicillins (oxacillin, cloxacillin, and dicloxacillin) have unpredictable activity and frequently are inferior to penicillin G against anaerobes.[3]

Carbenicillin and Ticarcillin

Carbenicillin has good in vitro activity against most strains of the *B. fragilis* group, as well as against other penicillin-sensitive anaerobes,[1, 2] and is effective in the treatment of clinical infections.[4] Ticarcillin is a newer semisynthetic penicillin similar in structure to carbenicillin. Like carbenicillin, it has good in vitro activity against many anaerobic organisms[1] and was found to be effective also in the treatment of anaerobic infections.

Clinical trials of carbenicillin in the treatment of pulmonary and intraabdominal anaerobic infections in adults suggest that the drug is efficacious when given in a dose of 400 to 500 mg/kg/day.[5,6] Carbenicillin has also been found to be effective alone or in combination with an aminoglycoside in treatment of aspiration pneumonia[7] and chronic otitis media[8] in children. Carbenicillin has a particular advantage in these infections because of its synergistic quality with aminoglycosides against *Pseudomonas aeruginosa*, which was also present in these infections.

Sutter and Finegold[4] reported that carbenicillin inhibited 96% of *B. fragilis* strains at a concentration of 100 µg/ml; however, Tally and colleagues[9] found that only 60% of strains were inhibited by 128 µg/ml. Carbenicillin was shown to be effective in the treatment of anaerobic infections even where resistant *B. fragilis* was involved.[6,8] This drug also has the advantage of possessing a wide spectrum of activity against Gram-negative aerobic bacilli, making single-drug therapy of mixed infections possible in some instances.

Ticarcillin also has been shown to be active against *B. fragilis*,[10] and clinical trials suggest that it is effective in the treatment of anaerobic infections. Ticarcillin is similar in pharmacology and spectrum of activity to carbenicillin, and it is effective at only half of the daily dose of carbenicillin. Because of the high sodium content in both of these drugs, the ability to give ticarcillin disodium at a lower dose may represent an advantage. Another adverse effect of these drugs is the induction of a thrombocytic malfunction noted especially with carbenicillin.

Because of the need to achieve high serum levels, the daily dosage of these drugs is high. Carbenicillin and ticarcillin therapy is expensive.

Cephalosporins

The antimicrobial spectrum of cephalosporins against anaerobes is similar to penicillin G, although they are less active on a weight basis. Similar to penicillin G, most strains of the *B. fragilis* group and many of the *B. melaninogenicus* group are resistant to these agents by virtue of cephalosporinase production.[1,2] Cefoxitin is relatively resistant to this enzyme and is therefore effective against the *B. fragilis* group. Cefoxitin is active in vitro against at least 95% of strains of *B. fragilis* at a level of 32 µg/ml,[1,2] but cefoxitin is relatively inactive against most species of *Clostridium* (including *Clostridium difficile*), other than *Clostridium perfringens*. Early clinical experiences with cefoxitin in anaerobic infections showed it to be effective in eradication of these infections.[11] Because of the poor penetration of cephalosporins into the cerebrospinal fluid, however, they may not be effective in the treatment of central nervous system infections.

Moxalactam disodium is a new semisynthetic beta-lactam antibiotic for parenteral treatment of various infections by susceptible pathogens. Moxalactam is highly active against beta-lactamase-producing strains of *Neisseria gonorrhoeae* and *Haemophilus influenzae* and has a broad spectrum of activity against enteric Gram-negative bacilli and most strains of *B. fragilis*.[12] Moxalactam is comparable in vitro to cefoxitin against anaerobic Gram-negative bacilli such as *B. fragilis*. Because of its activity against *B. fragilis*, moxalactam is being promoted for treatment of intraabdominal and gynecologic infections; how the drug compares in effectiveness with established regimens such as clindamycin and gentamicin, or with cefoxitin, is undetermined.

Chloramphenicol

Chloramphenicol is one of the antimicrobial agents most active against anaerobes.[1, 2] Resistance to this drug is rare, although it has been reported in some *Bacteroides* species.[13] Although several failures to eradicate anaerobic infections, including bacteremia, with chloramphenicol have been reported,[14] this drug has been used for over 25 years for treatment of anaerobic infections. It is regarded as the drug of choice for treatment of serious anaerobic infections when the nature and susceptibility of the infecting organisms are unknown and in infections of the central nervous system. The toxicity of chloramphenicol must be borne in mind, however. The risk of fatal aplastic anemia with chloramphenicol is estimated to be approximately one per 30,000 patients treated. This serious complication is unrelated to the reversible, dosage-dependent leukopenic side effect. Other side effects are the production of the potentially fatal "gray syndrome" when given to neonates and optic neuritis in individuals who take the drug for a prolonged time.

The absorption of orally administered chloramphenicol base is good with peak serum levels of 8 to 15 µg/ml at two to three hours following a dose of 7 mg/kg, and peak levels of 10 to 20 µg/ml following a dose of 15 mg/kg.[15] Multiple dosing at six- to eight-hour intervals provides somewhat higher levels on the second day with no subsequent increase. The palmitate is slowly hydrolyzed to active drug by pancreatic lipases in the duodenum so that the peak serum level is somewhat lower and delayed compared to the base. The sodium succinate preparation used for intravenous administration, like the palmitate, has no intrinsic antimicrobial activity, and the ester must be hydrolyzed in vivo. Kinetics of this hydrolysis appear to be slow and incomplete and show considerable individual patient variability.[15] Peak levels with the usual doses generally range from 10 to 25 μg/ml at one to two hours after infusion.[15]

Free chloramphenicol is metabolized primarily in the liver by glucuronide conjugation in the presence of normal hepatic function. The glucuronide metabolite is nontoxic and inactive as an antimicrobial. Urinary products with administration of chloramphenicol sodium succinate include inactive forms, primarily the unhydrolyzed succinate ester and the metabolized glucuronide, and only 5% to 15% appears as biologically active chloramphenicol.[16] With impaired renal function, there is a delay in the excretion of the nontoxic glucuronide and unhydrolyzed succinate ester, but this has no significant effect on serum levels of the biologically active and potentially toxic form.[16] Chloramphenicol glucuronyl transferase activity appears to be a function of prenatal and postnatal age, being very low prior to birth and at birth.[17] It also appears to be reduced with serious hepatic dysfunction, leading to increased serum levels of biologically active drug with the usual doses. The approximate half-life as a function of age is as follows: children over one month and adults, 4 hours; neonates two to four weeks, 12 hours; and neonates from birth to 15 days, 24 hours.[17] These observations account for the variations in recommended maintenance regimens based on age noted above.

The rate of chloramphenicol metabolism in the liver may also be influenced by drug interaction, as with phenobarbital, which increases the rate of glucuronide conjugation owing to enzyme induction.[18]

Serum level measurements are often advocated for infants, young children, and occasionally for adults, owing to wide variations noted.[19] The usual objective is therapeutic levels of 10 to 25 μg/ml. Levels exceeding 25 μg/ml are commonly considered potentially toxic in terms of reversible bone marrow suppression, and levels of 40 to 200 μg/ml have been associated with the gray syndrome in neonates or encephalitis in adults.[17]

Chloramphenicol is widely distributed in body fluids and tissue, with a mean volume distribution of 1.4 L/kg.[19] The drug has a somewhat unique property of lipid solubility to permit penetration across lipid barriers. A consistent observation is the high concentrations achieved in the central nervous system, even in the absence of inflammation. Levels in the cerebrospinal fluid, with or without meningitis, usually are one-third to three-fourths the serum concentrations.[18] Levels in brain tissue may be substantially higher than serum levels.[20] The drug also shows rather unique properties for penetration across the blood-ocular barrier. Joint fluid levels are generally low in the absence of inflammation, but are relatively high—50% or more of serum concentration—in the presence of septic arthritis.[21] The drug readily crosses the placenta to provide cord blood levels. Studies in experimental animals with subcutaneous abscesses show peak levels within abscesses that approximate 15% to 20% of the peak serum concentration.[22] This is comparable to the levels achieved with multiple other antimicrobials, including virtually all beta-lactam compounds, and it is substantially lower compared to abscess levels achieved with clindamycin.

Erythromycin

Erythromycin, which possesses low human or animal toxicity,[23, 24] has moderate to good in vitro activity against anaerobic bacteria other than *B. fragilis* and fusobacteria.[1] Erythromycin is active against *B. melaninogenicus,* microaerophilic and anaerobic streptococci, Gram-positive non-spore-forming anaerobic bacilli, and certain clostridia. It shows relatively good activity against *C. perfringens* and poor or inconsistent activity against Gram-negative anaerobic bacilli.

Emergence of erythromycin-resistant organisms during therapy has been documented.[25] Erythromycin is effective in the treatment of mild to moderately severe anaerobic soft tissue and pleuropulmonary infections when combined with adequate debridement or drainage of infected tissue. Phlebitis is reported to develop in one-third of the patients receiving intravenous erythromycin, but the oral preparation is well tolerated.

Lincomycin and Clindamycin

The in vitro susceptibility of various anaerobic bacteria to lincomycin was initially demonstrated in 1966.[26] Subsequently, several groups of workers[1] found that the 7-chloro-7-deoxylincomycin analogue, clindamycin, is even more active against anaerobes than the parent compound. Lincomycin is highly active against a variety of anaerobic bacteria; however, clostridia, *B. fragilis,* and *F. varium* are relatively resistant to lincomycin.[1]

Clindamycin has a broad range of activity against anaerobic organisms and has proven its efficacy in clinical trials. Approximately 96% of anaerobic bacteria isolated in clinical practice are susceptible to easily achievable levels of clindamycin.[1, 2] *B. fragilis* is generally sensitive to levels below $3\mu g/ml$. There are, however, reports of resistant strains associated with clinical infections, although these are uncommon. Among the other resistant anaerobes are various species of clostridia. Approximately 20% of *Clostridium ramosum* are resistant to clindamycin, as are a smaller number of *C. perfringens*. Many strains of *F. varium* are resistant, but this organism is uncommon in clinical infections. Recently, a few strains of peptococci were found to be resistant.[2]

Clindamycin hydrochloride is rapidly and virtually completely absorbed from the gastrointestinal tract. Absorption is not decreased by food.[27] In children receiving 2 mg/kg, the mean peak serum concentrations were 2.1 $\mu g/ml$ at 30 minutes and 0.3 $\mu g/ml$ at six hours.[27]

Clindamycin palmitate is also absorbed rapidly and efficiently after oral administration, but serum concentrations are slightly lower than after clindamycin hydrochloride. Food does not affect absorption. In healthy children, doses of 2, 3, and 4 mg/kg gave mean peak serum concentrations of 0.2 to 0.3, 0.4, and 0.5 µg/ml, respectively, with a half-life of 1.5 to 2.2 hours.[28] After repeated doses, the serum concentrations increased until they reached equilibrium. Infants under six months of age who received doses of 3 mg/kg had serum concentrations up to 2.7 µg/ml.[29]

Clindamycin phosphate given intravenously to infected children who received 7 mg/kg over a one-hour infusion had mean serum concentrations of 9 and 2 µg/ml at one and eight hours, respectively.[30] Repeated intravenous treatment with any dosage did not increase these concentrations, regardless of whether the drug was administered every 6, 8, or 12 hours.[30] Continuous intravenous infusions of 900 to 1350 mg per day maintained serum concentrations of 4 to 6 µg/ml.

Only about 10% of active clindamycin is excreted unaltered in the urine, and only small quantities are found in the feces. Most of the drug is inactivated by metabolism to N-demethyl clindamycin, which has three times the bioactivity of the parent compound and clindamycin sulfoxide, both of which are excreted in the urine and bile.[31]

Clindamycin is rapidly removed from serum to body tissues and fluids and it penetrates well into saliva, sputum, respiratory tissue, pleural fluid, soft tissues, prostate, semen, bones, and joints,[32] as well as into fetal blood and tissues. There are no data to show that significant concentrations are achievable in the human brain, cerebrospinal fluid, or eye.

Several reports[33] described the successful use of this drug in the treatment of anaerobic infection. Clindamycin does not cross efficiently the blood-brain barrier and should not be administered in central nervous system infections. Because of the effectiveness of its activity against anaerobes it is frequently used in combination with aminoglycosides for the treatment of mixed aerobic-anaerobic infections of the abdominal cavity and obstetric infection.[33] The primary manifestation of toxicity with clindamycin is colitis.[34] It should be kept in mind that colitis has been associated with a number of other antimicrobial agents, such as ampicillin and many cephalosporins, and has been described in seriously ill patients in the absence of previous antimicrobial therapy. Colitis following clindamycin therapy[34] was associated with recovery of *C. difficile* strains in adults and children receiving clindamycin therapy.[35] The occurrence of colitis in pediatric patients is very rare, however.[36] Clinical studies using clindamycin in a pediatric population showed it to be effective in the treatment of intraabdominal infections,[37] osteomyelitis,[38] aspiration pneumonia,[39] and chronic otitis media.[40]

Metronidazole

Metronidazole is active against anaerobic protozoa, including *Trichomonas vaginalis, Entamoeba histolytica,* and *Giardia lamblia.* This drug also shows excellent in vitro activity against most obligate anaerobic bacteria, such as *B. fragilis,* other species of *Bacteroides,* fusobacteria, and clostridia.[1, 41] Occasional strains of anaerobic Gram-positive cocci and nonsporulating bacilli are highly resistant. Microaerophilic streptococci, *Propionibacterium acnes,* and *Actinomyces* species are almost uniformly resistant.[1, 41] Aerobic and facultative anaerobes, such as coliforms, are usually highly resistant. Over 90% of obligate anaerobes are susceptible to less than 2 μg/ml metronidazole.[41]

For anaerobic bacterial infections, the most frequently employed oral doses are 250 to 750 mg two or three times daily.[42] Peak serum levels following a single dose of 250 mg or 500 mg are approximately 6 μg/ml and 12 μg/ml, respectively. Multiple 500-mg oral doses given four times daily result in peak serum levels of 20 to 30 μg/ml.[43] The recommended dose of the intravenous preparation for serious anaerobic infections is 15 mg/kg infused over one hour (approximately 1 g for a 70-kg adult) with maintenance dosage of 7.5 mg/kg every six hours (approximately 500 mg for a 70-kg adult). The peak blood levels achieved with intravenous administration approximate those noted with oral administration, indicating that the oral formulation is nearly completely absorbed.[43] Thus, parenteral administration appears to offer no additional benefit for patients who can receive oral treatment; furthermore, the intravenous form is substantially more expensive. The serum half-life is approximately eight hours.[42] The drug diffuses well into nearly all tissue, including the central nervous system, abscesses, bile, bone, pelvic tissue, breast milk, and placenta.[43] Metronidazole is extensively metabolized in the liver by oxidation, hydroxylation, or conjugation of side chains on the imidazole ring. The major metabolic products are the acid or alcohol metabolites that have antibacterial and mutagenic potential.[44] The kidney is the major excretory route for the parent compound and its metabolites in the presence of normal renal function.[42] The clearance of metronidazole is not altered in renal failure, but accumulation of metabolites may be noted with repeated doses. The manufacturer recommends the usual dose in anuric patients. Reduced dosage is recommended in patients with severe hepatic disease, but precise recommendations are not available.

Adverse reactions to metronidazole therapy are rare and include central nervous system toxicity symptoms of peripheral neuropathy, ataxia, vertigo, headaches, and convulsions. Gastrointestinal side effects include nausea, vomiting, metallic taste, anorexia, and diarrhea. Other adverse reactions include neutropenia, which is reversible with discontinuation of the drug, phlebitis at intravenous infusion sites, and drug fever. The tolerance of metronidazole in patients treated was excellent, and none developed an adverse reaction.

Some studies in mice[42] have shown possible mitogenic activity associated with administration of large doses of this drug. It should be noted that in these animal toxicity studies, the drug has generally been administered for the lifetime of the animal, a situation that may not be relevant for humans. Other experiments[43] have shown that administration of metronidazole to rats and hamsters does not induce any pathology. Furthermore, evidence of mutagenicity was never found in humans despite metronidazole use for over two decades for other diseases.[45] Despite this perplexing issue, the Food and Drug Administration (FDA) approved the use of metronidazole for the treatment of serious anaerobic infections in adults. Clinical experiences in adults[44] indicate it to be a promising agent in the treatment of infections caused by anaerobes, especially central nervous system infections.[46, 47]

There is limited experience at present in the use of metronidazole in pediatric patients, and only a few cases are reported in the literature.[46-50] Brook[51] recently studied the tolerance and efficacy of metronidazole in 15 pediatric patients who had anaerobic infection. Five patients had soft tissue abscess, four had aspiration pneumonia, three had chronic sinusitis, and three had intracranial abscess. No local or systemic adverse reactions were noted. A good response to therapy with a complete cure occurred in 14 of the 15 children.

There are several anaerobic infections in children for which the use of metronidazole seems advantageous. This is especially true in central nervous system infections because of the excellent penetration of the drug into the central nervous system.[45] Until the FDA approves the use of this drug for children, however, it should be used only in seriously ill patients, following the FDA regulations.

Other serious infections for which this drug would be advantageous are anaerobic endocarditis or infections in a compromised host, where the bactericidal activity of the drug is important.

Tetracyclines

Tetracycline, once the drug of choice for anaerobic infections, is presently of limited usefulness because of the development of resistance to it by virtually all types of anaerobes. Only about 45% of all *B. fragilis* strains presently are susceptible to this drug.[1, 2] The newer tetracycline analogues, doxycycline and minocycline, are more active than the parent compound. There is still significant resistance to these drugs, however, so that they are useful only when susceptibility tests can be done or in less severe infections in which a therapeutic trial is feasible. The use of tetracycline is not recommended before eight years of age because of the adverse effect on teeth.

Other Agents

Bacitracin is active against *B. melaninogenicus* but is inactive against *B. fragilis* and *Fusobacterium nucleatum*.[1, 2]

Vanocmycin is effective against all Gram-positive anaerobes, but is inactive against Gram-negative ones. Little clinical experience has been gained in the treatment of anaerobic bacteria using this agent.

Clavulanic acid is a new beta-lactamase inhibitor that resembles the nucleus of penicillin but differs in several ways. Clavulanic acid irreversibly inhibits beta-lactamase enzymes produced by some Enterobacteriaceae, staphylococci,[52] and beta-lactamase-producing *Bacteroides* species (*B. fragilis* group and strains of *B. melaninogenicus* and *B. oralis*).[53] When used in conjunction with a beta-lactam antibiotic, it may prove to be effective in treating infections caused by beta-lactamase-producing bacteria. Its usefulness in the chemotherapy of human infections is currently being evaluated. Clavulanic acid and other beta-lactamase inhibitors have weak antibacterial activity alone, but may prove to be effective adjuncts to penicillins in the treatment of resistant organisms.

Synergistic Antimicrobial Combinations

Combinations of antibiotics are continually being studied in attempts to discover more effective therapy for serious infections. Combined therapy might delay emergence of antimicrobial resistance, provide broad spectrum coverage for infections of unknown or mixed etiology, or generate a greater antibacterial effect against specific pathogens than is achievable with a single drug. The improved killing, as expressed by effective bactericidal activity, of the offending anaerobic organisms is especially important in the treatment of endocarditis and bacteremia. Another situation in which combination therapy may be valuable is the treatment of closed space infections, such as brain or lung abscesses, that cannot be surgically drained either because of location or the patient's clinical condition. Combination therapy should not be used indiscriminately: risks of adverse reactions are increased when multiple drugs are administered, and combination therapy is sometimes less effective than a single drug against a specific pathogen.[54] Of the antimicrobial agents effective in vitro against *B. fragilis*, only metronidazole has been consistently inhibitory and bactericidal at achievable concentrations.[55] Thus, the possibility of synergistic combinations against *B. fragilis* and other anaerobic organisms is clinically important.

Several reports[56] have suggested the presence of an in vitro activity of the combination of metronidazole and spiramycin against anaerobic organisms other than *B. fragilis* and have indicated the clinical efficacy of this combination in certain anaerobic infections.

Fass, Rotilie, and Prior[57] reported in vitro synergism of the combination of clindamycin and gentamicin against a single strain of *B. fragilis*. Busch, Sutter, and Finegold,[58] however, did not find synergism against *B. fragilis* with the combination of clindamycin and amikacin. Leigh[59] found an indifferent interaction (neither synergism nor antagonism) of clindamycin and gentamicin against *B. fragilis*. Brook and coworkers[60] have observed in vitro and in vivo synergisms between penicillin and gentamicin against all strains of the *B. melaninogenicus* group.

Synergistic interaction between aminoglycosides and penicillins was observed and studied in aerobic organisms. This combination was found to be effective in the treatment of enterococcal and staphylococcal diseases. It is postulated that the penicillins, which inhibit the cell wall synthesis, enhance the penetration of aminoglycosides, which have lethal action on the ribosomes. *B. fragilis,* which is a strict anaerobe, is resistant to aminoglycosides because of their ineffective transport into facultatively anaerobic bacteria under anaerobic conditions.[58] A recent study,[61] however, demonstrated that the ribosomes of the strictly anaerobic bacteria *C. perfringens* and *B. fragilis* are susceptible to the action of streptomycin and gentamicin. The susceptibility of *Bacteroides* ribosomes to aminoglycosides, combined with the ability of penicillin to impair the organism's membranes, suggests a possible explanation for the synergistic combination between the agents against *B. melaninogenicus*. Busch, Sutter, and Finegold[58] studied the activity of combinations of different antimicrobial agents against *B. fragilis*. A synergistic effect was observed only with the combination of clindamycin and metronidazole. These authors suggested that this combination may prove useful in the treatment of selected infections such as endocarditis, septic thrombophlebitis, and osteomyelitis, in which *B. fragilis* is implicated as a single or primary pathogen and for which maximal antibacterial activity is desired. The combination might also become useful in the event of increased resistance of *B. fragilis* to individual antimicrobial agents.

Significance of Beta-Lactamase

Many *Bacteroides* species produce beta-lactamase, which enables them to resist penicillin.[62] *B. fragilis* has been known to produce this enzyme. Until recently, most *B. melaninogenicus* and *B. oralis* strains were considered to be susceptible to penicillin. Within the last decade, however, penicillin-resistant strains have been reported with increasing frequency.[62]

The appearance of penicillin resistance among *Bacteroides* species has important implications for chemotherapy. Many penicillin-resistant bacteria can produce enzymes that degrade penicillins or cephalosporins. Such organisms, present in a localized soft tissue infection, release the enzyme into the environment, thus degrading penicillin in the area of the infection, thereby protecting not only themselves but also other pathogens that are penicillin-sensitive. Thus, penicillin therapy directed against a susceptible pathogen might be rendered ineffective by the presence of a penicillin-producing organism.

Several studies demonstrated the activity of this enzyme in aerobic infection. De Louvois and Hurley[63] demonstrated degradation of penicillin, ampicillin, and cephaloridine by purulent exudates obtained from 4 of 22 patients with abscesses. Studies by Masuda and Tomioka[64] demonstrated possible beta-lactamase activity in empyema fluid. Most infections studied were polymicrobial and contained both *Klebsiella pneumoniae* and *P. aeruginosa*. O'Keefe and associates[65] demonstrated inactivation of penicillin G in an experimental infection model in the rabbit peritoneum. These studies suggest that local infection with *B. fragilis* may modify penicillin content of abscess fluid by enzymatic degradation in vivo.[65]

The importance of this phenomenon in anaerobic infections was first demonstrated in animals by studies[66] of mixed infections of penicillin-resistant and penicillin-susceptible bacteria in rabbits. Subsequently, Hackman and Wilkins[67] were able to show that penicillin-resistant strains in mice of *B. fragilis*, *B. melaninogenicus*, and *B. oralis* could protect *Fusobacterium necrophorum*, a penicillin-sensitive pathogen, from penicillin therapy.

Brook and colleagues[68] recently tested the hypothesis that beta-lactamase-producing strains of *B. fragilis* and *B. melaninogenicus* can protect group A beta-hemolytic streptococci (GABHS) in mice from penicillin. A mixed infection was induced in mice in the form of a subcutaneous abscess involving a penicillin-susceptible GABHS and a beta-lactamase-producing strain of either *B. melaninogenicus* or *B. fragilis*. The infected animals were treated for seven days with parenteral penicillin, penicillin and clavulanic acid, or clindamycin. All modes of treatment prevented the formation of abscesses in animals inoculated with GABHS alone, but not in those inoculated with GABHS and *Bacteroides* species. There was, however, a marked reduction in size of the abscesses and the total number of viable GABHS in the pus from the animals treated with penicillin and clavulanic acid or clindamycin as compared to untreated controls and to those treated with penicillin alone. Thus, protection of GABHS from penicillin by beta-lactamase-producing strains of *Bacteroides* species was demonstrated in infected mice. Clindamycin or the combination of penicillin and clavulanic acid, which are active against both GABHS and *Bacteroides* species, were more effective in the treatment of the infection.

Also observed was the protective effect of beta-lactamase production by aerobic organisms (such as *K. pneumoniae* or *Staphylococcus aureus*) on *B. melaninogenicus*. Penicillin was ineffective in eradicating the penicillin-susceptible anaerobe in the presence of the aerobic beta-lactamase producer. The phenomenon is supported further by the ability to treat the infection when clavulanic acid is administered in addition to the penicillin. Bryant and co-workers[69] have studied the beta-lactamase activity in human pus obtained from 12 patients with polymicrobial intraabdominal abscesses or polymicrobial empyema. Pus supernatant of six specimens rapidly inactivated penicillin, cephalothin, and cefazolin. Carbenicillin and ticarcillin were similarly degraded by supernatant of certain pus specimens. Cefoxitin, chloramphenicol, and clindamycin were not appreciably inactivated by pus supernatant. Degradation of penicillin and cephalosporin congeners in pus was due to the presence of beta-lactamase. Pus supernatant containing only beta-lactamase reduced the bactericidal activity of carbenicillin against *B. fragilis* in an abscess model. Bactericidal acitivity of clindamycin or cefoxitin was not impaired in pus containing beta-lactamase.

The ability of beta-lactamase-producing organisms to protect penicillin-sensitive microorganisms has been demonstrated in vitro. When mixed with cultures of *B. fragilis,* the resistance of GABHS to penicillin increased at least 8500-fold.[70] Simon and Surai[71] have demonstrated the ability of *S. aureus* to protect GABHS from penicillin.

The results of all of these studies raise questions concerning the efficacy of beta-lactamase-susceptible antibiotics against beta-lactamase-producing anaerobic bacteria present in abscesses. This problem may be important in circumstances where surgical drainage is delayed or incomplete.[72] In seriously ill patients who suffer from mixed infection where beta-lactamase-producing bacteria are also present, the clinician should consider administering antibiotics effective also against these beta-lactamase producers. The recent development of potent enzyme inhibitors like clavulanic acid, and the study in animal models of polymicrobial infection, may facilitate a new approach to this problem.

REFERENCES

1. Sutter, V. L., and Finegold, S. M. Susceptibility of anaerobic bacteria to 23 antimicrobial agents. *Antimicrob. Agents Chemother.* 10:736, 1976.

2. Finegold, S. M. *Anaerobic bacteria in human disease.* New York: Academic Press, 1977.

3. Busch, D. F. et al. Susceptibility of respiratory tract anaerobes to orally administered penicillins and cephalosporins. *Antimicrob. Agents Chemother.* 10:713, 1976.

4. Sutter, V. L., and Finegold, S. M. Susceptibility of anaerobic bacteria to carbenicillin, cefoxitin, and related drugs. *J. Infect. Dis.* 131:417, 1975.

5. Fiedelman, W., and Webb, C. D. Clinical evaluation of carbenicillin in the treatment of infection due to anaerobic bacteria. *Curr. Ther. Res.* 18:441, 1975.

6. Thadepalli, H., and Huang, J. T. Treatment of anaerobic infections: carbenicillin alone compared with clindamycin and gentamicin. *Curr. Ther. Res.* 22:549, 1977.

7. Brook, I. Anaerobic isolates in chronic recurrent suppurative otitis medical treatment with carbenicillin alone and in combination with gentamicin. *Infection* 5:247, 1979.

8. Brook, I. Carbenicillin in treatment of aspiration pneumonia in children. *Curr. Ther. Res.* 23:136, 1978.

9. Tally, F. P. et al. In vitro activity of penicillins against anaerobes. *Antimicrob. Agents Chemother.* 7:413, 1975.

10. Roy, I.; Bach, V.; and Thadepalli, A. In vitro activity of ticarcillin against anaerobic bacteria compared with that of carbenicillin and penicillin. *Antimicrob. Agents Chemother.* 11:258, 1977.

11. Heseltine, P. N. R. et al. Cefoxitin: clinical evaluation in 38 patients. *Antimicrob. Agents Chemother.* 11:427, 1977.

12. Brook, I. In vitro activity of moxalactam (LY-127935) against anaerobic microorganisms. *J. Antimicrob. Chemother.* 6:676, 1980.

13. Kagnoff, M. F.; Armstron, D.; and Blevins, A. *Bacteroides* bacteremia. Experience in a hospital for neoplastic disease. *Cancer* 29:245, 1972.

14. Gorbach, S. L., and Bartlett, J. G. Anaerobic infections. *N. Engl. J. Med.* 290:1177, 1237, 1289, 1974.

15. DuPont, H. L. et al. Evaluation of chloramphenicol acid succinate therapy of induced typhoid fever and rocky mountain spotted fever. *N. Engl. J. Med.* 282:53, 1980.

16. Lindberg, A. A. et al. Concentration of chloramphenicol in the urine and blood in relation to renal function. *Br. Med. J.* 2:724, 1966.

17. Lietman, P. S. Chloramphenicol and the neonate—1979 view. *Clin. Pharmacokinet.* 6:151, 1979.

18. Windorfer, A., Jr., and Pringsheim, W. Studies on the concentrations of chloramphenicol in the serum and cerebrospinal fluid of neonates, infants and small children. Reciprocal reactions between chloramphenicol, penicillin, and phenobarbitone. *Eur. J. Pediatr.* 124(2):129, 1977.

19. Sack, C. M.; Koup, J. R.; and Smith, A. L. Chloramphenicol pharmacokinetics in infants and young children. *Pediatrics* 66:579, 1980.

20. Kramer, P. W.; Griffin, R. S.; and Campbell, R. J. Antibiotic penetration of the brain: a comparative study. *J. Neurosurg.* 31:295, 1969.

21. Druz, D. J. et al. The penetration of penicillin and other antimicrobials into joint fluid. *J. Bone Joint Surg.* 49:1415, 1967.

22. Joiner, K. A. et al. Antibiotic levels in infected and sterile subcutaneous abscesses in mice. *J. Infect. Dis.* 143:487, 1981.

23. Shoemaker, E. H., and Yow, E. M. Clinical evaluation of erythromycin. *Arch. Intern. Med.* 93:397, 1954.

24. Finegold, S. M. et al. Management of anaerobic infections. *Ann. Intern. Med.* 83:375, 1975.

25. Lewis, P. et al. Erythromycin therapy of anaerobic infections. In *Current chemotherapy* Washington, D.C.: American Society for Microbiology, 1978, p. 653.

26. Finegold, S. M.; Harada, N. E.; and Miller, L. G. Lincomycin activity against anaerobes and effect on normal human fecal flora. *Antimicrob. Agents Chemother.* 6:659, 1966.

27. DeHaan, R. M. et al. Pharmacokinetic studies of clindamycin hydrochloride in humans. *Int. J. Clin. Pharmacol.* 6:105, 1972.

28. DeHaan, R. M., and Schellenberg, D. Clindamycin palmitate flavored granules: multidose tolerance, absorption, and urinary excretion study in healthy children. *J. Clin. Pharmacol.* 12:74, 1972.

29. Twin, N., and Coilipp, P. J. Absorption and tolerance of clindamycin-2-palmitate in infants below 6 months of age. *Curr. Ther. Res.* 12:648, 1970.

30. Deigin, R. D. et al. Clindamycin treatment of osteomyelitis and septic arthritis in children. *Pediatrics* 55:213, 1975.

31. Wagner, J. G. et al. Absorption, excretion and half-life of clindamycin in normal adult males. *Am. J. Med. Sci.* 256:25, 1968.

32. Panzer, J. D. et al. Clindamycin levels in various body tissues and fluids. *J. Clin. Pharmacol.* 12:259, 1972.

33. Gorbach, S. L., and Thadepalli, H. Clindamycin in the treatment of pure and mixed anaerobic infections. *Arch. Intern. Med.* 134:87, 1974.

34. Tedesco, F. J.; Barton, R. W.; and Alpers, D. H. Clindamycin associated colitis: a prospective study. *Ann. Intern. Med.* 81:429, 1974.

35. George, W. L. et al. Aetiology of antimicrobial agent-associated colitis. *Lancet* 1:802, 1978.

36. Randolph, M. F., and Morris, K. E. Clindamycin associated colitis in children. A prospective study and a negative report. *Clin. Pediatr.* 26:722, 1977.

37. Berlatzky, Y. et al. Use of clindamycin and gentamicin in pediatric colonic surgery. *J. Pediatr. Surg.* 11:943, 1976.

38. Rodriguez, W. et al. Clindamycin in treatment of osteomyelitis in children. A report of 29 cases. *Am. J. Dis. Child.* 131:1088, 1977.

39. Brook, I. Clindamycin in treatment of aspiration pneumonia in children. *Antimicrob. Agents Chemother.* 15:342, 1979.

40. Brook, I. Bacteriology and treatment of chronic otitis media in children. *Laryngoscope* 89:1129, 1979.

41. Chow, A. W.; Patten, V.; and Guze, L. B. Susceptibility of anaerobic bacteria to metronidazole: relative resistance of non-spore forming gram-positive bacilli. *J. Infect. Dis.* 131:182, 1975.

42. Rustia, M., and Shubik, P. Experimental induction of hematomas, mammary tumors and other tumors with metronidazole in noninbred Sas: WRC (WT)BR rats. *J. Natl. Cancer Inst.* 63:863, 1979.

43. Cohen, S. M. et al. Carcinogenicity of 5-nitrofurans 5-nitromidazoles, 4-nitrobenzenes and related compounds. *J. Natl. Cancer Instit.* 51:403, 1973.

44. Tally, P.; Sutter, L.; and Finegold, S. M. Treatment of anaerobic infections with metronidazole. *Antimicrob. Agents Chemother.* 7:672, 1975.

45. Beard, C. M. et al. Lack of evidence for cancer due to use of metronidazole. *N. Engl. J. Med.* 301:519, 1979.

46. Berman, B. W. et al. *Bacteroides fragilis* meningitis in a neonatal successfully treated with metronidazole. *J. Pediatr.* 93:793, 1979.

47. Rom, S.; Flynn, D.; and Noone, P. Anaerobic infections in a neonate. Early detection by gas liquid chromatography and response to metronidazole. *Arch. Dis. Child.* 52:740, 1977.

48. Brook, I. Bacteriology of intracranial abscess in children. *J. Neurosurg.* 54:484, 1981.

49. Law, B. J., and Marks, M. I. Excellent outcome of *Bacteroides* meningitis in a newborn treated with metronidazole. *Pediatrics* 66:463, 1980.

50. O'Grady, L. R., and Ralph, E. D. Anaerobic meningitis and bacteremia caused by *Fusobacterium* species. *Am. J. Dis. Child.* 130:871, 1976.

51. Brook, I. Metronidazole in the treatment of anaerobic infections in children. *Proceedings,* First United States Metronidazole Conference, Tarpon Springs, 1982, p. 319.

52. Reading, C., and Cole, M. Clavulanic acid: a beta-lactamase inhibiting beta-lactam from *Streptomyces clavuligerus. Antimicrob. Agents Chemother.* 11:852, 1977.

53. Wust, J., and Wilkins, T. D. Effect of clavulanic acid on anaerobic bacteria resistant to beta-lactam antibiotics. *Antimicrob. Agents Chemother.* 13:130, 1978.

54. Rahal, J. J. Antibiotic combinations: the clinical relevance of synergy and antagonism. *Medicine* 57:179, 1978.

55. Whelan, J. P. F., and Hale, J. H. Bactericidal activity of metronidazole against *Bacteroides fragilis. J. Clin. Pathol.* 26:393, 1973.

56. Laufer, J.; Mignon, H.; and Videau, D. L'association métronidazole-spiramycine: concentrations et synergie in situ comparées aux CMI de la flore buccale. *Rev. Stomatol. Chir. Maxillofac.* 74:387, 1974.

57. Fass, R. J.; Rotilie, C. A.; and Prior, R. B. Interaction of clindamycin and gentamicin in vitro. *Antimicrob. Agents Chemother.* 6:582, 1974.

58. Busch, D. F.; Sutter, V. L.; and Finegold, S. M. Activity of combinations of antimicrobial agents against *Bacteroides fragilis. J. Infect. Dis.* 133:321, 1976.

59. Leigh, D. A. *Bacteroides* infections. *Lancet* 2:1081, 1973.

60. Brook, I. et al. In vitro and in vivo synergism between aminoglycosides and penicillin against *Bacteroides melaninogenicus* group (abstr. 653). *Proceedings,* 22nd Interscience Conference on Antimicrobial Agents and Chemotherapy, Miami Beach, Fla., 1982, p. 181.

61. Bryan, L. E.; Kowand, S. K.; and Van Den Elzen, H. M. Mechanism of aminoglycoside antibiotic resistance in anaerobic bacteria: *Clostridium perfringens* and *Bacteroides fragilis. Antimicrob. Agents Chemother.* 15:7, 1979.

62. Brook, I.; Calhoun, L.; and Yocum, P. Beta lactamase-producing isolates of *Bacteroides* species from children. *Antimicrob. Agents Chemother.* 18:164, 1980.

63. de Louvois, J., and Hurley, R. Inactivation of penicillin by purulent exudates. *Br. Med. J.* 2:998, 1977.

64. Masuda, G., and Tomioka, S. Possible beta-lactamase activities detectable in infective clinical specimens. *J. Antibiot.* (Tokyo) 30:1093, 1977.

65. O'Keefe, J. P. et al. Inactivation of penicillin G during experimental infection with *Bacteroides fragilis. J. Infect. Dis.* 137:437, 1978.

66. Tacking, R. Penicillinase producing bacteria in mixed infections in rabbits treated with penicillin. *Acta Pathol. Microbiol. Scand.* 35:445, 1954.

67. Hackman, A., and Wilkins, T. D. Influence of penicillinase production by strains of *Bacteroides melaninogenicus* and *Bacteroides oralis* on penicillin therapy of an experimental mixed anaerobic infection in mice. *Arch. Oral Biol.* 21:385, 1976.

68. Brook, I. et al. In vitro protection of Group A beta hemolytic streptococci by *Bacteroides* (abstr. 109). *Proceedings,* 21st Interscience Conference of Antimicrobial Agents and Chemotherapy, Chicago, 1981.

69. Bryant, R. E. et al. B-lactamase activity in human pus. *J. Infect. Dis.* 142:594, 1980.

70. Brook, I., and Yokum, P. In vitro protection of group A beta-hemolytic streptococci from penicillin and cephalothin by *Bacteroides fragilis. Chemotherapy* 29:18, 1983.

71. Simon, H. M., and Sukair, W. Staphylococcal antagonism to penicillin group therapy of hemolytic streptococcal pharyngeal infection: effect of oxacillin. *Pediatrics* 31:463, 1968.

72. Tally, F. P. Factors affecting antimicrobial agents in an anaerobic abscess. *J. Antimicrob. Chemother.* 4:299, 1978.

INDEX